# CORONARY
# NURSING
# CARE

*Consultant:*

WILLIAM F. FOWKES, M.D.
*Coordinator for Heart*
*Regional Medical Programs, Area III*
*Stanford University Medical Center*
*Palo Alto, California*

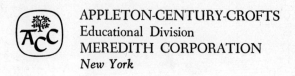

APPLETON-CENTURY-CROFTS
Educational Division
MEREDITH CORPORATION
*New York*

# CORONARY NURSING CARE

**C. Luise Riehl, R.N., B.A.**
*Program Coordinator of Health Professions, Lecturer and Clinical Instructor, Cardiovascular Nursing, University Extension, University of California, Santa Cruz; Director of Nursing Education, Coronary Care Instruction, Vocational Nursing Programs, San Jose Unified School District, San Jose, California*

Library of Congress Catalog Card Number:
79-133175

*Second Printing*

PRINTED IN THE UNITED STATES OF AMERICA
390-74042-X

# PREFACE

The increasing number of texts and manuals on coronary care nursing forces the author of a new one to justify her own efforts, if only to herself. To the cries of the young graduate nurses joining with other young people saying "Tell it like it is," the question arises that what we *teach* is often different from what we *tell*. Sometimes we teach of the miracles involved in saving a life and the importance of the subject we teach. Sometimes, we teach students to dislike, and then to avoid, the very subject we are teaching by being vague and nonaction oriented. Yes, instructors do influence students, for students are people and it has long been proven that people influence people. Once an instructor, whether in an academic or health institution, realizes this fact, he (or she) will realize that the best of his efforts must be directed toward the universal objective of all instruction: the intent to send students away from the instruction with at least as favorable an attitude toward the subject or experience as they had when they first arrived.

Allow me to clarify this point further. The demands for competent trained coronary nurses far exceed the supply. This creates staffing problems for many hospitals. Yet, trained and competent nurses leave the coronary nursing units because they have been exposed to too much too soon and have been placed in a role of conflict between what they have been taught is their role and what hospital policy will permit. Others are sent from other areas to "relieve" the regular staff on their days off or as vacation relief, without any previous instruction in coronary concepts or exposure to electronic monitoring equipment. They are expected to learn as they go, so to speak. Aside from the legal implications inherent in such situations, one cannot help question the moral values involved when patients are placed in an area designed to provide specialized, intensive care and then not ensuring that they receive such care.

We must recognize that the success of a coronary care unit depends upon the qualifications, preparation, and ability of the nursing personnel rather than the use of new electronic instrumentation. Yet, it is not unusual to find those planning a coronary care unit emphasizing the electronic instrumentation and overlooking the fact that the effectiveness of any equipment depends upon the ability of the personnel to use it. Any nurse put into this "new unit" will soon become consumed with anxieties and fears. She strives to educate herself by several means—local educational institutions offering courses in coronary care nursing, through the literature supplied by the manufacturer who promised instruction and servicing 24 hours a day, or through her own resources of self-education by overzealous reading. More frequently she is forced to request transfer, or resign, from such an overwhelming negative environment. The point here is that how the story of an experience with new equipment or nursing activities does end is the result of the things that happen to the nurse or student while she (or he) is in the presence of those pieces of equipment or nursing activities. Experience has shown the history of an attitude toward a subject to be influenced by the events that occur in relation to it. And that brings us back to our original point. If this book can enable the nurse or student to better approach the concept of working in the coronary care unit as well as the medical and surgical units to which the coronary patient progresses with rehabilitation, and enables her to use the skills and knowledge she already knows, yet instills the desire to learn more, the goal of the author will have been achieved.

The request to tell it like it is can best be met by a description of the two related aims that govern the writing: 1) to provide a clear and realistic picture of contemporary aggressive management of the cardiac patient, and 2) to offer in simplified form a plan for recognition of life-threatening cardiac arrhythmias. Both of these aims should meet the requirements of the nurse already possessing considerable knowledge and skill in the care of medical and surgical patients, and still meet the requirements of the new student.

The text is not intended to take the place of a comprehensive text in the subjects to which it refers frequently. The brief outlines covering recognition and treatment of some disorders and arrhythmias are such that they may be clipped out and added to the nurse's own quick reference file. To the student who has been encouraged to keep a current medication index file, this is no new idea.

As one might guess, once the suggestion came to the author to put her notes into the form of a text, many offers of help soon followed. Since it began with Dr. Hondorp and the students, it was to them that the author first presented the contents, individually and in groups, noting their reactions, questions, and suggestions. The object was to see what would keep them wanting to hear more and then to keep on wanting more.

The second stage began when the content was in written form. It consisted in asking teachers and consultants to use it in the classroom or hospital setting and mark down anything that broke their train of thought, turned them off, or turned them on; to describe the reactions of students or personnel; to keep a record of questions and suggestions; to keep a record of discussions which necessitated additional material required for clarity, or less material to avoid the "overkill" approach.

In short, I asked for help . . . and did I get it! I got more than I bargained for. What I thought was going to be a small notebook, or pocketbook, on recognition and treatment of arrhythmias soon was torn apart, added to, questioned, and trampled! One of my best chapters on developing objectives was thrown out entirely because I had gotten too "theoretical" to be telling it straight. Examples that did not "exampt" were vetoed. Patient assessment and nursing diagnosis fared badly. Some of my best efforts (I thought) were tossed aside in the quest to "tell it like it is."

Such unheralded encouragement (or discouragement) should not go unrecognized. So the author wishes to acknowledge a great debt of gratitude to Dr. Gordon Hondorp, cardiologist, who first suggested and urged the writing of the text; Dr. William C. Fowkes, Coordinator for Heart Disease, California Regional Medical Program, Area III, Stanford Medical Center; Miss Marjorie Keys, Assistant Director and In-service Coordinator, Stanford Hospital, Stanford Medical Center, Palo Alto; Dr. Harriet Schuttee, Research Nurse-Psychologist, Regional Medical Program, Area III, Stanford Medical Center; Dr. Irene Nasielski, In-service Director, Serra Medical Hospital; Dr. Malcolm Parker, chairman, education committee, Santa Clara County Heart Association; Dr. Robert Baer, lecturer in Cardiology, Valley Medical Center; Miss Marty Wolfinger, instructor, Coronary Care Nursing, West Valley Junior College, and supervisor, Coronary Care Unit, Good Samaritan Hospital, San Jose; Mrs. Jennie Bejuklian, head nurse, Coronary Care Unit, Kaiser Foundation Hospital, Santa Clara, California.

The author wishes to extend her thanks to Mr. Earl Lewis, Santa Clara County Heart Association, and to the American Heart Association for the hugh amounts of materials and literature made available; to Mrs. Susan Emig, registered nurse and art student, whose art sketches certainly lessened the anxiety of the author; to Tampa Tracings and Dr. J. L. Marriott, cardiologist, who provided many of the ECG tracings. And finally, my sincere appreciation to Charles Bollinger, editor-in-chief, Nursing Education Books, Appleton-Century-Crofts, for his patience throughout the preparation of the manuscript.

*C. Luise Riehl*

# CONTENTS

PREFACE / v

**PART I   THE PATIENT AND CORONARY CARE**

1. AN EMERGING PATTERN / 1

> MODERN TECHNOLOGY . . . 1   THE CHALLENGE . . . 3
> EMOTIONS AND PSYCHOLOGIC FACTORS . . . 3   PHYSIO-
> LOGIC FACTORS . . . 5   SUMMARY . . . 7   REVIEW
> AND ADVANCE . . . 7

2. BASIC DESIGN AND EQUIPMENT / 10

> GUIDING PRINCIPLES . . . 10   DEVELOPING A UNIT
> . . . 11   UNIT EQUIPMENT . . . 14   MEMORY LOOPS
> AND RECORDING EQUIPMENT . . . 21   THOROUGH
> RECORDING OF EMERGENCY EVENTS . . . 21   IMPORT-
> ANCE OF CARDIAC NURSE SPECIALIST . . . 21   TRAIN-
> ING OF CARDIAC NURSE SPECIALIST . . . 22   METH-
> ODS OF RESUSCITATION . . . 22   CESSATION OF RE-
> SUSCITATIVE EFFORTS . . . 24   POSTRESUSCITATION
> CARE . . . 24   AV BLOCK . . . 25   FUTURE DE-
> VELOPMENTS . . . 25   SUMMARY . . . 26   REVIEW
> AND ADVANCE . . . 26

3. REVIEW OF PERTINENT RELATIONSHIPS
   OF CERTAIN ANATOMIC FUNCTIONS
   AND SYSTEMS / 28

> CIRCULATORY SYSTEM . . . 28   MUSCLES . . . 37
> AIR PASSAGES . . . 40   NERVOUS SYSTEM . . . 44
> SUMMARY . . . 47   REVIEW AND ADVANCE . . . 47

**ix**

4. THE PATH LEADING TO MYOCARDIAL
   INFARCTION / 51

ETIOLOGY . . . 51  SPECTRUM OF CORONARY ARTERY
DISEASE . . . 53  ANGINA PECTORIS . . . 54  MYO-
CARDIAL INFARCTION . . . 54  LEARNING FROM
STUDY . . . 54  GENERAL DISCUSSION OF ARTERIO-
SCLEROTIC HEART DISEASE . . . 55  ASYMPTOMATIC
CORONARY DISEASE . . . 58  ACUTE CORONARY IN-
SUFFICIENCY . . . 58  FURTHER ASPECTS OF MYO-
CARDIAL INFARCTION . . . 59  THERAPY . . . 61
SUMMARY . . . 63  REVIEW AND ADVANCE . . . 64

5. CONSIDERATIONS ON STAFFING A CORONARY
   CARE UNIT / 68

PERSONALITY OF THE CORONARY CARE NURSE . . . 68
INFORMAL RELATIONSHIP DEVELOPS . . . 69  PER-
SONNEL AND THE CORONARY CARE UNIT . . . 70
PLANNING COMMITTEE . . . 71  UNIT STAFF-
ING . . . 72  TRAINING PROGRAMS FOR NURSES . . . 73
TRAINING PROGRAMS FOR PHYSICIANS . . . 78  RE-
VIEW AND ADVANCE . . . 80

6. INTEGRATING OBJECTIVES / 84

OBJECTIVES . . . 84  NURSE'S ROLE ON ADMISSION
OF PATIENT . . . 85  DELEGATION . . . 89  AC-
TIVITY . . . 90  NUTRITION . . . 92  OXYGEN
THERAPY . . . 93  PAIN, ANXIETY, AND REST . . . 95
ANTICOAGULANT THERAPY . . . 96  GASTROINTES-
TINAL PROBLEMS . . . 97  SUMMARY . . . 98  RE-
VIEW AND ADVANCE . . . 99

7. LABORATORY IN EVALUATION
   OF HEART DISEASE / 103

PRINCIPLES OF DIAGNOSTIC SERUM ENZYMOLOGY
. . . 104  TRANSAMINASES . . . 105  LACTIC DEHY-
DROGENASE . . . 107  CREATINE PHOSPHOKINASE
(CPK) . . . 109  OTHER ENZYMES . . . 109  SUM-
MARY . . . 110  REVIEW AND ADVANCE . . . 111

8. ELECTROLYTE DISTURBANCES / 114

WHAT ELECTROLYTES ARE . . . 114  THE CATION
SODIUM . . . 116  THE CATION POTASSIUM . . . 117
THE CATION CALCIUM . . . 119  THE CATION MAG-
NESIUM . . . 120  THE ANION BICARBONATE . . . 121
THE ANION CHLORIDE . . . 123  ACID-BASE DISTURB-
ANCES . . . 123  SUMMARY . . . 125  REVIEW AND
ADVANCE . . . 126

9. THE NUTRITIONAL NEEDS OF THE
   CORONARY PATIENT / *129*

   CARDIAC DYSFUNCTION AND COMPENSATORY MECH-
   ANISMS . . . *129*   OBESITY FACTORS . . . *130*   PRIN-
   CIPLES OF DIET . . . *131*   COUNSELING THE PA-
   TIENT . . . *133*   LOW CHOLESTEROL . . . *134*   PRAC-
   TICAL APPLICATION . . . *136*   SUMMARY . . . *136*
   REVIEW AND ADVANCE . . . *139*

10. ANTICOAGULATION / *144*

   INDICATIONS FOR USE OF ANTICOAGULANTS . . . *144*
   CONTRAINDICATIONS TO ANTICOAGULANT THERAPY
   . . . *145*   HEPARIN . . . *146*   COUMARIN DERIVA-
   TIVES AND RELATED COMPOUNDS . . . *149*   LABORA-
   TORY TESTS AND DISCUSSION . . . *153*   SUMMARY
   . . . *155*   REVIEW AND ADVANCE . . . *155*

11. X-RAY IN THE EVALUATION OF HEART DISEASE / *158*

   BACKGROUND INFORMATION . . . *158*   ROUTINE SETS
   . . . *159*   FLUOROSCOPY . . . *161*   SELECTIVE
   CORONARY ARTERIOGRAPHY . . . *161*   MYOCARDIAL
   REVASCULARIZATION . . . *164*   SUMMARY . . . *164*
   REVIEW AND ADVANCE . . . *164*

12. ASSOCIATED PROBLEMS IN CORONARY
    HEART DISEASE / *166*

   CONGESTIVE HEART FAILURE . . . *166*   THROM-
   BOEMOBLIC DISEASE . . . *175*   CARDIOGENIC SHOCK
   . . . *178*   CARDIAC ARRHYTHMIAS . . . *182*   POST
   MYOCARDIAC INFARCTION SYNDROME . . . *183*   RUP-
   TURE OF THE VENTRICLE . . . *183*   SUMMARY
   . . . *183*   REVIEW AND ADVANCE . . . *183*

**PART II   ELECTROCARDIOGRAM AND
            ELECTRICAL TRACINGS**

13. THE ELECTROCARDIOGRAM / *187*

   ELECTRICAL CONDUCTIVITY . . . *187*   THE CONDUC-
   TIVITY PATHWAY . . . *188*   SUMMARY OF ACTIVITY
   AT THIS POINT . . . *200*   PRECORDIAL LEADS . . . *201*
   V LEADS . . . *202*   DIRECTIONAL FORCES . . . *203*
   SUMMARY . . . *206*   REVIEW AND ADVANCE . . . *206*

14. INTERPRETING THE ELECTROCARDIOGRAM / *208*

   CONDUCTIVITY PATHWAY IN BRIEF . . . *208*   RHYTHM
   . . . *209*   RATE OF TIMING . . . *209*   P WAVE

. . . *210* COMPLEX . . . *212* T WAVE . . . *214*
Q-T DURATION . . . *214* SUMMARY . . . *215* RE-
VIEW AND ADVANCE . . . *215*

15. MYOCARDIAL INFARCTION AND ECG TRACINGS / *218*

CLINICAL INFARCTION . . . *220* OTHER CONSIDERA-
TIONS . . . *226* SUMMARY . . . *226* REVIEW AND
ADVANCE . . . *227*

16. DRUGS USED IN ARRHYTHMIAS / *232*

ANTIARRHYMIC DRUGS . . . *232* DIGITALIS INTOXI-
CATION OR TOXICITY . . . *242* TREATMENT OF
DIGITALIS-INDUCED ECTOPIC RHYTHMS . . . *243*
TREATMENT OF DIGITALIS-INDUCED BLOCKS . . . *243*
SUMMARY . . . *243* REVIEW AND ADVANCE . . . *244*

17. SA NODE AND ATRIAL ARRHYTHMIAS / *247*

TYPES OF ARRHYTHMIAS . . . *247* INTERPRETING A
RHYTHM STRIP . . . *248* THE SPONTANEOUS DIS-
CHARGE CYCLE . . . *249* NORMAL SINUS RHYTHM
*253* SINUS BRADYCARDIA . . . *254* SINUS TACHY-
CARDIA . . . *255* SINUS ARRHYTHMIA . . . *255*
SINUS BLOCK OR SINUS ARREST . . . *256* WANDER-
ING PACEMAKER . . . *257* PREMATURE ATRIAL CON-
TRACTION (APC) OR (PAC) . . . *258* ATRIAL TACHY-
CARDIA . . . *260* PAROXYSMAL SUPRAVENTRICULAR
TACHYCARDIA . . . *261* PAT WITH BLOCK . . . *263*
ATRIAL FLUTTER . . . *265* ATRIAL FIBRILLATION
. . . *267* CARDIOVERSION . . . *271* SUMMARY
. . . *274* REVIEW AND ADVANCE . . . *275*

18. AV NODE AND VENTRICULAR ARRHYTHMIAS / *281*

NODAL RHYTHM . . . *282* CORONARY SINUS RHY-
THM . . . *284* NODAL TACHYCARDIA . . . *284* PRE-
MATURE NODAL CONTRACTION (PNC) OR NPC
. . . *285* ATRIOVENTRICULAR HEART BLOCKS . . . *286*
AV DISSOCIATION . . . *295* LEFT AND RIGHT
BUNDLE BLOCKS . . . *296* VENTRICULAR PREMA-
TURE CONTRACTIONS . . . *297* PARASYSTOLE AND
FUSION BEATS . . . *299* VENTRICULAR TACHYCAR-
DIA . . . *302* VENTRICULAR FIBRILLATION . . . *304*
INDICATIONS FOR COUNTERSHOCK . . . *307* SUM-
MARY . . . *308* REVIEW AND ADVANCE . . . *308*

19. CARDIAC ARREST / *312*

REVIEW OF THE TERM "SUDDEN DEATH" . . . *312*
HISTORY OF TREATMENT OF CARDIAC ARREST . . . *313*

THE NURSE'S RESPONSIBILITY . . . 315   CARDIAC
ARREST . . . 318   ADAMS-STOKES ATTACKS . . . 323
SUMMARY . . . 324   REVIEW AND ADVANCE . . . 326

## PART III   APPENDICES

A. TERMINOLOGY COMMON TO CARDIOVASCULAR DISEASE / 329

B. BIBLIOGRAPHY / 361

C. CASE STUDY OF L. H. / 365

D. CASE STUDY OF W. J. / 372

E. CASE STUDY OF M. Y. / 378

F. REFERENCES FOR APPENDICES A, B, AND C / 383

G. BASIC ORIENTATION COURSE IN CORONARY CARE FOR NURSES / 385

H. POSITION DESCRIPTION: CLINICAL SPECIALIST IN CARDIAC
NURSING / 395

I. POSITION DESCRIPTION: STAFF NURSE IN CORONARY CARE
NURSING / 397

J. PHYSICIAN'S ORDERS / 399

INDEX / 403

# CORONARY NURSING CARE

# I The Patient and Coronary Care

# ∥ AN EMERGING PATTERN

One can scarcely pick up a newspaper, magazine, or journal that he does not see an article on the impact of technologic change on the field of medicine. The concern over health is no longer the exclusive concern of the health professions. A few years ago, a common cry shared by all the health professions was: "The 'public' must be educated to their health needs for their own sake." But, now, the avenues of public media have caught up the "public," who is now turning to the health professions, saying: "Tell us."

## *Modern Technology*

Our generation of health professionals, aided and supported by the public we serve, has an opportunity that is unique.[1] We have at our disposal the tools that can reshape health patterns of a nation. There are limits imposed upon us by still-uncrossed frontiers of biologic science; but those frontiers are rapidly receding. In the meantime we have a great deal of room in which to move forward.

In general, pioneering has pressed on in the field of technology; developments are taking two forms: the adaption of modern technology to specific disease problems, and the reexamination and reorientation of programs to meet present and future needs. Some trends are significant in themselves, such as application of modern technology to problems of early diagnosis, detection, treatment, and restoration. Examples of these would include mammography in cancer diagnosis, computer-screening statistical coordination in diabetes, and the development of the artificial kidney. It is a safe assumption that we can anticipate the discovery of a workable artificial heart in time.

1. Aaron W. Christensen. The Disease Pattern of the Next Decade. Delivered at the annual meeting of Western Branch American Public Health Association, Phoenix, Arizona, May 29, 1963.

1

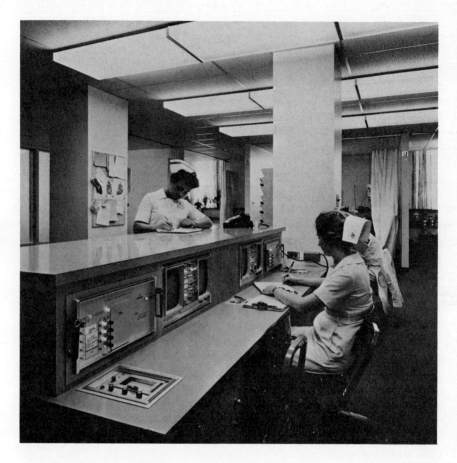

*FIG. 1* Nurses' central station in an eight-bed coronary care unit is equipped with electronic instruments for continuous simultaneous surveillance of all patients in the unit. Central station cardioscopes display ECG and heart rate for each of the patients. "Memory Loop" recorders are constantly recording on a five-minute length of magnetic tape, and enable a physician *after* an emergency situation to play back ECG information recorded *prior* to the emergency. This information helps explain why a heart attack occurred, for example, and can lead to corrective treatment to prevent a reoccurrence.
(Courtesy of Corbin-Farnsworth, Division of Smith Kline Instruments, Inc., Palo Alto, Calif.)

Other trends are significant in that they are meaningful as guideposts to the future. Computer systems are being used in a number of ingenious ways to speed the application of health knowledge and to economize on time and effort of scarce health professionals. It has been shown experimentally, and is now a real fact, that a computer system can successfully classify electrocardiograms using statistical techniques. Heart signals taken on patients in one part of the country can be relayed by standard telephone line to a central computer. The signals are analyzed electronically and the results automatically returned to their origination point in 30 seconds. The potential of this kind of project will mean that speedy and accurate evaluation of electrocardiogram tracings can be made widely accessible to physicians through electronics (Fig. 1).

Also in the heart disease field, recording the heart sounds [2] of children as a screening technique for congenital and rheumatic heart disease is being tested. Here the basic tool is an inexpensive, portable adaptation of high-fidelity recording equipment available on the open market. Such a system will clearly have widespread value, especially in communities where one or two cardiologists are expected to serve many thousands of people. A further refinement, now under study, indicates that a computer system can successfully separate normal and abnormal heart sounds, thereby adding the computer to the array of devices for screening heart abnormalities in children.

## The Challenge

Nurses have been enthusiastic about their increased responsibilities in coronary care units and are stimulated by the unique combination of direct patient care and cardiac monitoring. A new aspect of the nurses' role is detecting and evaluating early signs of circulatory failure and arrhythmias. They must know when to call the physician and how to evaluate drug and other therapy. In cases of death-producing arrhythmias, the nurse proceeds with defibrillation or cardiopulmonary resuscitation and then works with the physician, as a team, to further definitive therapy.

No doubt, new techniques in the detection and treatment of circulatory failure are on the horizon. As these take their place within the scope of the coronary care unit, nurses will continue to be responsive to the ideals of improved patient care and the saving of lives through team effort. But, as these new ideas are presented, they are not introduced without their toll in stress and "anxiety syndrome" upon the nurse.

## Emotions and Psychologic Factors

Routine nursing care in the coronary care unit is based on the individual needs of the patient. The nurse must be able to identify and evaluate these needs and meet them as far as she possibly can. They are all equally important,

2. *Ibid.*

whether physical, emotional, dietary, educational, or rehabilitative. When indicated, the nurse should utilize interdisciplinary resources to meet these needs.

As the nurse learns the values and norms of nursing, her behavior changes; sometimes, in the enculturation of the student nurse—as with the older nurse experiencing change within the profession—she will encounter a number of stress factors. It is helpful to know that most other students or nurses who are expected to "float" from one unit to another are also experiencing stress. They are also experienced by other disciplines in the health professions.

The nurse makes up a part of the patient's immediate environment. When she encounters stress, she is affected in some way, and these behavioral changes are reflected in her work with patients.

It seems appropriate to define several terms with which the coronary care unit nurse will soon become familiar. *Stress* and *frustration* are two closely related terms that need clarification since they have many influences and implications on behavior in general. Stress occurs in a situation where pressures are felt by a person and, in turn, these pressures change his current behavior patterns. If the individual's behavior at the time he experiences the pressures is *goal-directed,* he will keep his goal in sight in such a way that his need-satisfaction sequence will usually be completed even under a high degree of stress. On the other hand, if the pressures become too great and reach a point above the stress threshold of the individual, he may then experience frustration. When this tolerance level is reached and frustration occurs, his behavior will no longer be goal-directed and his need-satisfaction sequences will be either temporarily or permanently interrupted.[3]

In addition to these changes, there are many other physiologic changes that may occur, such as an increase in muscle tension, a change in the pulse rate or palpitations, an increase in respiration, and an unpleasant feeling. The person who experiences frustration also usually feels that he is being punished by somebody, since he is being denied the satisfaction of his needs.

Another basic element of behavior is *anxiety*, which is a feeling state experienced when a person is in some way threatened or believes himself to be in danger. Anxiety has been defined as a state of dread or apprehension with respect to some anticipated danger. It serves as a signal which alerts the individual to the possibility of excessive excitation, from within or without, that might upset his equilibrium and create a painful, unpleasant state. As a warning, the anxiety acts as a stimulus to defensive action to handle the excitation. Anxiety, as such, consists of an unpleasant affect, felt as fear, and concomitant physiologic signs which are interpreted as preparation for action,

3. Martha M. Brown and Grace R. Fowler. *Psychodynamic Nursing: A Biosocial Orientation.* Philadelphia, W. B. Saunders Company, 1966, p. 20.

either flight or fight. Even when the actual threat remains unknown, the individual responds as though the danger came from the external environment and can only be dealt with by attacking it or running away from it. The unpleasant feeling gives way to hopelessness. In our culture, anxiety seems directly related to the anticipation of a loss of esteem, either by oneself or by others. Whenever anything happens that threatens to disturb one's usual pattern of interacting with others, one tends to experience anxiety. It is generally agreed that to experience anxiety is inevitable; therefore, the important thing is how the individual learns to cope with it.

## *Physiologic Factors*

The various organs and special senses respond in specific ways to stress; this is known as the "adaptive syndrome." Within seconds every part of the body is responding to the stress signal.

Of the special senses, the skin experiences pilomotor contraction, that is, the hair stands up and "goose bumps" emerge. The pupils dilate. Hearing becomes more acute.

As mentioned before, the rate of respiration changes and shifts from clavicular to diaphragmatic breathing. The rate increases with a short rapid panting rhythm. There is a change in the carbon dioxide-oxygen ratio. Tetany may be present due to the alkaline condition of the body caused by hyperventilation.

In the gastrointestinal tract the flow of saliva stops. Gastric secretions diminish with fear and increase with anger. Food digestion stops. Frequently, there will be spasm of the digestive tract with intense pylorospasm. This is what causes the nausea, and possibly, vomiting. There may also be diarrhea. The liver causes an increase in glyconeogenesis, that is, it produces carbohydrates from molecules which are not themselves carbohydrates—such as fats and proteins—in order that sufficient energy be present for flight or fight.

Consider the cardiovascular implications of stress. Injury causes the peripheral vessels to constrict in response to sympathetic nervous system stimulation. Reservoirs of blood release extra sequestered blood in response to the constriction. The various parts of the body which act in response are listed below.

| | |
|---|---|
| Spleen | 150 ml |
| Liver | 700–1000 ml |
| Abdominal veins | 300 ml |
| Venous plexus | 500 ml |
| Heart | 100 ml |
| Lungs | 100–350 ml |

Venous blood vessel stress reaction, or relaxation, is the phenomenon basic to this reservoir system. If a vessel is exposed to the increased pressure from increased volume, it adjusts, for a time, by distending. This allows for the stored blood to increase volume without overtaxing the heart by inordinate pressure. When the constriction stops, the volume returns to normal and the vein also returns to normal.

Pulse pressure is affected by stroke volume and resistance. A heart that is distended by an increased volume has a beat of greater strength. If the arterial walls have lost distensibility, from disease or injury such as atherosclerosis, the increased pressure may cause rupture.

What, then, are the causes of a weak, thready pulse? For one, a rapid heartbeat will give a drop in pressure. Low cardiac pressure may be the cause. If the beat is normal, one suspects the heart is normal and the cause may be pooling of blood or hemorrhage. When the pulse alternates between being strong then soft, the heart is suspect as either experiencing a myocardial infarction or drug intoxication as in digitalis accumulation.

The sympathetic nervous system regulation responds whenever there is a drop in blood pressures and/or an increase in carbon dioxide. The effect is generalized throughout the body. The effect of vasoconstriction (epinephrine or norepinephrine) is so strong that circulation to the kidneys, gastrointestinal tract, or the hands and feet may be occluded for minutes at a time. This ischemia is followed by a period of reactive hyperemia which is an increase of two to six times the normal blood flow to the area that has been hypoxic; the purpose is to reestablish nutritional balance. Sympathetic vasodilation occurs when the sympathetic nerve impulses diminish or when vasodilator fibers are stimulated.

Areas graphically affected by blood flow are the heart, lungs, and the gastrointestinal tract. For example, in coronary occlusion the damage that ensues is dependent upon the rapidity with which the occlusion and subsequent ischemia occur. If the occlusion is a long time in developing, collateral circulation can compensate and symptoms may be minimal. Any ischemia will diminish tissue function; therefore, contraction by the myocardium will be lessened. Death occurs because of diminished cardiac output with damming up of blood in the pulmonary or systemic veins and subsequent pulmonary edema. Cardiac fibrillation or rupture then ensues.

In the lungs, the alveoli will remain dry until capillary pressure becomes greater than colloid osmotic pressure. When this occurs, the fluid will cross the membrane and pulmonary edema occurs.

As you can see, the stress cycle can work to the detriment of the patient. The psychologic reactions of patients to their heart attacks vary depending upon the individual. Fear of death is inherent in most patients, and when they are admitted to the coronary care unit where monitoring equipment is used and special procedures performed, this fear is increased even more. Such emotion may take the form of denial, hostility, anxiety, frustration, depression, and dependency. The nurse learns to meet the patient's emotional problems by:

- Understanding the individual temperament of each patient
- Orienting the patient and family to the coronary care unit and the plans for transfer, when necessary
- Explaining the purpose of cardiac monitoring and other procedures
- Allowing for expression of feeling
- Showing an interest in the family as well as in the patient

The nurse also recognizes her own reactions to the unit and identifies the causes of her own stress, such as:

- Inadequate staffing and frequent rotation of shift
- Feeling of isolation from other hospital personnel
- Conflicts among doctors or indecision in emergency situations
- Prolonged resuscitation of terminal patients
- Experimentation on patients
- Reponsibility for completion of detailed data forms
- Increased responsibility requiring quick judgment and action
- Keeping patients in the unit unnecessarily long after the acute phase of the illness, or transferring them out too soon

## Summary

In this opening chapter the author has discussed some of the changes and predicted changes likely to occur in the health professions through advances made in modern technology. Recognizing that many nurses are hampered from effective performance, some views of stress factors which may affect her as well as the patient are discussed and some of the physiologic implications to the stress syndrome are presented. It is important for the nurse to remember that the initial physiologic insult may not be as important as what occurred and continues to occur as stress and strain. Thus, the nurse must observe, analyze, anticipate, and predict.

## Review and Advance

1. *What were the primary purposes of the first coronary care units?*
   The primary purpose in establishing the first coronary care units was that

they should serve as resuscitation centers. Experimental research indicated that many patients could be resuscitated if they were monitored electronically following a myocardial infarction. With quick recognition of signs of ventricular fibrillation, up to 70 percent of the patients suffering from primary cardiac arrest due to ventricular fibrillation could be resuscitated.

2.  *Should all registered nurses be trained to defibrillate patients?*
    No, not all registered nurses; only those who are assigned to the coronary care unit and their relief personnel. To best achieve the goals of the coronary care unit, the nurse must be capable of immediately detecting and identifying disturbances of heart rate and rhythms, and qualified to perform cardiopulmonary resuscitation including defibrillation.

3.  *How can a nurse become proficient before faced with such an emergency alone?*
    Experience in a "dog laboratory" originally was the only course available for both the physician and nurse to practice defibrillation techniques. However, recently, "Resusci-Annie" has been improved to enable much more elaborate techniques to be demonstrated. If your hospital or local heart association does not have such a practice mannequin available, inquiries should be made to the American Heart Association, who compiles a continuous index on all current aids and equipment to teaching coronary care unit personnel.

4.  *Then, the goals of current coronary care units are still the same as the original objective?*
    The principal purpose of the new coronary care unit is still the prevention of serious arrhythmias and "primary" cardiac arrest by immediate detection and adequate suppression of premonitory arrhythmias.

5.  *Is stress a common phenomenon?*
    Yes. Stress is commonly defined as exertion—strain and effort. For example, a businessman who worries continually about office problems while he is at home or about home problems while he is at the office is under stress. The doctor who treats patients all day and remains "on call" through his exchange service all night is under stress. A nurse who supports patients, hospital, and nursing personnel for eight or twelve hours a day, racing against time and "paperwork," is under stress. And the sick person whose body is working feverishly to regain health is under stress.

6.  *Then, nobody can escape stress?*
    I think this could be turned into a statement: To a certain degree, nobody can escape stress. But there are varying degrees and different forms of stress—mental, emotional, physical—all having some impact upon health. Some of these are good, some are harmful. Stress can often be the stimulus that spurs an individual on to success, or, depending upon the circumstances and a person's capacities or reactions, it may have damaging side effects which may lead to a diseased state, cause us to age prematurely, or—sometimes—even shorten life. For all these reasons, nurses should learn more about stress and how it touches and affects their own, as well as their patient's, life.

7.  *How can anxiety be "triggered"?*
    Anxiety is provoked by a sense of helplessness, a sense of isolation, a sense of insecurity, or a threat to the self-image. Anxiety is most likely to be associated with illness and hospitalization. In mild forms, it contributes to the patient's discomfort. In its more severe forms, the anxiety may seriously interfere with the patient's treatment and his response to it.

8.  *Can guilt be a source of anxiety and pain?*
    I would like to quote a passage from Frank Edmund See's book *Feeling Kind of Temporary* (Westwood, N.J., Fleming H. Revell Company, 1968):

    > Guilt is the mother of all anxieties. Her children are many. Some to which we have given names include the fear of telling the truth, the fear of public opinion, the fear of being oneself, the fear of poverty, the fear of failure, the fear of an incurable disease, the fear of death, the fear of fear itself. They are an all too common part of today's fouled-up situations. The price of fear is the price man must pay in order to be human.

# 2 BASIC DESIGN AND EQUIPMENT

Our manner of perceiving makes life interesting, if sometimes exasperating. In *Through the Looking Glass,* Lewis Carroll's beautiful book on perception, among other things Alice says:

"I see nobody on the road."

"I only wish *I* had such eyes," the King remarked in a fretful tone. "To be able to see Nobody! And at that distance, too!"

Fortunately for the nurse embarking on an educational program for her role within a coronary care unit, we need not ask her to look through a looking glass. The guidelines have already been laid by concerned groups. Reprinted here through permission of the American College of Cardiology are guidelines for the basic design and equipment for the coronary care unit.[1]

## Guiding Principles

The established and widespread popularity of the coronary care unit has been due primarily to the fundamental fact that management of patients with acute or suspected myocardial infarction in such a facility saves lives.

The greatest saving has most often been during the first three to five days following sudden electrical failure (arrhythmia). Heart failure or shock requiring intensive treatment has responded less successfully to presently available intensive care measures.

The coronary care unit provides two principal types of service. One is constant, intensive surveillance of the patient who initially appears to have few if any complications and whose circulatory status seems stable. If such a

1. Training technics for the coronary care unit, Second Bethesda Conference of the American College of Cardiology, December 11, 12, 1965, Washington, D.C.

patient should experience an unexpected, sudden electrical failure, chances of successful resuscitation are good in a properly operating coronary care unit. Thus, the constant surveillance has a secondary role of anticipating, and acting, should an emergency occur—but the primary purpose of preventing them from occurring is paramount (Fig. 1).

The second basic service is the intensive care of the seriously ill patient with complications. There is, of course, an intermediate service for those patients who require continuous surveillance and therapeutic measures, but not necessarily of an intensive degree.

## Developing a Unit

Exact and detailed planning that includes an acute sense of future needs must precede the development of a coronary care unit. Needless waste of ex-

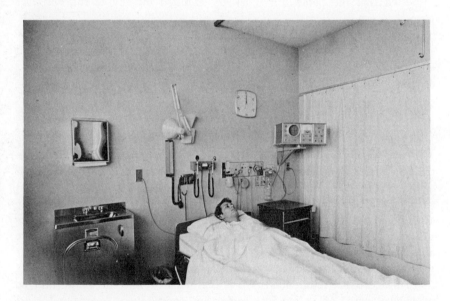

FIG. 1 Typical bedside coronary care installation. Mounted on the wall is a patient monitoring unit consisting of a cardioscope (for display of the patient's ECG), a heart rate meter with automatic alarm system, and a cardiac pacemaker to stimulate a faltering heart. Electrodes taped to the patient's chest relay his ECG signal to the cardioscope. A miniaturized photoelectric device attached to his ear senses each pulse beat, and relays this information to the bedside heart rate meter. The bedside instrument combination also relays the patient information to instruments at the nurses' central station, which is monitoring all patients in the unit simultaneously.

(Courtesy of Corbin-Farnsworth, Division of Smith Kline Instruments, Inc.
Palo Alto, Calif.)

penditures and equipment can be avoided if careful consideration is given to the needs of the individual hospital before elaborate units are designed and installed. While it is possible to define general principles of design the specific circumstances of every locale will determine and modify unit form and function; factors of basic importance certainly should include the size of the hospital and the number of patients to be accommodated.

It is recommended that various hospital personnel cooperate in designing the unit. Joint planning should at least include the hospital administrator, physicians, nurses, architects, and an electrical engineer.

Before costly construction of special new facilities is undertaken, the initial use of existing facilities should be encouraged insofar as is possible. Above all, it must be emphasized that a hospital should not initiate the *operation* of special facilities for coronary care until properly trained personnel are available to staff them.

To promote the most efficient use of the coronary care unit, it has been suggested that the patient in shock be admitted initially to the hospital's general intensive care area. There such patients will receive adequate treatment while, at the same time, unit facilities will be made more available to the seemingly stable patient and the one needing less intensive bedside care, both of whom have good chances of successful resuscitation should complications occur.

## LOCATION IN HOSPITAL

Location of the coronary care unit in a hospital will depend upon the general design of the hospital itself. While the unit should have its own supplies, equipment, and nurse cadre, it cannot be isolated; and ideally, it should be adjacent to a general medical facility within the institution, easily accessible from both the emergency and admitting rooms. There are advantages to having the unit in close proximity to the hospital's general intensive care area, one of which is possible use of the latter for treatment of certain patients with myocardial infarction if the coronary care unit is at full capacity.

An additional recommendation is that an area adjacent to the unit be made available to physicians for sleeping and consultation. A comfortably appointed room for the family located reasonably near the unit, while optional, serves both to enhance a quiet surrounding for the patient and prevent unnecessary interference with unit staff.

## GENERAL ENVIRONMENT

While the unit should provide as attractive an atmosphere as is feasible, the patient's desire for well-fitted accommodations must in no way compromise the need for adequate facilities of medical and nursing care. The principle of privacy has not been clearly established. The patient under surveillance should be placed in a private or semiprivate room according to the acuteness of his condition. The design of such a room should avoid total physical and emotional isolation from the outside environment. Although some patients with myocardial infarction must be protected to an appropriate extent from outside stimuli, such items as television sets, radio, clocks, and calendars should be available for use as medically indicated so the patient can maintain some degree of external contact.

The suggestion has been made that under certain circumstances patients requiring intensive treatment (e.g., those in shock) might be cared for in an

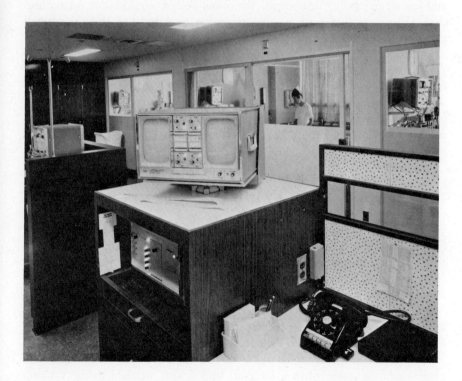

*FIG. 2* Typical elements in a fully instrumented coronary care unit. The nurses' central station (foreground) is equipped with a Lifeguard Central Station for monitoring both electrical and mechanical cardiac activity for four patients simultaneously. Mounted in the cabinet is a Tape Loop Recorder and an ECG (electrocardiogram) Direct Writer. The patients' rooms (background) can be curtained for privacy. Mounted on the wall in each room is a bedside monitor combined with a cardiac pacemaker.

(Courtesy of Corbin-Farnsworth, Division of Smith Kline Instruments, Inc. Palo Alto, Calif.)

open recovery room rather than in one large room per patient. While this proposal may have merit, it is difficult to make a specific recommendation on the basis of present experience.

### PHYSICAL DESIGN

The intensive care area should be arranged to allow optimal surveillance of all patients in the unit at all times from the central nurses' station. It is desirable, though not always feasible, for the arrangements to permit the nurse or physician at the bedside of one patient to maintain observation of the other patients in the unit and of equipment for resuscitation and defibrillation (Fig. 2). Adequacy of space is essential for proper surveillance of the patient and use of emergency equipment. The room design should allow for no less than 150 square feet, with no dimension less than ten feet. It is suggested that rooms for patients under intensive treatment be at least three feet larger in each dimension than those for patients whose primary need is surveillance.

Tomorrow's developments in therapeutic devices and techniques may bring a pump support, as well as sensing devices other than those now in use. Extra conduits in the wall should be considered for future monitoring or other such equipment. To meet the space requirements for such developments, it is of great importance to avoid initiating operation in an already inadequate area.

## *Unit Equipment*

*Monitors.* It is the consensus of the subcommittee * that the continuous electrocardiogram is the sole variable which presently lends itself to consistent and reliable monitoring (Fig. 3). The monitoring of other indices, such as central venous pressure or central venous oxygenation content, while possible, has been neither entirely satisfactory nor necessarily useful.

Instruments for rapid, direct recording of electrocardiograms should be available in each unit. These may be operated by a manually activated switch in the central nursing station console or at the bedside.

The electrocardiogram should be monitored through a standard frontal plane electrode system with a standard lead system attached to the patient. Plugs and connectors of the lead system should be completely compatible and interchangeable with other equipment, such as the electrocardiographic monitor and direct-writing electrocardiogram.

*Electrodes.* Several types of electrodes are available, though none are uniformly satisfactory. Problems to be solved include high-frequency static,

* The Subcommittee on the Coronary Care Unit of the American College of Cardiology.

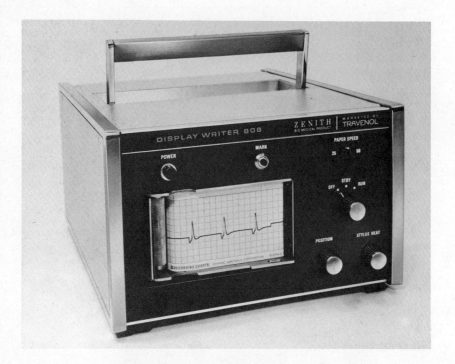

*FIG. 3* Instruments for rapid, direct-writing-recording of electrocardiograms should be available in each unit. These may be operated by a manually activated switch in the central nursing station or at the bedside.

(Courtesy of Travenol Laboratories, Inc., Morton Grove, Ill.)

artifacts, and the lack of a consistently successful means of maintaining continuous electrode attachment to the patient. For the registration of chest leads, the American Heart Association, in specifying the physical size or area of a chest lead electrode, states that it may be 3 cm in diameter, or smaller.

*Oscilloscope.* It is suggested that an oscilloscope be available in each patient's room to display whatever signals are being monitored (Fig. 4). This oscilloscope need not be in continuous operation. The screen should be so situated as to be out of the patient's view. It is strongly recommended that a remote or "slave" oscilloscope at the nurses' station continuously display the monitored signals for each patient.

*Alarm System.* Every unit should be equipped with both audible and visual alarm signals, installed in such a manner as to prevent inadvertent turn-off. The system will require modulations of tone and audible signal volume, and must be so constructed that any of the unit staff is able at a moment's

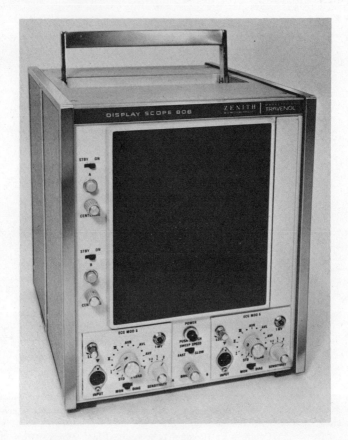

*FIG. 4* An oscilloscope can display whatever signals are being monitored.
(Courtesy of Travenol Laboratories, Inc., Morton Grove, Ill.)

notice to determine the source of the alarm. At present, the effectiveness of the adjustable delay is uncertain. Every alarm system should include a means of adjusting and varying the upper and lower heart rate limits which serve to produce the alarm. In addition, there should be an alarm at the patient's bedside by which the nurse may call or summon assistance should a crisis occur when she is alone in the unit.

*Pulse Signals.* While the visual pulse signal is apparently useful, it is the consensus that the audible signal or "beeper" is disturbing to the patient and not completely reliable. If the audible pulse signal is contained in the unit equipment, it should be provided with a turnoff switch. Such a signal will be most useful when employed selectively for more seriously ill patients.

### PLACEMENT OF EQUIPMENT

To conserve a maximum of floor space, it is recommended that as many devices as possible be hung from walls and ceiling. They should at least include the sphygmomanometer and oxygen and suction equipment hung from the wall, as well as intravenous hanging rods suspended from the ceiling, and an oscilloscope and other monitoring equipment suspended from shelves or ceiling.

### ELECTRICAL REQUIREMENTS

Each room in the unit should contain an absolute minimum of eight electrical outlets. To avoid total power loss in the event of equipment failure, two independent electrical circuits with circuit breakers should be available in each room.

Three-ground wiring is mandatory for all electrical equipment in the unit. The third ground wire and the "hotline" ground should be of the same potential.

It is strongly suggested that the director of the coronary care unit have an electronics expert examine all grounding upon installation to verify its adequacy. Experience has indicated that maintenance of satisfactorily grounded equipment requires close inspection and supervision. Ungrounded equipment, except for the mobile defibrillator, should never enter the unit, and precautions must always be taken to prevent incorrect installation and resultant inadequate grounding of instruments.

Again, with a look to the future, the facility should be designed with conduits of adequate size to accommodate unforetold needs for power lines not initially included in unit equipment.

Finally, in common with the needs of the hospital as a whole, the requirement of auxiliary power for the coronary care unit is obvious.

### SPECIALIZED SUPPORTIVE EQUIPMENT

*Defibrillators.* Electrical reversion of cardiac arrhythmias became clinically practical with the development of the defibrillator capable of terminating episodes of ventricular fibrillation. The time factor is of vital importance in the application of defibrillation. Because of the urgent nature of this service, it is obvious that the defibrillation apparatus should be immediately available from nearby within the unit.

As to the type of apparatus, there is evidence which favors the efficacy of the so-called DC defibrillator. Nonsynchronized equipment is adequate for

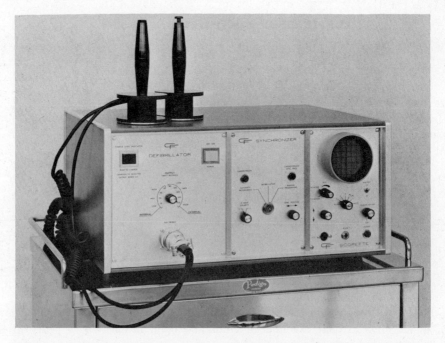

*FIG. 5* Defibrillator, Cardiac Synchronizer and three-inch Scopette cardioscope are combined in this model bedside unit. It is shown mounted on a stainless steel cart for mobility from one unit to another, but may be mounted on the wall above the patient's bed.

(Courtesy of Corbin-Farnsworth, Division of Smith Kline Instruments, Inc., Palo Alto, Calif.)

defibrillation; a device which applies the simplest shock is sufficient to deliver a satisfactory defibrillating pulse during the shortest time period. Synchronization is recommended, however, for those devices that use elective termination of arrhythmias by electric shock (Figs. 5 and 6).

As with all equipment essential to optimal function of the unit, there should be duplication of defibrillators in each unit.

*Pacemakers—External and Internal.* The term "electrical cardiac pacemaker" or "electrical pacemaker" is applied to an electrical device which can substitute for a defective natural pacemaker and control the beating of the heart by a series of rhythmic electrical discharges (Fig. 7). If the electrodes which deliver the discharges to the heart are placed on the outside of the chest, it is called an "external pacemaker." If the electrodes are placed within the chest wall, it is called an "internal pacemaker."

*Respiratory Equipment.* Respiratory apparatus of various types should be available within the unit, as well as devices for intermittent positive pressure

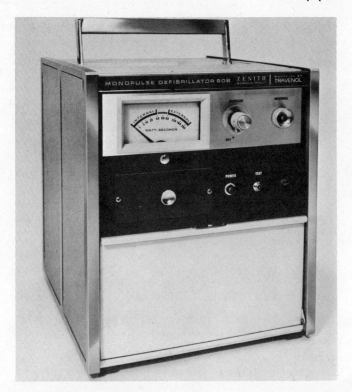

FIG. 6 The portable-type defibrillator can be easily transported to the patient unit when the need arises. It can be kept easily available within the CCU.

(Courtesy of Travenol Laboratories, Inc., Morton Grove, Ill.)

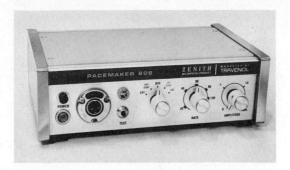

FIG. 7 The "electrical cardiac pacemaker" or "electrical pacemaker" can substitute for a defective natural pacemaker and control the beating of the heart by a series of rhythmic electrical discharges.

(Courtesy of Travenol Laboratories, Inc., Morton Grove, Ill.)

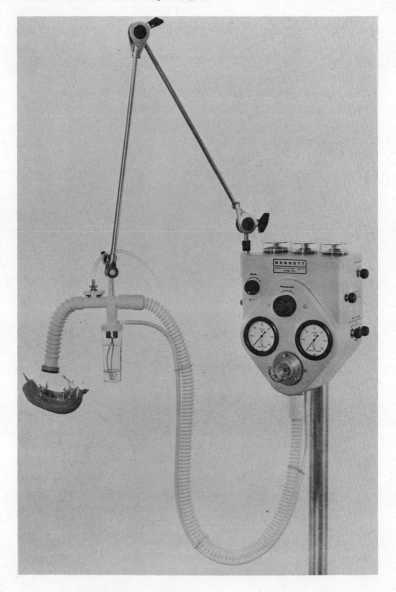

*FIG. 8* Respiratory apparatus.

(Courtesy of Puritan-Bennett Corp., Kansas City, Mo.)

breathing and for facilitating mouth-to-mouth breathing (Fig. 8). It is pointed out that respirators which are pressure-cycled do not function effectively in cardiopulmonary resuscitation. Cardiac compression activates such respirators, causing them to recycle without filling the lungs.

## Memory Loops and Recording Equipment

Experience to date has disclosed technical difficulties in the performance of "memory loops" for recording prealarm electrocardiograms. It is quite possible that in the future this device and the automatic write-out of arrythmias will be perfected to permit the development of frequency and type indexes of arrhythmias. Presently, however, such devices are applied largely in the research area and are most useful for on-the-spot study and review of unexpected complications.

A possible major development from the coronary care unit concept is an understanding of progress of complications. Certain arrhythmias may be found to predispose to certain later complications. It may also be possible some day to extend presently known correlations between anatomic locations of the injury to certain later complications. A routine of treatment based on automatically recorded data may be developed as well.

### Emergency Supply Cart

An emergency cart well stocked with drugs and appropriate instruments should be available for immediate utilization at the bedside. An inventory should be made daily to ensure that it is complete.

## Thorough Recording of Emergency Events

It is recognized that all information which becomes available during cardiac arrest or other emergency situations should be recorded (i.e., electrocardiogram, "memory loop," etc.). Thus events leading to the complication are identified and may be of great importance from a medicolegal standpoint.

Electrocardiographic evidence, however, should not be the sole criterion used to confirm or deny the occurrence of cardiac arrest and to initiate the process of resuscitation. Neither should it be the only means of establishing medicolegal documentation.

## Importance of Cardiac Nurse Specialist

The coronary care unit contains the basic elements for superior care of patients with myocardial infarction and arrhythmic complications and for the prompt recognition and treatment of cardiopulmonary arrest.

Of these elements, the most vital is the cardiac nurse specialist. She offers excellence in intensive nursing procedures through her familiarity with the particular physical and emotional needs of the coronary patient and through her training in the recognition and emergency management of such complications as congestive heart failure, shock, systemic and pulmonary embolization, cardiac arrest, and other arrhythmic catastrophes.

At the present state of medical knowledge, any hoped-for reduction in the high mortality associated with myocardial infarction must rely heavily on the prevention and correction of arrhythmic catastrophes. Cardiac resuscitation, therefore, centers around the nurse's recognition of premonitory disturbances and management of arrhythmic cardiopulmonary arrest.

## Training of Cardiac Nurse Specialist

The value of the expertly trained cardiac nurse specialist to the coronary care unit cannot be overemphasized. The range of skills required of her is broad. A partial listing includes thorough training in the prompt recognition of the following:

1. Basic rhythm in the electrocardiogram and significance of changing events.
2. Signs of unconsciousness, unresponsiveness, and ceased respiration as well as presence or absence of heartbeat by feeling the carotid or femoral pulse.
3. Signs of arrhythmic catastrophic events from the face of the monitor.
4. Ventricular asystole, ventricular fibrillation, atrial and ventricular ectopic arrhythmias, and atrioventricular block.

The nurse must be expected to master the principles of cardiopulmonary resuscitation, closed-chest massage and assisted ventilation. It is especially important that she be trained to administer DC countershock when no member of the house staff is immediately available.

The survival rates of several established units dramatically improved after the nurses staffing the units were fully trained in the recognition of complications and in immediate institution of resuscitative efforts.

In the smaller community hospitals where the house staff and trained cardiac nurse specialists are not available, the nurse on duty must continue assisted ventilation and assisted circulation until the attending physician arrives. Under such conditions, however, it must be pointed out that the rate of successful cardiac resuscitation following arrhythmic arrest will be materially lowered.

## Methods of Resuscitation

The following discussion pertains to resuscitative procedures rather than to roles of unit personnel. It is assumed that the trained nurse or physician will be available and upon recognition of the catastrophe will take immediate action. The methods outlined here require implementation by a highly alert and keenly trained team to achieve optimal results.

### Ventricular Fibrillation

Following recognition of ventricular fibrillation, transthoracic shock using DC or AC equipment should be instituted immediately. Although the subcommittee has recommended the use of DC current for fibrillation, hospitals now using AC equipment should realize that it will provide effective countershock for ventricular fibrillation.

The DC defibrillator should be set at 400 watt-seconds or joules. If an AC defibrillator is employed, 440 volts or above should be used immediately, preferably at 0.25-second duration. The shock should be activated by the individual who administers it. If, following the initial countershock discharge, the patient has not returned to adequate rhythm, a second countershock should be administered immediately. If this is ineffective, assisted ventilation and circulation should be attempted.

Should the immediate application of these countershocks not result in conversion, assisted ventilation and circulation must be maintained and measures adopted which will increase the so-called cardiac tone. Thus, the fibrillatory pattern is improved in order that the next countershock may be effective. Correction of acidosis and administration of epinephrine or isoproterenol are possible means of improving cardiac tone before countershock is reapplied.

An antiarrhythmia drug, such as procainamide, quinidine, or lidocaine, should also be employed if defibrillation does not immediately occur or reversion to ventricular fibrillation occurs.

It should be remembered that acidosis develops rapidly during treatment for fibrillation. Therefore, patients in cardiac arrest ought to receive 40 mEq of sodium bicarbonate every five minutes to ten minutes. Anticipating the physician's steps will greatly prove to the patient's benefit. After treatment of the acidosis and administration of vasopressor and cardiotonic drugs (epinephrine, isoproterenol), countershock may successfully terminate previously unresponsive ventricular fibrillation.

### Ventricular Standstill

If the immediate catastrophe is ventricular standstill, it is the opinion of the subcommittee that as the initial step, a prompt, hard blow should be given the anterior chest. This will, in some instances, return electrical activity immediately. Should this fail, external pacing is recommended for only 15 to 20 seconds. If return to nodal or sinus rhythm with a palpable pulse does not then ensue, immediate assisted ventilation and closed-chest message should be instituted. Epinephrine or isoproterenol with Neo-Synephrine or other vasopressor agent should be administered and acidosis corrected. When a matter of minutes in controlling the arrhythmia may mean life or death, and *when cardioversion techniques are not available,* propranolol hydrochloride may be given intravenously slowly and in low dosage. Although risks must necessarily be taken to control the arrhythmia in these cases, the cautious use of the drug will reduce them to a minimum. Care in the administration of propranolol hydrochloride and constant monitoring is essential, as the failing heart requires some sympathetic drive to maintain myocardial tone.

While the use of intravenous calcium chloride or gluconate may occasionally be helpful, caution must be exercised in the administration of calcium to the patient who has received digitalis or has exhibited any evidence of digitoxic arrhythmia. A concentrated calcium solution will cause necrosis if injected intramuscularly. Patients in whom standstill does recur are most likely acidotic, and this must be combated with suitable drug therapy.

## *Cessation of Resuscitation Efforts*

The decision to stop the resuscitative procedure must be made by the physician in charge when he believes that irreversible complications exist or when cardiac or central nervous system death is evident. The nurse specialist must continue resuscitative efforts until otherwise directed by the physician. A decision to cease procedures may be facilitated by electroencephalographic evidence.

## *Postresuscitation Care*

The next step in the basic resuscitation plan may be termed postresuscitation care, a service as important as the resuscitation procedures themselves. Such care proceeds as follows:

- The underlying cause of the arrest must be treated.
- Arterial pH determinations should be secured and continuous treatment of acidosis provided.
- Vasoconstrictive and cardiotonic drugs should be used as necessary.
- Assisted ventilation should be provided if needed.
- Immediate hypothermia may be instituted if the patient is not awake when the arrest is terminated. Hypertonic solutions such as urea, mannitol, or hypertonic glucose may be used as well to decrease cerebral edema.

## AV Block

The mode of treatment for atrioventricular block will be determined by the degree of AV block present. Appropriate action for the various degrees consists of:

- First-degree–close observation for progression to more serious grades.
- Second-degree–positioning of a transvenous, battery-powered pacemaker in the right ventricle, attached to a transistorized unit. If the patient has satisfactory hemodynamics, the catheter may be left in place and the patient not paced unless cardiac output and rate decrease.
- Third-degree–internal pacing with a transvenous pacemaker. Whether the catheter should be bipolar or unipolar and whether it should be positioned by fluoroscopy or by blind technique are matters of individual preference.

## Future Developments

It is hoped that the establishment of coronary care units in large institutions equipped with basic research and clinical facilities will lead to development of studies which will ultimately provide improved forms of therapy, chiefly for power failure of the heart.

Untold challenges remain in the field of cardiac care for the coronary patient. Much worthwhile research will no doubt be forthcoming from highly motivated, enterprising units using such modalities as coronary arteriography, left ventricular angiograms, radioisotope scanning techniques, precise acid-base fluid electrolyte studies, measurement of cardiac output, intracardiac systemic and venous pressures, paired pulse pacing, diastolic augmentation by assisted circulation, and partial left heart bypass.

The nurse will play a prominent role in most or all of the above procedures. Being aware of chemical, vagal, electrical, or hypoxic mechanisms that can promote ventricular fibrillation or cardiac asystole, the coronary care unit nurse will act to prevent such conditions from occurring. In order to do this, she must be skilled in identifying arrhythmias. But recognition will not be enough. For therapy, the nurse will have atropine in readiness for a patient observed to be in bradycardia; she will have lidocaine or propranolol in readiness for the patient in whom she observes developing premature contractions. For the patient experiencing conduction defects, she will have a pacemaker and specially prepared wires for intrathoracic placement of a pacemaker in anticipation of the physician's actions. And, when the nurse recognizes ventricular fibrillation, she will deliver DC countershock. Many of these procedures are already being carried out in research medical centers. However, it should be anticipated that within a time span of a few years, all of these procedures plus many more will be commonplace nursing procedures.

## Summary

In this chapter, the basic design and equipment of the coronary care unit have been presented. In addition, recognition has been given to the role of the cardiac nurse specialist. The nursing administrator must be thoroughly familiar with the basic concepts of the coronary care unit. The unit's nurse-in-charge and the members of the nurse cadre of the unit should be proficient in all the services the unit provides. Beyond this, there are two important groups of nurses whose training requirements and functions differ and whose relations to the operations of the unit should, therefore, be clearly understood.

Every unit should have a reserve or "back-up" pool of nurses who are considered basic members of the cadre of coronary care unit registered nurses. These nurses substitute for regular members of the cadre when the latter are absent because of illness, vacation, or other causes. This reserve group must be fully trained in all the techniques applied in the unit and be kept at peak proficiency.

## Review and Advance

1. *When is the most critical period of the coronary patient?*
   Within the first four days following the acute attack.
2. *What are the two principal types of services provided by the coronary care unit?*
   The first type of service is constant surveillance of the patient who initially appears to have few if any complications and whose circulatory status is stable. The constant surveillance has a secondary role of anticipating and acting should an emergency occur—but the primary purpose of preventing one from occurring is paramount. The second type of service is provided for the seriously ill patient with associated complications.
3. *Why is it important that nurses expecting to work in the coronary care unit be "in on the planning stage"?*
   As with all changes planned within the hospital—or any other business organization—it is a sociologic fact that individuals who are asked to contribute to a project while it is still in the planning stage feel a certain commitment to see it through to its completion. A certain amount of pride and self-satisfaction derived from participation in the decision-making appears to be a necessary factor in personal morale. However, aside from these factors, it makes logical sense; since nurses will be working in the unit, they should be

thoroughly familiar with certain needs of the patients in regard to the placement of equipment. Space arrangements must be allotted with an eye to meeting the patient's needs and providing an environment which will supply his needs in the most efficient manner.

4. *For the small hospital that wishes to set up a coronary care unit, where may specifications be obtained?*
The American Heart Association or the local, state, or county Heart Association is the best source of information. Other sources include Regional Medical Program Area Offices and the United States Printing Office.

5. *Are all the monitoring devices practical when they are often "out of order," or aren't working?*
In answer to this and many similar questions:
Bethesda, Maryland, was the site in the fall of 1969 of a two-day conference to untangle legal, financial, and semantic bottlenecks related to the present status and future development and use of medical devices. The conference was sponsored by the Association for the Advancement of Medical Instrumentation (AAMI) and supported in part by the National Heart Institute of NIH. In environmental diseases and medical device problems, it was pointed out that it was vital to protect the patient. But it is also important to trace the cause or source of difficulties with devices. Participants at the conference coined the phrase "periontogenic disease" to describe disorders in the environment of the patient and in the device. They may be caused by faulty design of the device, inability of the body to absorb foreign matter, toxicity, or tissue incompatability. Or the problem could arise from the patient's psychologic inability to accept a life-sustaining or monitoring device. These must be recognized. And it is equally important to recognize that sometimes problems which are deemed to have been caused by device failure or malfunction are, in fact, a consequence of human error or other factors unrelated to the efficiency or reliability of the device tself.

6. *What about electrical hazards in modern hospitals—with so many of the new devices tied into one circuit?*
The conferees at the conference named above stressed the need for more control and research in this area. Yes, a patient can be jolted pretty badly if he is "hooked up" simultaneously to several different pieces of equipment plugged into different power sources without equal ground potentials. Exactly what constitutes a dangerous threshold of leakage current? What are the safest approaches to power distribution in hospitals? How can the operator of an electrical device be sure that it's functioning properly? One possibility might be to set up a mechanism for frequent inspections of electrical gadgets and equipment; another is to get all medical and nursing personnel to establish a routine of testing any device at the bedside before it's connected to or directed at a patient.

7. *Why should nurses have to accept this responsibility?*
Because the line must be drawn somewhere and nurses are dedicated individuals. One of the reasons for electrical problems in hospitals is that in some areas of the United States, construction of a hospital demands no special electrical safety considerations. The contractor is required merely to follow the building codes that are applied to an apartment building, for example, or any other facility. The possibility of developing new and more comprehensive architectural codes which would provide greater electrical protection in hospitals will no doubt be a major development of the future.

# 3 REVIEW OF PERTINENT RELATIONSHIPS OF CERTAIN ANATOMIC FUNCTIONS AND SYSTEMS

There is an increasing trend in certain states to have physicians engage in continual medical education throughout their professional careers as a requirement for maintaining membership in their state association. Failure to keep abreast of rapid advances taking place in medicine could not only result in expulsion from the association but the loss of hospital staff privileges under the ruling. The motivation is a sense of responsibility to ensure the public that a member of the association is competent throughout his life, not just at the time he was initially licensed.

It is good to see that the medical profession has joined the nursing profession in its efforts to stimulate the individual to be responsible for his own individual self-development. Nothing remains static in today's world; in fact, the only certain thing in itself is the constant change factor. This chapter is included to refresh your memory on aspects of anatomy and physiology that you will need to recall in your depth study of coronary care.

## Circulatory System

A nurse must thoroughly understand the basic physiology of circulation in order to be alert to any changes that might affect the patient.

The circulation of blood is a simple mechanical process consisting of a pump, the heart, and vessels necessary for the conveyance of oxygenated blood from the heart to the periphery, and unoxygenated blood from the periphery to the heart. The circulatory system is divided into two separate circulations: a low-pressure, smaller pulmonary circulation and a high-pressure, larger systemic circulation.

In the development of these two separate circulations in the fetus the pulmonary circulation is bypassed by various shunts. These shunts close soon after birth; not infrequently they remain open, which is one of the causes giving rise to babies with *diseased hearts*. Less than one month after conception the heart of an embryo normally begins to beat and continues for a lifetime (Fig. 1).

### HEART

The heart is a four-chambered muscular organ lying in the anterior, inferior portion of the mediastinum. It is cone-shaped and made up of interwoven and interlaced striated involuntary muscle. The heart is contained

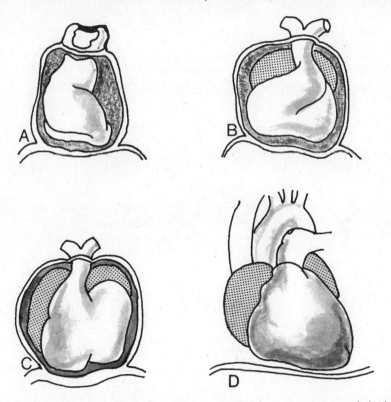

*FIG. 1* In the embryo, the heart develops from a tube that twists, turns, and divides in complex ways to form a four-chambered, fully-mature heart. The developmental stages are shown from the simple tube to the four chambers of the heart represented by the left atrium and ventricle in the foreground, while the right atrium and ventricle are slightly obscured and to the posterior side.

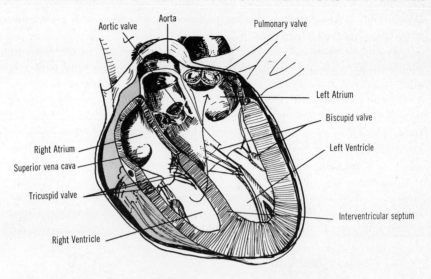

FIG. 2 Blood enters the right atrium from the venae cavae, goes to the right ventricle, and from there to the lungs via the pulmonary artery. It returns to the left atrium, passes down to the left ventricle, and from there through the aorta to the body.

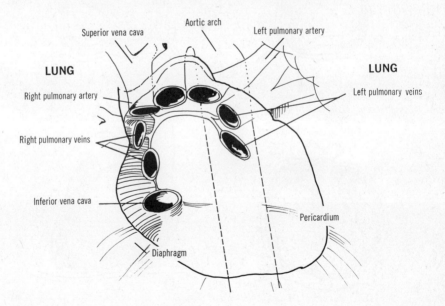

FIG. 3 The pericardial sac is attached to the diaphragm and to the necks of the great vessels. The points of entry of the various vessels are shown. Note that the left pulmonary veins pass behind the inferior vena cava and the right atrium to enter the rear of the left atrium.

within a sac termed the pericardium and its surface is bathed by pericardial fluid. The blood supply to the heart itself is by the coronary arteries, a left anterior and a right posterior artery arising from the aortic sinus or coronary sinus (Figs. 2 and 3). The blood is collected in anterior and posterior veins which empty into the coronary sinus and then into the right atrium.

The nerve supply to the heart is effected through the vagus and sympathetic nerves. The vagus can be considered the more important of the two. It exerts a continuous restraining influence on the heart. The sympathetic nerve control of the heart is considered subordinate to the vagus control because under normal resting conditions it is inactive, and on stimulation of the sympathetic supply, acceleration of the heart begins only after a considerable latent period. The sympathetic and vagus centers in the medulla, together, form a functional area termed the *cardiac center*. The quantity and quality of

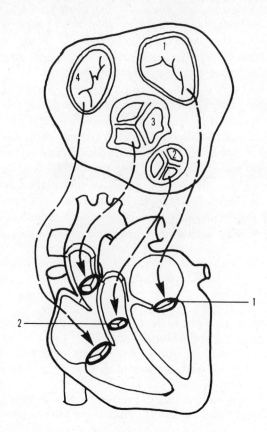

FIG. 4  Upper part of drawing shows view of heart from top looking down on valves. Arrows lead to corresponding valves in sectional view below: 1. mitral, or bicuspid valve; 2. pulmonary, or semilunar valve; 3. aortic, or semilunar valve; 4. tricuspid valve.

blood that bathes this area affects the heart rate. A slight anoxia, small excesses of carbon dioxide, and an increase in temperature will produce an increase in heart rate. A severe lack of oxygen or excess of carbon dioxide will slow the heart and even produce heart block.

Venous blood enters the right atrium and passes through the tricuspid valve into the right ventricle. From here it passes through the pulmonary valve into the pulmonary circulation where, in the alveoli of the lung, carbon dioxide is removed and oxygen is absorbed (Fig. 4). This involves a complicated shift in ions brought on largely by the changes in partial pressures and pH. The blood is collected in the pulmonary veins and is returned to the left atrium. This is a low pressure system of 30/10 mm mercury (the pulmonary artery pressure, as opposed to the aortic pressure of 120/80). From the left atrium it passes through the mitral valve into the left ventricle. The left ventricle is thicker than the right due to the fact that it must produce the force necessary for systemic circulation. The blood then passes out of the aortic valve to the systemic circulation at a pressure of 120/80 mm mercury. This is termed aortic pressure. Venous blood returns to the right atrium through the superior and inferior vena cava and the coronary sinus.

The cardiac cycle is made up of two phases: diastole and systole. The former is the filling and relaxation phase of the cycle during which the diastolic blood pressure is recorded normally at 80 mm of mercury. There will be more discussion of this later. During diastole, the arterial pressure is maintained by elastic recoil of the great arteries (Fig. 5). The average rate of this cycling is approximately 70 times a minute.

You can see from the foregoing discussion that the left ventricle-aortic pressure is about four to five times higher than the right ventricle-pulmonary artery pressure. These pressures are relationships that can be markedly altered in many diseases. Some such disturbances can be summarized as follows:

- Generalized constriction of arterioles, as in arterial hypertension, causes elevation of arterial diastolic pressure, and in order to preserve adequate blood flow the left ventricular systolic and arterial systolic pressures also rise.
- Obstruction of the aorta, as in coarctation, causes elevation of pressures in the aorta proximal to the obstruction.
- Relaxation of arterioles reduces arterial pressures, as in neurogenic syncope (fainting) or with the use of certain drugs like nitroglycerin or hexamethonium.
- Acute blood loss reduces venous pressures and ultimately prevents normal cardiac filling; therefore, cardiac output and arterial pressures finally decrease.
- Congestive heart failure produces a rise in ventricular diastolic pressures and, in combination with increased total blood volume, results in increased capillary, venous, and atrial pressures. The rise in venous pressure

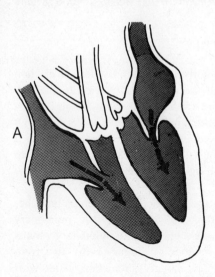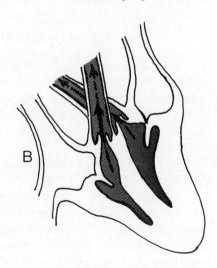

*FIG. 5* The heart pumps by alternately contracting and relaxing. Contraction begins at the top, in the atrii, and passes downward to the ventricles. It is followed by an instant's rest. A shows the heart in diastole, that is, in a condition of relaxation when the ventricles are filling with blood. The walls of the heart are thick and powerful as they must be since B shows the centricles in systole, or forcefully contracting, ejecting the blood to the entire body and to the lungs for reoxygenation. Diastole, or relaxation, and systole, or contraction, make up the beat of the heart.

is necessary for the preservation of blood flow since, if ventricular diastolic pressure rises and venous pressure does not rise, the blood will not arrive in time to fill the heart ventricles before the next ventricular contraction.

- Narrowing or stricture of the valvular openings in the heart causes obstruction or increased resistance to blood flow from one chamber to the next. Flow can only be maintained by a rise in pressure in the chamber behind the obstruction. This may be measured by observing a "pressure gradient" or abnormal drop in pressure from one chamber to the next.
- "Insufficiency" of a valve, or failure to close properly, allows backflow of blood through the valve, loss of pressure in the chamber or artery ahead, and increase in pressure of chamber behind.
- Abnormal communications between areas of different pressures allow flow of blood from the high-pressure area to the low-pressure area. If this flow is sufficient the pressure will drop in the high-pressure area and rise in the low-pressure area. Examples are ventricular septal defects (flow from high-pressure left ventricle to low-pressure right ventricle) and patent ductus arteriosus (flow from high-pressure aorta to low-pressure pulmonary artery through the persistent congenital connecting vessel).[1]

1. Walter Modell et al. *Handbook of Cardiology for Nurses,* 5th ed. New York, Springer Publishing Co., Inc., 1966, pp. 52–53.

### PULMONARY CIRCULATION

Pulmonary circulation begins with the pumping action, or ejection of blood from the right ventricle through the pulmonary valve into the pulmonary conus or trunk. This splits or bifurcates after a short distance into a right and left pulmonary artery which enter their respective lungs (Fig. 6). The blood contained in these arteries is venous or unoxygenated and under a low pressure (30/10 mm of mercury). Due to the fact that the resistance to the flow of blood is slight, the work of the right ventricle is less; consequently, the muscular wall is thinner.

The right and left pulmonary artery then divide into numerous branches and the smallest capillaries are intimately associated with the pulmonary alveoli. At this point oxygenated blood is collected into the pulmonary venous system and returned to the left atrium via four pulmonary veins, two from each lung. The amount of blood in the pulmonary circulation varies with

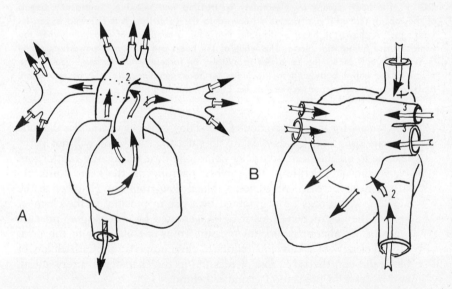

*FIG. 6* A. Arrows show directional blood flow in great vessels that carry the blood from the heart. The pulmonary artery carries blood to the lungs for oxygenation; the aorta carries blood to the rest of the body through its many branches. From the arch of the aorta, blood leaves by way of the innominate artery, left common carotid artery, and the left subclavian to nourish the top parts of the body; the aorta then doubles back down behind the heart where it branches into other large arteries which are a major part of the vast 75,000 miles of arteries, arterioles, capillaries, venuoles, and veins. B. Rear view of the heart showing the great vessels that bring the blood to the heart: the superior and inferior vena cava return venous blood to the right atrium, while the pulmonary veins bring freshly oxygenated blood to the left atrium.

the phases of respiration. There is approximately 9 percent of the total blood volume during inspiration and approximately 6 percent of the total blood volume during expiration in the pulmonary system. In conditions such as mitral stenosis the flow of blood from the pulmonary veins to the left ventricle is obstructed at the mitral valve. The left atrium does not empty properly and there is an increase to 20 percent or more of the total blood volume in the lungs. The lungs become engorged, ventilate poorly, and contain less air. This is termed *pulmonary congestion.*

Arising from the aorta (systemic circulation) are bronchial arteries which supply the lung parenchyma and then for the most part empty into the pulmonary circulation. This is the blood supply to the bronchi down to the terminal bronchioles. They are the vasa vasorum of the pulmonary arteries and supply the walls of the bronchi. Under normal conditions, the anastomoses between the bronchial artery and the pulmonary circulation occurs only at the capillary level and the amount of blood transferred is small. In pathologic conditions such as *pulmonary stenosis* there are large anastomoses which shunt a considerable amount of blood into the pulmonary circulation.

### SYSTEMIC CIRCULATION

The oxygenated blood received into the left ventricle is forced out of the aorta into the peripheral vessels under a pressure of 120/80 mm of mercury. Branching from the aortic branch (arch) is the innominate artery which divides into the right subclavian and right common carotid artery branches, and at the most distal portion of the arch, the left subclavian artery arises. From the descending thoracic aorta there arise pericardial arteries, bronchial arteries, mediastinal arteries, paired intercostal arteries and branches to the esophagus. These arteries are usually small and varied in number.

Immediately beneath the diaphragm, from the abdominal aorta arises the celiac (coeliac) artery which branches into the splenic artery, the left gastric artery and the hepatic artery. Immediately distal to the celiac artery arises the superior mesenteric artery which supplies the small intestine. Further distally, the renal (paired) arteries arise and provide the blood supply to the kidneys. At approximately this same level, the inferior mesenteric artery branches and carries blood to the terminal colon. The aorta then splits into right and left common iliacs at the promontory of the sacrum. The common iliacs bifurcate into the internal iliac arteries. The external iliac continues beneath the inguinal ligament as the femoral artery, which subsequently divides into the superficial and deep femoral arteries. At the knee the superficial femoral artery is termed the popliteal. This divides into an anterior and posterior tibial artery. The anterior tibial artery as it passes on to the dorsum of the foot is called the dorsalis artery. At the ankle the posterior tibial is behind the medial malleolus.

The other branches of the aorta which are primarily concerned in vascular surgery are the carotids, which divide to form the internal and external carotids (carotis) supplying the face and skull. The subclavian artery courses into the arm to become the axillary and brachial arteries which then divide into the radial and ulnar arteries.

The venous return from the extremities and viscera is via the corresponding vein into the superior and inferior vena cava. This returns the unoxygenated blood to the right atrium. The blood from the viscera is routed through the liver via the splenic, inferior mesenteric veins. These form the portal vein which enters the liver and subsequently, through the hepatic vein, empties into the inferior vena cava.

## VASOCONSTRICTOR CENTER

The pressure maintained in this vast network falls from 120 mm in the arteries to approximately 5 mm of mercury in the veins. The most marked decrease in the gradient of pressure is in the arterioles which offer the most peripheral resistance and are the most adjustable. The smooth muscles in the walls of the arterioles alter the caliber of the vessel in accordance with physiologic needs. They are easily controlled by nervous influences and chemical factors. The vasomotor system supplies the nervous control for the arterioles and is the most important single factor in the control of the peripheral resistance. It is dominated by a center in the medulla which is chiefly the vasoconstrictor center. It is questionable whether a vasodilator center exists and dilation of the arterioles is achieved mainly through the inhibition of the vasoconstrictor center.

The vasomotor center receives afferent impulses from all parts of the body and is influenced by certain reflexes which control the heart. Its effects are mediated over the sympathetic system and result in peripheral vasoconstriction. It is this vasoconstricting property of epinephrine, or adrenalin, which is utilized extensively in maintaining blood pressure during extensive cardiovascular surgery.

## COLLATERAL CIRCULATION

The various portions of the body are supplied by specific arteries, most of which have been enumerated. However, there are other channels through which blood may reach a particular area; this is termed *collateral circulation*.

Collateral circulation is established where two or more arteries supply the same organ. The capillary networks of these arteries communicate and the blood from the functioning artery is forced into the capillaries or capillary network of the occluded one, eventually producing dilation of these capillaries sufficient to maintain the viability of the affected body area.

The establishment of collateral circulation is a prolonged process and in many instances may be unknown until demonstrated by an arteriogram. In other instances it is not sufficient, and as a result of the decreased blood supply gangrene results. When gangrene develops in an extremity, amputation is often necessary. At the present time, surgeons are able to establish collaterals in the form of prosthetic grafts to "bypass" occluded arteries. It is known that such a collateral system can occur in the heart, but, so far, prosthetics have been unsuccessful here. Successful transplanting or rerouting of the internal mammary arteries to the heart has been accomplished. This is termed the "Vinberg" after its founder.

# *Muscles*

Muscle, commonly referred to as "flesh," is the tissue by which, because of its power of contraction, movements are made in the higher animals. You remember that muscular tissue is divided, according to its function, into two great groups: voluntary and involuntary. The former is under the control of the will, while the latter changes its actions independently of thought.

The voluntary muscles are often referred to as the "striped" muscles because, under the microscope, all the voluntary muscles have a striped (striated) appearance; the involuntary muscles, for the most part, appear "unstriped" or plain. There are several exceptions to the last statement. The heart muscle, which is involuntary, is partially striped as are certain muscles of the throat and inside the ear.

## VOLUNTARY MUSCLE

Muscle classed as voluntary is arranged in a regular method over the body, being mainly attached to the skeleton. Because of this arrangement, it is sometimes called the skeletal muscle.

Each muscle is enclosed in a sheath of fibrous tissue known as fascia, or "epimysium," and from this, partitions of fibrous tissue, known as "perimysium," run into the substance of the muscle dividing it into small bundles. Each of these bundles consists of a collection of fibers which form the unit of the muscle. Each fiber is enclosed in an elastic sheath of its own which allows it to lengthen and shorten. At the ends of the elastic sheath, a minute bundle of connective tissue fibers joins it to the neighbor or to one of the connective tissue partitions in the muscle. By means of this connection, the fiber produces its effect upon contracting.

Now how does this system hold itself in check? The elastic sheath is pierced by a nerve fiber, which breaks out upon the surface of the muscle fiber, thereby bringing each small muscle fiber under the control of the nervous system. This controls the discharge of energy which produces muscular contraction.

Between the muscle fibers run many capillary blood vessels. They are so placed that the contractions of the muscle fibers empty them at once of blood, and thus the active muscle is ensured of an especially good blood supply. However, none of these blood vessels pierce the elastic sheath, so that the blood does *not* come into direct contact with the muscular tissue. Where, then, do these muscles get their nourishment? From the lymph that exudes from the blood vessels. The lymph circulation is also involuntarily controlled—as required—by the muscular contractions. Between the muscle fibers and surrounded by a sheath of connective tissue lie, here and there, special structures known as "muscle-spindles." Each of these contains thin muscle fibers, numerous nuclei, and the endings of sensory nerves. They appear to be the sensory —or touch—organs of the body.

## INVOLUNTARY MUSCLE

Involuntary muscle includes, as already stated, the heart muscle and unstriped muscle. The heart muscle actually stands in structure between the striped and unstriped muscle. Each fiber is short, has a nucleus in its center, communicates with neighboring fibers by short branches, shows a faintly striped appearance near its exterior, and has no elastic sheath.

Plain, or unstriped, muscle is found in the following areas: the inner and middle coats of the stomach and intestines; the ureters and the urinary bladder; the windpipe and bronchial tubes; the ducts of the glands; the gall bladder; the uterus and the Fallopian tubes; the middle coat of the lymph and blood vessels; the iris and ciliary muscle of the eye; the tunic of the scrotum; and in association with various glands of the hairs and skin. The fibers are very much smaller than the striped variety, although they vary greatly in size. Each is pointed at its end, has one or more oval nuclei in the center, and has a delicate sheath of elastic enveloping it. The fibers are grouped in bundles, much the same as the striped fibers, but they adhere to one another by cement material, *not* by the tendon bundles found in voluntary muscle.

## ORIGIN AND DEVELOPMENT OF MUSCLE

All of the muscles of a developing individual originate from the central layer, or mesoblast, of the embryo, each fiber taking origin from a single cell. Later on in life, muscles have the power of increasing in size—as the result of use—and healing after parts have been destroyed after injury. This healing process takes place partly by the growth and splitting of the original fibers to form new fibers, and partly from reserve cells which lie in every muscle between the muscle fibers. An example showing to what extent the unstriped muscle can expand is given by the uterus, which greatly increases in size during the months of pregnancy and yet returns to normal, or near normal, in the course of a month to six weeks after childbirth.

## MUSCULAR ENERGY

The combination of the chemical and physical properties of muscle combine to form the basis for producing heat and mechanical work. The energy of muscular contraction is derived from a complicated series of chemical chain reactions. Complex substances are built up then torn down again, supplying each other with energy for this purpose. The immediate energy for contraction is supplied by high energy phosphate bonds, the first chemical action breaking down adenyl-pyrophosphate (adenosine triphosphate) into phosphoric acid and adenylic acid. Next is the phosphocreatine which breaks down into creatine and phosphoric acid, giving energy for the rebuilding of adenyl-pyrophosphate. Creatine is a normal nitrogenous constituent of muscle. Then, glycogen (glucose) is burned through a series of steps to water and carbon dioxide. Under conditions of low oxygen tension, lactic acid accumulates —the stored sugar, through the intermediary stage of sugar bound to phosphate, breaks down into lactic acid to supply energy for the rebuilding of phosphocreatine. Finally, part of the lactic acid is oxidized to supply energy for building up the rest of the lactic acid into glycogen again. If there is not enough oxygen, lactic acid accumulates and fatigue results.

There are several points to notice in this version of muscular activity. First, muscle contraction and relaxation take place in the absence of oxygen— the anaerobic phase. Secondly, oxygen comes into the picture in the phase of recovery, and by oxidizing some of the lactic acid winds up the contracting mechanism once more. Lastly, the energy of contraction does not come directly from the breakdown of glycogen as is so commonly believed. All of the chemical changes are accomplished by indirect means by the action of several enzymes. *It is important to keep these enzymes in mind; we will pick them up again when discussing diagnostic tests.*

Involuntary muscle has several peculiarities of contraction. In the heart, *rhythmicity* is an important feature—one beat appearing to be, in a sense, the cause of the next beat. This partial, steady contraction of muscle which determines tonicity or firmness, referred to as "tonus," is a characteristic of all muscle but particularly of unstriped muscle in some localities, as in the walls of the arteries. The arteries owe their elasticity and strength mainly to this fact. The involuntary muscle forming the middle coat of the bowels, gland ducts and other tubes, contracts in a peristaltic movement—which means that a ring of contraction passes slowly along the tube, the muscle relaxing as the ring of contraction passes on.

Fatigue, although mentioned briefly above, comes on when a muscle is made to act for some time. It is due to the accumulation of waste products, especially sarcolactic acid produced by the muscle's activity. As these wastes are carried away by the blood, the muscle recovers.

Rigor mortis is a condition which comes on in the muscles after death, and to which the general stiffening of the body is due. It consists of a state of permanent, wasteful contraction, beginning in the muscles of the neck and lower jaw at a period which varies from ten minutes to seven hours after death, and spreading gradually over the whole body. It comes on more quickly after death by exhaustion or from some weakening disease; occasionally, it comes on instantaneously after violent injuries causing death so that the body is fixed in the position in which death occurs. The rigidity lasts usually from sixteen to twenty-four hours, but it varies.

## Air Passages

These are the nose, pharynx or throat, larynx, trachea or windpipe, and bronchi or bronchial tubes.

The air, on entering the nose passes through a high narrow passage on each side, the outer wall of which projects along three lines (the turbinate processes) so as almost to touch the dividing septum between the nostrils, thus making on each side three passages in which the air is warmed, moistened, and filtered of dust particles. Mouth breathing is a bad habit because the air is not prepared for entrance to the lungs. In the pharynx, the air and food passages meet and cross. The larynx lies in front of the lower part of the pharynx and is the organ where the voice is produced by means of the vocal cords. The opening between the two cords is called the glottis, and shortly after passing this point, the air reaches the trachea. This leads into the chest and divides above the heart into two bronchi, one of which goes to each lung. Here they split into finer tubes. The bronchi divide within the chest at the level of the second rib. The texture of the lungs is very highly elastic, so that when the chest is opened surgically or by injury, each lung collapses to about one-third of its normal bulk.

The larynx is enclosed in two strong cartilages, the thyroid and the cricoid. Beneath this, the trachea, which is stiffened by rings of cartilage so that it never closes no matter what position the body may be in, is traced down until it disappears behind the breastbone, or xyphoid.

Each lung is roughly conical in shape with an apex projecting into the neck and the base resting upon the diaphragm. The rounded outer surface of each is in contact with the ribs of its own side, while the heart, lying between the lungs, hollows out the inner surface of each to some extent (Fig. 7). There

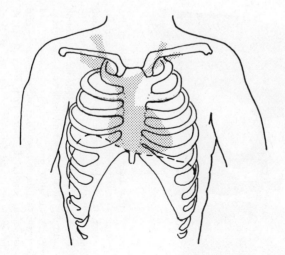

FIG. 7 A person's heart is approximately the size of his own fist clenched. It is well protected within the rib cage, above the diaphragm. Its apex is pointed downwards and to the left, but the mass of the heart lies in the cenral part of the chest behind the sternum, rather than to the left as one would imagine.

is an outer border, along which the outer and inner surfaces meet, and the borders of the two lungs touch one another for a short distance behind the middle of the breastbone. The apex, which is blunt, extends into the neck approximately one and a half inches above the clavicle and is covered here by the muscles of the neck. The base is deeply hollowed, corresponding to the domed shape of the diaphram, which is pushed up by the liver on the right side, and by the stomach and spleen on the left. The right lung is split by two deep fissures into three lobes; the left has two lobes divided by a single fissure.

Each lung is covered by a membrane, the pleura or pleural membrane, in such a way that one layer of the membrane is closely adherent to the lung, from which it cannot be separated; the other layer lines the inner surface of one half of the chest wall. These two layers form a closed cavity, "the pleural cavity," which surrounds the lungs except at the point where the bronchi and vessels enter it. This cavity is merely the potential state, the two layers being separated by a thin layer of fluid which enables them to glide with very little friction over one another as the lung expands and retracts in breathing.

It has been stated that the heart lies between the lungs. Thus it would follow that not only does the heart lie in contact with the two lungs, but that changes in the volume of the lungs cannot fail to have an effect upon the heart's action. The heart is also connected by vessels to both lungs. The pulmonary artery passes from the right ventricle and divides into two branches,

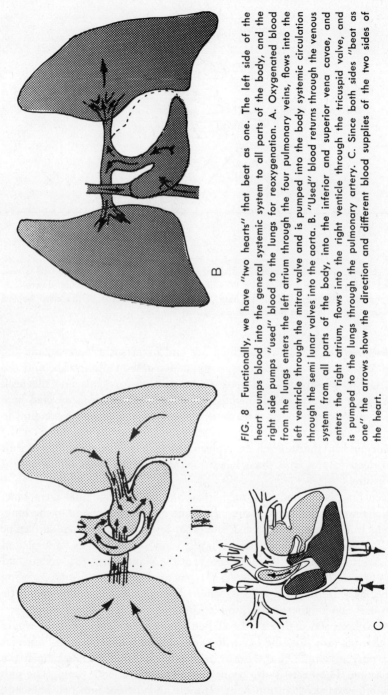

FIG. 8 Functionally, we have "two hearts" that beat as one. The left side of the heart pumps blood into the general systemic system to all parts of the body, and the right side pumps "used" blood to the lungs for reoxygenation. A. Oxygenated blood from the lungs enters the left atrium through the four pulmonary veins, flows into the left ventricle through the mitral valve and is pumped into the body systemic circulation through the semi lunar valves into the aorta. B. "Used" blood returns through the venous system from all parts of the body, into the inferior and superior vena cavae, and enters the right atrium, flows into the right ventricle through the tricuspid valve, and is pumped to the lungs through the pulmonary artery. C. Since both sides "beat as one" the arrows show the direction and different blood supplies of the two sides of the heart.

42

one of which runs straight outward to each lung, entering along with the bronchial tube at the hilum, or root of the lung. From this point also emerge the pulmonary veins which carry the blood purified in the lungs back to the left atrium (Fig. 8).

Each main bronchial tube entering the lung at the root divides into branches, which divide again and again and are distributed all throughout the lung substance. These are very minute tubes and are known as the bronchioles, or "capillary bronchi." All these tubes consist of a mucous membrane surrounded by a fibrous sheath. The sheaths have the function of preventing the tubes from being closed and so obstructing the passage of air. The larger and medium-sized bronchi are richly supplied with glands secreting mucus, which is poured out upon the surface of the membrane. This surface is composed of columnar epithelial cells, which are provided with cilia, small hair-like processes credited with the power of moving expectoration upward toward the throat. The wall of the bronchial tubes is very rich in fibers of elastic tissue, and immediately beneath the mucous membrane is a layer of circularly placed unstriped muscle fibers. This muscular layer plays an important role in the removal of mucus by coughing.

The smallest divisions of the bronchial tubes open out into a number of dilatations and these are covered with minute sacs known as the "alveoli." Each alveoli consists of a delicate membrane composed of flattened platelike cells, strengthened by a wide network of elastic fibers to which the great elasticity of the lung is due. In these thin-walled air cells the important function of the lungs is carried on (Fig. 9). The average adult breathes more than

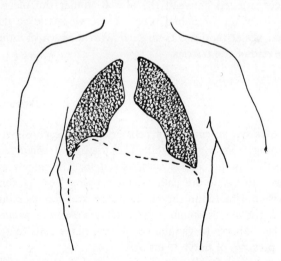

*FIG. 9* The lung bases rest on a dome-shaped transverse muscle, the diaphragm, and their top parts, the apices, are in the root of the neck.

12,000 quarts of air a day. We can go without food for several days and water for many hours without disastrous results, but life without air terminates within a very few minutes. The two lungs lie on either side of the chest cavity. In gross appearance, they are cone-shaped, and grayish in color (almost black for people living in urban areas).

At birth, the lungs are solid and contain no air. The baby's first breath establishes pressure within the lungs essentially the same as atmospheric pressure. As the infant's chest cage enlarges faster than the lungs, this internal pressure forces the lungs to expand to fill all of the available space within the baby's chest, gently surrounding the heart.

Let us see how this takes place. You have already seen how the lungs and the heart work together; now let us go further. The branches of the pulmonary artery accompany the bronchial tubes to the farthest recesses of the lung, dividing like the latter into finer and finer branches, and ending in a dense network of capillaries, which lie everywhere between the alveoli. The capillaries are so closely placed that they occupy an area much greater than the spaces between them. The air in the alveoli is separated from the blood only by two delicate membranes—the wall of the alveoli and the capillary wall—through which an exchange of air readily takes place. The blood from the capillaries is collected by the pulmonary veins, which also accompany the bronchial tubes to the root of the lungs.

Another much smaller set of bronchial blood vessels runs upon the walls of the bronchial tubes; these serve the purpose of nourishing the lung tissue.

Also there is in the lung an important system of lymph vessels, which begin in spaces situated between the alveoli, under the pleural membrane and in the walls of the bronchial tubes. These vessels leave the lung along with the blood vessels and are connected with a chain of bronchial glands lying near the end of the trachea.

## Nervous System

The nervous system consists of cells and fibers, each of which is a long process extending from a nerve cell. The brain and spinal cord are often spoken of together as the *central nervous system*. The nerves which proceed from them on either side are called "cerebrospinal" or "peripheral nerves." The third division, situated in the neck, thorax, and abdomen, and intimately connected with the cerebrospinal nerves, is known as the *autonomic nervous system*. This last consists of ganglia containing nerve cells that are profusely connected by plexuses of nerve fibers.

The nerve cells originate or receive impulses through afferent nerves coming from the skin, organs of sense, joints, and so on, and these are passed from them to muscles, blood vessels, and other tissue. The autonomic system is concerned mainly with the movements and other functions of the internal organs, secreting glands, and blood vessels—activities which proceed independently of the will.

Nerve cells, from one of which springs each nerve fiber, are found in the grey matter of the brain and spinal cord. They also exist in the ganglia of the sympathetic system, in connection with some of the nerves of special sense, and on the *posterior roots* of the spinal nerves. The shape of these nerve cells varies. The most common appearance is that of a large, clear cell, containing an oval nucleus, and running out at various points into long processes which, as a rule, branch again and again. These "dendrite processes" meet with similar processes from neighboring cells; the points of contact are called *synapses*. The state of closure or openness of these synapses is believed to be of great importance in quickening or blocking nerve impulses. See also FUNCTIONS OF NERVES, p. 46. The body of the cell has a mottled appearance, owing to its containing many bodies, known as "Nissl's granules," which appear to be of the nature of food material that will be used up when the cell is called to action.

Each nerve fiber proceeds from a nerve cell to a definite organ, to or from which it carries a special form of nerve impulse; the manner in which the fiber ends in the organ varies in different cases. The simplest mode of ending is that of the nonmedullated fibers which proceed to involuntary muscle such as the intestines, and form a complex network between the layers of the muscle, from which fine nerve fibers pass between the muscle fibers. In the heart, the nerves end in a similar manner. In voluntary muscles the arrangement is more complicated. Each nerve fiber splits up into numerous branches, which go to neighboring muscle fibers. Each branch pierces the membrane surrounding its muscle fiber, and ends by spreading out into a plate composed of granular material and numerous nuclei. The endings of sensory nerves in the skin have a special arrangement. Most of these end, not in the cuticle as would be supposed (this is without feeling), but in the projection of the skin beneath it. Here each nerve fiber enters a small rounded bulb.

## DEVELOPMENT AND REPAIR OF NERVE FIBERS

The whole nervous system is developed from the epiblast, or outer layer of the embryo, the brain and spinal cord arising from an infolding on the surface along the back to form a tube and all the nerves being formed directly or indirectly as outgrowths from this tube, increasing in length until they reach the muscle, skin, or other structure for which they are destined. As already mentioned, each nerve fiber is the process of a nerve cell. If this nerve is cut, that part of its fibers which is separated from the cells immediately starts to degenerate. Within a few days a bundle of small new fibers grows out from the cut end of each fiber in that portion which has not been cut off from connection with the nerve cells, and these grow through the scar and down the sheath of the degenerated portion until they reach the organs to which the nerve originally proceeded. Thus the nerve is restored. This process is quickened when the cut ends have been carefully brought together. It is believed that when this is done no degeneration takes place at all, but the nerve heals and again transmits the impulse at once.

### FUNCTIONS OF NERVES

The greater part of the body activity originates in the nerve cells, food materials being used up in the process. As the result of this process impulses are sent down the nerves, which simply act as transmitters. The impulse that passes from a nerve cell along a nerve fiber to a muscle may be compared to an *electric spark* (current) that explodes in a mine since the nerve impulse causes sudden chemical changes in the muscles as the latter contracts. The anterior fiber roots from the spinal cord are the motor fibers to muscles; the posterior roots consist of sensory fibers from the skin. In addition to motor fibers, through which blood vessels are contracted and relaxed, fibers which control secreting glands leave the cord in the anterior roots; in addition to the sensory fibers that bring in impulses from the muscles, joints, and other organs, fibers that mediate the sense of locality, as well as the sense of feeling, also enter the cord by the posterior roots.

The connection between the sensory and motor systems of nerves is important. The simplest kind of nerve action is known as *automatic action*. In this part of the system controlling goes on rhythmically, such as in the lungs, making discharges from its motor cells sufficient to keep the muscles of respiration in regular action, influenced only by occasional sensory impressions and chemical changes from various sources, which increase or diminish its activity according to the needs of the body.

In reflex action the parts engaged are a sensory ending, say to the skin; a sensory nerve leading from it to the spinal cord, where it ends by splitting up into processes near the nerve cells; a nerve cell which is stimulated by the sensory impulse, and which immediately sends a motor impulse down its nerve; and a muscle which contracts as a result.

Voluntary acts are more complicated than reflex ones. The same mechanism is involved but, in addition, the controlling power of the brain is brought into play. This exerts first of all an *inhibitory*, or blocking, effect which prevents immediate reflex action; then the impulse, passing up to the two sides of the cerebrum, sets up activity in a series of cells there, the complexity of these processes depending upon the intellectual processes involved. Finally, the inhibition is removed and the impulse passes down to motor cells in the spinal cord, and a muscle, or set of muscles, is brought into play through the motor nerves.

The nourishment (tophic) function of nerves is another most important part of their integrity, for it appears that constant passage of nerve impulses down the nerves of any part is important for its nutrition. If sensory nerves are diseased or injured, ulceration of the skin, decubitus, and other changes are likely to occur, while muscles waste and disappear if their motor nerves are permanently destroyed.

## Summary

Just as it is artificial to separate the history from the physical, so it is equally illogical to separate the heart from the rest of the body and examine the cardiovascular system apart from the whole. Thus, this brief discussion of anatomy and physiology has been presented to show some of the relationships you are about to meet in your study of coronary care.

## Review and Advance

1. *Is the "visceral nervous system" the same as the "involuntary nervous system"?*
   Yes, these are two of the terms which refer to the autonomic nervous system. The term "autonomic" indicates that this system is autonomous, or that it functions independently of the central nervous system and peripheral nervous system. However, this is not so. The autonomic nervous system is functionally integrated with other nervous tissue of the body.
2. *What does the autonomic system control?*
   Involuntary actions—that is, contraction or relaxation of smooth and cardiac muscles and secretions of many of the glands—are regulated by the autonomic nervous system.
3. *Does the autonomic nervous system act as a unit?*
   There are two divisions of the autonomic nervous system referred to as the sympathetic and the parasympathetic nervous systems. In general, if one system stimulates a function, the other inhibits it. The systems oppose one another in governing the functions of smooth muscles, and glands. Some of the major effects of the two systems are:

| Sympathetic Effects | Parasympathetic Effects |
| --- | --- |
| Increase in cardiac rate and output | Decrease in cardiac rate and output |
| Constriction of blood vessels in skin and viscera | Dilation of blood vessels not pronounced |
| Elevation of blood pressure | Lowering of blood pressure |
| Elevation of blood sugar | No effect on blood sugar |
| Relaxation of smooth muscle in bronchi | Constriction of smooth muscle in bronchi |
| Decrease in peristalsis | Increase in peristalsis |
| Tightening of sphincters | Relaxation of sphincters |
| Promotion of urinary retention | Decrease in urinary retention |
| Dilation of pupils | Constriction of pupils |

From this comparison, it can be noted that the overall function of the autonomic nervous system is to maintain a constant environment for the cells of the body. This includes constant body temperature, regulation of the heart rate and respiratory rate, digestive functions (in fact, *all* the processes vital to cell integrity), and a constant fluid environment.

4. *How can one remember all the functions of the autonomic nervous system?*
   You are not expected to remember all the functions of both divisions of the autonomic system. However, it will help to remember that when your body is called upon to fight and your heart beats faster to provide more energy to the cells, it is the sympathetic division that induces the increased defensive action. After your body has met the challenge, it is the parasympathetic division that induces the restoration of used body energy and the conservation of the body's resources in preparation for other emergencies.

5. *What are considered the main causes of AV dissociation or first-degree heart block?*
   First-degree block may be due to vagal stimulation, digitalis, rheumatic fever, and various congenital and acquired heart disease. First-degree AV block may precede second-degree AV block, the most common two forms being Wenckebach and the 2:1 AV block, in which the ventricular rate equals one-half the atrial rate.

6. *Does a rapid atrial rate necessarily mean some form of AV block is present?*
   Various types of AV block are *usually* present when there is a rapid atrial rate, because the refractory period of the atria is shorter than the AV junction, and not all of the atrial impulses can be, or are, conducted to the ventricles.

7. *What is atherosclerosis?*
   Atherosclerosis is primarily a disease of the large arteries, of which the coronary arteries are a part, in which lipid deposits called atheromatous plaques appear in the subintimal layer of the arteries. These plaques contain an amount of cholesterol in large quantities. They are also associated with degenerative changes in the arterial wall. In a later stage of the disease, the fibroblasts infiltrate the degenerate areas and cause progressive sclerosis of the arteries. In addition, calcium sometimes joins the lipids to develop calcified plaques. When these two reactions occur, the walls of the arteries become extremely hard and inelastic. The disease is then referred to as "arteriosclerosis," or simply "hardening of the arteries."

8. *Atherosclerosis does not affect the smaller arteries or capillaries?*
   The arteries involved usually are the abdominal, thoracic, coronary, cerebral, and renal arteries. The arterioles and capillaries are not usually affected.

9. *Is impulse transmission along the nerve an electrical phenomenon?*
   In short, yes. However, an all-inclusive statement about nerve transmission would be one indicating that impulse transmission is a combined *chemical-electrical* phenomenon.

10. *Is a resting cell said to be "polarized"?*
    In the resting state—no impulse transmission—nerve fibers are polarized. In a simple example, a polarized fiber has positive ions located on the outer surface of the membrane that surrounds the fiber and an equal number of negative ions located on the inner surface of the nerve fiber membrane. Nerve fibers are surrounded by a semipermeable membrane. When an impulse is transmitted along a nerve fiber, the permeability of the fiber is increased, and the charged surface becomes depolarized or neutralized. An impulse permits the positive charges on the outer surface and the negative

charges on the inner surface of a neuron to unite. The depolarized action "runs" along the neuron until the impulse reaches the nerve endings. This is the electrical phenomenon. The transmission of an impulse from one neuron ending to the next neuron, or organ, is the chemical phenomenon.

11. *What is the cholinergic action?*

   At the nerve endings of all parasympathetic and sympathetic preganglionic fibers, all parasympathetic postganglionic fibers, sympathetic postganglionic fibers to sweat glands, and motor fibers to skeletal muscles, a chemical known as acetylcholine is produced. All these fibers are said to be cholinergic because they secrete acetylcholine at their nerve endings. The acetylcholine produced is rapidly destroyed by an enzyme called cholinesterase.

12. *Is this different from adrenergic action?*

   Yes. With the exception of the postganglionic sympathetic sweat-gland fibers, all sympathetic postganglionic fibers produce a chemical known as epinephrine or adrenalin. Nerve fibers that produce epinephrine are called adrenergic. Thus, there is a basic functional difference between the respective postganglionic neurons of the parasympathetic and sympathetic systems, one secreting acetylcholine and the other, principally epinephrine. These two chemicals secreted by the postganglionic neurons act on the different organs to cause the respective parasympathetic or sympathetic effects. Therefore, these chemicals, or substances, are called parasympathetic and sympathetic mediators, or cholinergic and adrenergic mediators.

13. *How does acetylcholine affect the heart?*

   Acetylcholine, classified as a hormone, has two major effects on the heart: it decreases the rate of rhythm of the SA node and decreases the excitability of the AV junctional fibers between the atrial muscles and the AV node, which slows the transmission of the cardiac impulse into the ventricles. This is vagal stimulation. Very strong vagal stimulation will completely stop the rhythm or cause complete blocking of impulse through the AV junction.

14. *What is the term used to describe the mechanisms for maintaining balance in the body?*

   Because of the importance of the internal environment to the activities of the cells, many adaptions are involved in maintaining the state of equilibrium within well-defined limits. Walter B. Cannon (*The Wisdom of the Body*, W. W. Norton & Co., Inc.) defines these mechanisms as "homeostasis." In describing his concept of how the constancy of the internal environment is maintained, he states: "The coordinated physiological processes peculiar to living things which maintain most steady states in the organism—involving as they may, the brain and nerves, the heart, lungs, kidneys and spleen, all working cooperatively—that I have suggested a special designation for these states, homeostasis."[2]

15. *What are "receptors"?*

   The regulation and integration of bodily processes require that the body have *receptors* that enable it to recognize disturbances in its internal and external environment. These structures communicate information about the disturbances to a center or centers which receive it, evaluate it, and initiate messages that are communicated to the appropriate effector cells. The effector cells are muscle or gland cells; upon stimulation, they act to correct the disturbance.

2. Walter B. Cannon. *The Wisdom of the Body*. New York, W. W. Norton & Company, Inc., 1932, p. 24.

16. *How are homeostatic mechanisms regulated?*

According to Cannon, the regulation of homeostatic mechanisms is primarily controlled by the sympathoadrenal system. We have already touched on some of these. Danger or its signs, whether inside or outside the body, result in activation of the sympathetic nervous system and the adrenal medulla. Cannon also states that the sympathoadrenal system is responsible for regulating the mechanisms whereby the resulting processes are repaired.

According to present-day knowledge, the autonomic nervous system, under the control of the hypothalamus, has an essential role in maintenance of homeostasis. In spite of some exceptions, sympathetic and parasympathetic divisions of the autonomic nervous system appear to have opposing functions. In addition to nervous control of homeostatic mechanism, hormones also play an important role. Their production is directly, or indirectly, subject to control by the hypothalamus. In some instances the action of a hormone enhances the action of the nervous system. For example, epinephrine and norepinephrine support the action of the sympathetic nervous system. Adrenal steroids are essential to the reaction of the body to changes in either the internal or external environment and to the response of the body to injury. The adrenal steroids have been demonstrated to play a role in the regulation of fluid, mineral, and glucose metabolism.

Other hormones, such as insulin, thyroxin, parathyroxin, and antidiuretic hormone also function in homeostasis. The suggestion is made to the reader to review the functions of the autonomic nervous system and the various hormones and their relationships to each other in a textbook of physiology.

17. *What part of the heart carries the main burden of function?*

From the standpoint of function, the essential part of the heart is the myocardium. It provides the power behind the force that keeps the blood moving throughout the system. Like all other tissues, the myocardium is dependent on a continuous blood supply. Since it cannot tolerate an oxygen deficit (as compared to skeletal muscle), the myocardium is more susceptible to hypoxia than is skeletal muscle. Death of cells occurs when oxygen deprivation continues longer than 30 minutes.

# 4 THE PATH LEADING TO MYOCARDIAL INFARCTION

Before the end of the next year, approximately 600,000 persons will have died due to coronary artery disease. Atherosclerosis causes at least 98 percent of myocardial infarctions, secondary to coronary occlusion.

Such statistics as these and many more are before us much these days. The new mass media drone out their hidden messages almost constantly, and we are exposed to small print which many of us do not see.

The fact that you as a nurse are concerned enough to want to know more about the present methods of treatment of heart disease is to your credit. But, as we strive to know more about the causes of heart disease, we find that there is much more here than meets the eye.

## *Etiology*

Atherosclerosis is the process whereby the lumen of an artery is gradually narrowed due to the deposits of lipid, or fatty, material not only on the wall of the vessel but actually penetrating it (Fig. 1A and B). One theory would suggest small thromboses on the intima of the vessel may be the initiating event in the atherosclerotic process. However, once formed, the atherosclerotic plaque may allow formation of platelet thrombi and, eventually, calcification and, ultimately, thrombosis.

We have learned several interesting factors concerning the coronary arteries. Male infants are born with coronary arteries whose lumen is much smaller than that of female infants; this difference is primarily in the width of the intimal layer of the artery. Perhaps this hidden factor is why men are more prone to this disease in later life. However, it has been learned that

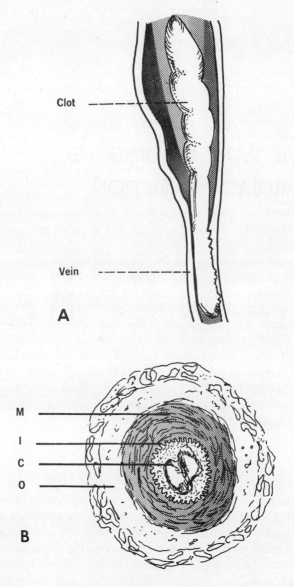

*FIG. 1* The coronary arteries (B) are not simple tubes as are the veins (A), but are complicated structures that grow and change with age. Their walls are three layers thick. The middle layer (M) is composed of muscle fibers which constrict the channel of the artery when they contract. The inner layer (I) lines the artery. The clotted blood (C) within the channel shows how the artery is obstructed in coronary thrombosis. The outer layer (O) consists of dense fibrous tissue.

50 percent of the soldiers who died in Korea within a median age of 22 years had grossly apparent atherosclerotic disease, although none of them had clinical signs of coronary heart disease at the time or a history of the disease any time prior.[1]

Multiple studies of population groups both within the United States and throughout the world have strongly suggested that there is a very high association between dietary intake of fat, serum lipid level, and the incidence of coronary heart disease. There are other rare causes that should be realized but not be covered here, such as anomalous coronary artery location, aortitis with occlusion of the coronary os, periarteritis nodosa, coronary embolism, sub-bacterial endocarditis of the aortic valve, Buerger's disease, and dissecting aneurysm of the coronary artery.

## *Spectrum of Coronary Artery Disease*

We have already hinted that there is more to heart disease than meets the eye. For this reason, clinical coronary heart disease is considered an "iceberg disease," because in most cases the pathologic changes in the coronary arteries antedate the clinical signs and symptoms. However, it can be shown that there is a wide spectrum both in pathologic changes in the arteries and also in the clinical manifestations. For instance, can it be stated that certain factors out of the person's past make him a "coronary-prone individual"? The following factors may indicate the possibility:

- Hereditary predisposition
- Elevated serum lipids
- Systemic hypertension
- Obesity
- Diabetes mellitus
- Tobacco smoking
- Chronic stress

It is noted that the death rate for myocardial infarction in middle-aged males is from 50 to 200 percent higher among cigarette smokers compared to non-smokers. In addition, it has been estimated that there are at least 60,000 deaths each year from coronary artery disease in smokers that could have been prevented had they not smoked. The "coronary personality" is described as an aggressive, compulsive, hard-working individual who is quite competitive and self-disciplining.

1. M. M. Weiss. Ten-year prognosis of acute myocardial infarction. *American Journal of the Medical Sciences,* January 1956, 231:9–12.

In latent coronary artery disease, patients do not have the typical symptoms of coronary heart disease, such as angina pectoris. However, they usually manifest many of the previously mentioned factors leading to coronary-prone individuals. On electrocardiogram examination, they may show an abnormal exercise pattern (Master's 2-step test or Treadwill test).

## Angina Pectoris

The original description of angina pectoris by Dr. Heberden in 1768 is a masterpiece of clinical observation and description. The term basically refers to a pain or tightness in the retrosternal area experienced by patients when they hurry, rush, exert themselves, or become emotionally stimulated. This is usually relieved within two to five minutes by rest or by some form of the nitrite or nitrate drug, e.g., nitroglycerin.

Physical signs of angina pectoris are few. One might see intermittent increased force of the apex beat, a late systolic murmur, and a "gallop" rhythm at the apex. Occasionally, the murmur of aortic valve stenosis or an arrhythmia might be heard on auscultation.[2]

## Myocardial Infarction

Myocardial infarction occurs when there is necrosis of heart muscle due to inadequate blood supply and is characterized by sudden onset of severe retrosternal chest tightness or pain, often accompanied by weakness, pallor, diaphoresis, dyspnea occasionally associated with hypotension and shock, arrhythmias, or pulmonary edema.

"Impending myocardial infarction" may be suspected in a patient who has a sudden onset of angina pectoris with frequent daily attacks increasing in severity and frequency, or in a patient who has had angina but in whom the frequency and severity is greatly increased. These patients may benefit from immediate bed rest, oxygen, and anticoagulant therapy; in other words, they are usually treated as an actual myocardial infarction case.

## Learning from Study

Although the details of this clinicopathologic study of coronary heart disease may be read in its entirety for those of you interested,[3] data is here

2. *Ibid.*
3. Howard F. Conn, ed. 1965. Current Therapy. Philadelphia, W. B. Saunders Company, 1965.

presented on an intensive study of 150 patients, all residents of Rochester, Minnesota, who suffered a myocardial infarction and later died. (These views are not stated as generalizations in all geographic areas.) It is pointed out that patients who experience angina pectoris for months or years prior to an initial acute myocardial infarction have a much poorer prognosis, with higher initial and late mortality than the patient who has an acute myocardial infarction without any previous chest pain or angina pectoris. Certain hypotheses seem evident:

- Greater stress should be put on the importance of recognizing and treating the coronary-prone individual.
- Stress the importance of always remembering the patient with acute myocardial infarction is an individual, who is very frightened and has needs of an emotional as well as a physical nature. In addition, the psychologic aspects of the recuperation and rehabilitation period are extremely important and a positive optimistic approach is most important.
- There is great value in the 10-hour constant electrocardiogram monitoring to determine how quickly ambulation can be recommended and how much exertion can be optimally tolerated by the recuperating heart.
- As far as anesthetic-surgical risk goes, no elective surgery should be carried out until at least six months following myocardial infarction. The mortality rate for all patients with a history of coronary artery disease is approximately three times as great as for those without such a history.
- A great weight of present information and evidence points to the fact that long-term anticoagulant therapy is of definite benefit in preventing re-infarction and death following an acute myocardial infarction. It is rather agreed that this treatment is helpful for 12 years following the infarction, but if the patient is otherwise doing well, it does not appear to be as beneficial following this period.

## General Discussion of Arteriosclerotic Heart Disease

This disease is confusing since it includes a combination of several disease entities which are really one disease in different degrees of severity. There usually is no progressive element from one to the next, so that the patient can begin at either end of the spectrum and move in any direction—angina to heart attack, sudden heart attack, etc. The distinction between the various forms of the entity is made more on the basis of the laboratory findings than on the clinical picture, despite the fact that the patient is probably getting more and more of the disease with the simple passage of time.

As has been already stated, to the best of our present knowledge the disease is produced by the creation of an atheromatous plaque of cholesterol and some fatty acids in the intimal lining of the arteries, in this case the heart. The result is a certain amount of organic obstruction of the blood flow as it

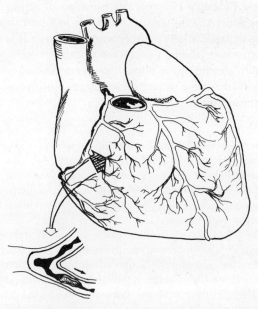

FIG. 2 A coronary thrombosis does not merely mean that a "plug" has suddenly clogged a coronary vessel. It may be a gradual process whereby protein or lipids have been deposited and have grown slowly over a long period of time. The arrow shows an area where a portion of heart muscle is dead or dying because its blood supply has been cut off. The enlarged view shows schematically how a thrombus shuts off flow of blood to area beyond it. Thrombi, or clots, tend to form or lodge, in areas where a blood vessel divides.

goes on to nourish the heart tissue itself. If any tissue in the body does not receive enough blood, it may object to the existing circumstances whether by pain, malfunction, or, if severe enough, actual death of the tissue (Fig. 2).

The main working definition of these conditions is that of an actual or a functional decrease in the amount of blood going to the heart relative to the needs of the heart muscle at the time. When we say "blood supply," we really mean the oxygen supply, since the main function of the blood is to carry oxygen to the myocardium. (See Chapter 3.) We are therefore dealing with a disproportion between the oxygen supply to the heart and the needs of the heart in order for it to continue its activity or the activity in which the rest of the body may be engaged.

As mentioned, this disproportion may be functional or organic, and some of the possible causes include the following:

- A "plug" in the artery—a thrombus, embolus, etc.
- Tachycardia—at a pulse rate of 200 beats per minute for one or two hours,

a normal heart will develop dysfunction. It requires a lot of blood to nourish the heart that is beating at such a rate; thus, if the heart does not get the blood, the person will either develop pain (ischemia), heart failure, or even death of the tissue since it is being poorly nourished. At very high rates the period of diastole is markedly reduced. It is in diastole that the heart fills with blood in preparation for the next beat and also when coronary flow to the left ventricle occurs (Fig. 3).

- Anemia—many times associated with a mild tachycardia, and in any case, the amount of oxygen-carrying capability is decreased because the amount of hemoglobin is low. This necessitates a higher cardiac output to keep up with the body's needs.
- Thyroid disease—especially overactive gland with resultant tachycardia and increased metabolic needs due to the increased metabolic rate.
- Chronic lung diseases with poor oxygenation of the blood due to poor gas exchange at the lung level.
- Congenital abnormalities of the heart and lung systems resulting in a combination of any of the above.

Although the disease is much more common in men at any given age, once the female has passed the menopause her vessels begin to look like that of the male. The disease appears to begin at about the age of 17 or 18 in our culture, and simply progresses with time. One of the helping factors in preventing the disease is the development of a good collateral circulation which occurs with age. This has nothing to do with the mortality of the disease—simply with the amount of tissue damage. Various diseases associated with high cholesterol levels seem to increase the frequency of heart attacks—diabetes mellitus, hypothyroidism, familial hypercholesterolemia—probably by hastening the arteriosclerotic process. Other diseases will increase the fre-

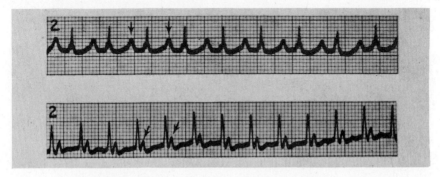

FIG. 3 Two examples of atrial tachycardia: in each the QRS is normally narrow and a P wave ( ↓ ) precedes every QRS.

(Reprinted with permission from Marriott, CCU Nursing Slides, 1967, Tampa Tracings, Oldsmar, Fla.)

quency, including obesity, hypertension, gout, or in similar family history. Arteriosclerotic process can be very localized symptom-wise, e.g., cerebrovascular accident versus myocardial infarction, mesenteric thrombosis, peripheral gangrene. Actually, there are really four main forms of the disease. We have already touched on angina pectoris and myocardial infarction. We will get back to them later.

## Asymptomatic Coronary Disease

This form of the disease seems to begin about the age 17 to 18, causes no symptoms, is undetectable by conventional means including the electrocardiogram and various blood tests (hemodynamics), and requires no therapy except to treat any of the possible predisposing factors including hypertension, obesity, thyroid, diabetes, hypercholesterolemia, etc., in an effort to tip the scales in favor of the patient and to try to slow down the progression of the process. There is no effective means to reverse the development of arteriosclerosis, although some of the above procedures will decrease the progression. Watch out for the personality of the person! Although it appears to be common knowledge that there is no known cause, some researchers and physicians feel they can characterize the type of person who has an increased predisposition to be a victim of a heart attack: the driver, rather than the physical worker, gets the disease—and this may be a good point for counterattack. Until we change many aspects of the way we live, such as our diet, our sedentary ways, and use of tobacco, we can expect this stage to be a widespread problem.

## Acute Coronary Insufficiency

This is really prolonged angina with electrocardiogram changes and inconclusive results of the enzyme studies, e.g., less than 50 percent rise in SGOT. (See Chapter 7.) These patients may be in the process of getting their heart attack and warrant more intensive therapy, including repeating the laboratory and electrocardiogram studies over a period of about seven to ten days before they can be cleared.

The patient will have a pain in the chest which does not stop when he stops to rest, or even with several doses of nitroglycerin. His clinical picture can be identical with that of an acute coronary occlusion and the diagnosis is really only made in a retrospective fashion when the results of all the tests are negative or equivocal as far as a true heart attack is concerned. It may take up to seven to ten days for the electrocardiogram to change; therefore, the enzyme tests are very important in the diagnosis.

Therapy for the disease stage is either that of an acute coronary until proven otherwise, or that of severe angina. It is important to prepare the patient for a rather long recuperative period, even though he may possibly return to work as soon as one week (usually two) after such an episode.

## Further Aspects of Myocardial Infarction

This represents the final stage of the whole process: death of cardiac muscle fibers in coronary ischemia, precipitating tachycardia.

Metabolic energy is necessary to build up ionic differentials across the membranes of the Purkinje fibers and the muscle fibers. If this metabolic energy is not available, appropriate polarization of the conductive membranes cannot occur and cardiac impulses cannot be conducted. Thus, ischemia of the cardiac muscle can cause local failure of the impulse conduction in the areas of the heart made ischemic by coronary occlusion.

It must be understood that muscular contraction requires energy, which must come from the nutrients carried in the blood. When the supply of blood is cut down or off, these nutrients are diminished or cut off; even though a depolarization wave may be conducted over the cardiac muscular fibers, there is not sufficient energy to cause normal contraction of the muscle fibers. In short, in order for cardiac muscle to live, a certain amount of basal metabolism must take place (Fig. 4A, B, C). If the blood flow to cardiac muscle is diminished beyond a critical level, the muscle not only becomes nonfunctional but actually begins to die. Death of the muscle fibers begins within about one hour in total ischemia and is complete in four to five hours.[4]

The patient will develop a chest pain, with or without activity, which radiates into the left arm and neck along the lines of the great blood vessels. There are usually subjective symptoms of a fear of impending death and malaise. The pain is severe, of crushing quality, does not clear with rest and nitroglycerin, and may be associated with nausea and vomiting, sweating, and, many times, complete collapse of the circulatory system—shock.

The basis of the therapy is to put the heart at rest and try to minimize any of the complications until the patient's heart is strong enough to support him in any activity. The usual outlook is good for about 80 percent of these patients to return to their previous activities with no restrictions, although they will remain under medical supervision for the rest of their lives.

Diagnosis depends largely upon the enzymes and electrocardiogram. The faster the changes, the worse the outlook—six hours for ECG, 250 units/ml or over for SGOT.

4. Arthur C. Guyton. *Textbook of Medical Physiology,* 3rd ed. Philadelphia, W. B. Saunders Company, 1968, p. 317.

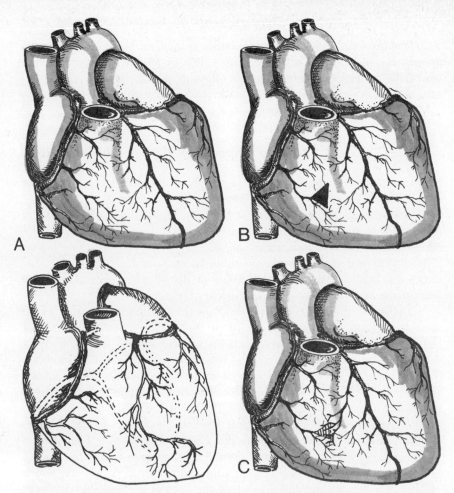

FIG. 4 A. The coronary arteries on the surface of the heart. The right coronary courses in the atrioventricular groove to the posterior ventricular surface. The left artery is short. Its circumflex branch extends to the posterolateral (around the side and back) surface of the ventricles. Notice how the right coronary artery leaves the aorta to encircle the right side of the heart. The left coronary artery also arises from the aorta and circles behind the pulmonary artery to reach the far side (left) heart. Branches are given off from both coronary arteries, the entire coronary system being arranged like a wreath around the heart. Thus, the heart's circulation is a small circuit, modeled largely after the greater circuit which services the whole body framework.

B. When blood supply is cut off in any part of the coronary artery or its branches, the tissue supplied by that particular blood supplier becomes malnourished, and eventually necrotic. The "infarcted" area may be limited to a small area, as shown here, or encompasses a massive area.

C. As healing progresses, scar tissue formed over and throughout the infarcted area. Meanwhile, a new network of small capillaries begins to form as the body begins to supply an alternative route in order to supply the injured area with a new blood supply necessary for its sustenance.

60

Not all coronary disease is painful and infarction may well be quite unrecognized by the patient. The incidence of painless myocardial infarction is probably about 25 percent. It is important to remember that coronary heart disease may present in one of its forms as insidious heart failure without angina, or the usual myocardial infarction syndrome.

## Therapy

Some aspects of the therapy and reasons for them are listed below.

*Bed rest.* Bed rest per se is not necessarily good since it interferes with blood return, and predisposes to thrombus formation in the leg veins. The *ideal* is to get the patient into a lounging type of chair (Fig. 5). No activities should be permitted and the use of the commode is recommended if it can be done with sufficient help; the patient must not be taxed. By and large, the patient should be gotten up into the chair as soon as possible.

*Oxygen.* This will assure a maximum supply of oxygen to the heart and should be used in an almost continuous fashion for at least several days. It may be of value in combating pain due to angina during the initial few days. Watch out for the patient who fights the oxygen; he simply may be fright-

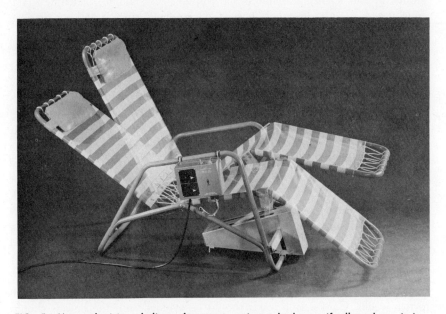

FIG. 5 Many physicians believe that most patients do better if allowed to sit in a lounge-type chair for a short time several times a day. The automatic tilt chair supports the arms, and the tilt position prevents venous congestion in the feet and legs.

(Courtesy of Jobst Institute, Inc., Toledo, Ohio.)

ened, in which case encouragement and explanation are in order, or he may have chronic lung disease and the oxygen is really sending him into a coma. He may be objecting to the coma in his own way by fighting the oxygen. The use of the cannula, tent, and the nasal tube, may be too traumatic in the really severe case. Oxygen will dry the patient's throat; give him liquids freely in sips.

*Relief of pain.* This should be done quickly and effectively since the neurogenic impulses involved in the pain mechanism are enough to produce shock, and the anxiety can produce a tachycardia. Demerol and morphia are considered the best drugs for this, although some physicians prefer morphia because it also provides some release of anxiety as well. Any of these medications may produce a fall in blood pressure, within one hour or so, which will usually last about three to five hours. This is to be expected and, as long as the patient is otherwise doing well, is no cause for alarm.

*Treat shock.* These patients do not require blood transfusions or large amounts of fluids, which may tax the circulation too much. An occasional patient with hypotension who has had vomiting and marked diaphoresis will respond to fluid replacement. The hallmark of this kind of patient is a low central venous pressure. At the same time, sweating can result in large fluid losses which must be replaced slowly, unless the loss becomes critical. Of the various pressor agents available, some consider metaraminol bitartrate (Aramine) better than levarterenol bitartrate (Levophed) since it will not produce any arrhythmias, has a direct cardiac action, and is easier and safer to give. (Aramine works by releasing stored norepinephrine and may deplete norepinephrine stores; it may not work in patients who have taken reserpine or guanethidine [Ismelin] and whose endogenous stores are depleted.) The patient should be watched carefully during this time, with frequent blood-pressure checks. Mephentermine sulfate (Wyamine) is also considered good for mild shock episodes and can be given via any route. Intravenous fluids should not include saline since the risk of fluid retention is so great in the early stages. In the past, some centers have used sympathetic blocks to reduce the circulatory return, especially in patients with pulmonary edema with or without prolonged shock. The best measure to evaluate the degree of shock is the urinary output on an hourly basis. If the kidneys are functioning adequately, it is good *direct* evidence that the cardiac output is adequate. The urine output should be at least 40 cc per hour. A trial with fluids may be used to assess this function. (Other pharmaceuticals are discussed in Chapter 16.)

*Diet.* Diet should be light for the first few days, and then essentially normal except for the sodium content, which should be low at least for one to two weeks. Gas-forming foods should be avoided, and the bowels should be given special attention in order to avoid straining at stool. There will be more discussion on diet in Chapter 9.

*Other Medications:*

1. Quinidine—to avoid arrhythmias which seem to occur in about 70 percent of the cases. Pronestyl may be used.
2. Aminophylline—of value in mild episodes of pulmonary edema and as a diuretic. It will also improve renal blood flow. Some type of diuretic is usually given for the first few days; however, if congestive failure is present, this may cause a low serum potassium. Call it to the attention of the physician if digitalis is being used. Low serum potassium may potentiate the action of the digitalis and result in arrhythmias secondary to a digitalis intoxication.
3. Digitalis—should be used for congestive heart failure or for its vagal effect in slowing the ventricular rate, and not to "perk up" the heart. It is a cardiac irritant and may produce arrhythmias. It should be used cautiously in atrial arrhythmias, such as atrial fibrillation.
4. Peritrate and other nitrates—evidence is conflicting when used in the early stages. Many physicians prefer to delay their use until patient is about to be discharged.
5. Anticoagulants—may be useful and are often used. The main contraindication is ulcer, open wounds, and some consider the development of a pericardial rub since the risk of bleeding into the pericardium is great, and anticoagulants may work by preventing thromboembolic complications. If the patient is on barbiturates, observe him closely, for when barbiturates and anticoagulants are used together, they will produce a false high prothrombin time and too much anticoagulant medication will be used. The latter means to avoid Luminal and any of the barbiturate-type sedatives and sleeping pills. Coumadin is preferred in this country among the anticoagulants because of the predictability of the response, but this, too, is variable. Certain drugs such as barbiturates, aspirin, and antibiotics may potentiate anticoagulants.
6. Sedation—some type of tranquilizer or sedative is necessary for these patients. In many cases, the physicians will advise heavy sedation for the first 24 to 48 hours to relieve anxiety.
7. Laxative—stool softeners or mild laxatives are used in order that the patient may have bowel movements at least every other day without strain.

## Summary

In this chapter is presented a brief coverage of atherosclerosis and arteriosclerosis and their relation to the path of cardiac involvement. This is not meant to be complete coverage of the diseases, because of the many aspects of their course. However, in the following chapters, the broad spectrum approach is essential as various modes of diagnostic and therapeutic treatment are presented. Depth content will be presented to enlarge your understanding as we move along. In other words, this is just the beginning. Now, let us move along to the expanding role of the nurse.

## *Review and Advance*

1. *Are coronary occlusion and myocardial infarction the same?*
   It is more accurate to specify an event, or "happening" when referring to coronary occlusion. However, the term is taken to mean a clinical disease associated with an acute thrombotic occlusion of a major coronary artery. *Acute* coronary thrombosis denotes the sudden obstruction of a coronary artery, either by development of a thrombus or by an intimal hemorrhage with swelling of the arterial wall or by an embolus. However, thrombosis is almost always a complication of coronary atherosclerosis and is an intrinsic stage of the atherosclerotic process. Myocardial infarction signifies the death or necrosis of a part or specific area of heart muscle because of an interference or interruption of its blood supply. The difference lies in the fact that although it may be a result of coronary occlusion, myocardial infarction may also occur without any obstruction of a coronary artery, following any sharp reduction in the volume or oxygen content of the conorary blood due to circulatory or blood disturbances.

2. *Are there any other names by which myocardial infarction is known?*
   There are many synonyms; among them are heart muscle disease, diffuse myocardial disease, noncoronary myocardial infarction, uncommon myocardial disease, idiopathic myocardial disease, idiopathic cardiac hypertrophy, idiopathic myocarditis, asymmetrical cardiac hypertrophy, cardiomyopathy, and myocardiopathy.

3. *In other words, anything that involves the myocardium can be safely called a myocardial infarction?*
   No, such a statement would be too all-inclusive. The *infarction* is the important difference: the death or necrosis of the myocardium.

4. *What is the correct term to use in referring to all the synonyms that do not refer to actual myocardial infarction?*
   They are usually referred to as the primary myocardiopathies, indicating that the emphasis is on the primary nature of the myocardial disease. As the term implies, myocarditis is characterized pathologically by inflammatory changes. In other words, primary myocardial disease consists of a group of diseases of varied etiology that primarily involve the myocardium and only minimally involve other important structures of the heart and the cardiovascular system.

5. *Is myocardial infarction always the outcome of angina pectoris?*
   The question would be better reworded to read: Is angina pectoris always a forerunner of myocardial infarction? And the answer would be "no." A patient suffering a myocardial infarction may never experience angina pectoris.

6. *Are changes immediately seen on ECG tracings after myocardial infarction?*
Not always. Development of electrocardiographic changes following an episode of myocardial infarction may be delayed for up to seven days.

7. *If electrocardiogram shows no immediate changes, why is it so important to get an immediate electrocardiogram done as soon as the patient is admitted to the coronary care unit?*
An admitting ECG tracing, as are all ECG tracings which the patient may have had in the past, is important to the physician in following the course of the disease and patterns seen. Serial ECG's in myocardial infarction will display a specific pattern, and assist the physician in locating the area of the heart muscle involved, as well as indicate if the injury area involves a layer or several layers of the muscle.

8. *When are the changes seen on the monitor or ECG following myocardial infarction?*
The earliest changes affect the RS-T segments and are usually seen within 24 hours. However, they may not be seen for 48 or 72 hours.

9. *Do most patients have a decrease in blood oxygen?*
A significant decrease in arterial $pO_2$ has been demonstrated in all patients with acute myocardial infarction, irrespective of whether complications are present or not.

10. *Are intravenous solutions usually given all cardiac patients?*
This will depend upon the severity of the illness and the physician. However, it is generally the feeling among physicians that it is essential to maintain an open and direct route for prompt administration of drugs in emergency circumstances for at least the first three days. When antiarrhythmic therapy is needed, it can be instituted immediately. In the event of cardiac arrest, bicarbonate and other drugs can be given immediately.

11. *What is a diastolic "gallop"?*
This refers to a rhythm with an accentuated "extra" sound besides the two sounds normally heard when one listens to the heart. The three sounds together create an auscultatory sound resembling that of a canter. As a rule, gallop rhythm is heard only in the patient with a rapid heart rate.

12. *Is there only one type of gallop rhythm?*
No, there are three main types of gallop rhythm: the protodiastolic, presystolic, and summation gallop. There are also other sounds or clicks but none of them resemble the usual form of gallop rhythm. The gallop rhythm may be heard best with the patient lying on his back or on his left side. At times gallop sounds are associated with a palpable or even a visible outward thrust, the result of vibrations of the heart striking the chest wall.

13. *What other signs and symptoms should be expected?*
A rapid fall or gradual fall in blood pressure within the first few days and a slight elevation of temperature are not unexpected. The blood studies usually reveal an elevated white blood count and the accelerated rate of sedimentation of red blood cells, and an increase in the activity of certain serum enzymes frequently associated with the heart. The patient may be experiencing dyspnea on mild exertion, with extreme fatigue, periods of syncope or dizziness, pallor or cyanosis, and palpitations.

14. *If the patient has persistent vomiting and his blood pressure is low, what medication can be safely given?*
It must be assumed that the physician has taken this into consideration in his

orders. Usually, vomiting or associated nausea can be lessened by giving atropine, 0.4 mg, although some physicians prefer antiemetic agents which do not have a hypotensive effect, such as Phenergan or Dramamine.

15. *Don't some of the analgesics cause a hypotensive effect?*
Yes, since analgesics may occasionally cause hypotension as well as hypoventilation, this can be minimized by giving small doses more frequently. In other words, it is recommended that the minimum effective dosage be used.

16. *Does complete bed rest mean no activity at all?*
Usually the physician indicates whether the patient may satisfactorily progress to early ambulation, or he may permit the patient the use of a bedside commode for bowel movements. Frequent movement of the lower extremities and regular periods of deep breathing or hyperinflation of the lungs should be encouraged. Many physicians agree with experimental research studies which stress early ambulation and some activity. The patient may be allowed to feed himself immediately, or sit in a chair one to two hours a day.

17. *How long should the myocardial infarction patient be kept at bed rest?*
It seems unreasonable for a protracted period of bed rest to be initiated on all myocardial infarction patients for the same fixed period. Each patient must be evaluated individually. The physician considers such factors as whether the patient is critically ill or asymptomatic after a brief episode of pain, whether fever is present for a protracted time or whether there is slight fever for a short time, whether the patient suffers from shock, congestive heart failure, pulmonary edema, or serious complications. The objective remains to diminish the work of the heart, thereby restricting myocardial anoxia caused by coronary occlusion and lessen the risk of serious arrhythmias. Therefore, the period of bed rest, depending upon the conditions surrounding the patient, may be from as short a period as two or three days to six weeks or longer.

18. *It seems that so much emphasis is put on the nurse's responsibility to the monitor, is there no other physical sign which suggests a change in the patient's condition?*
The emphasis on monitors should in no way belittle the value of other signs suggesting problems. For instance, electrolyte imbalances and acidosis are usually discovered by frequent blood studies, although respiratory changes such as rapid, shallow breathing may be indicative of either. Arrhythmias and generalized muscle weakness both are indicative of excessive potassium in the blood. Another example would be the mental confusion, excessive thirst, and tachycardia indicating hypokalemia.

19. *What type of pain is typical of myocardial infarction?*
*Severe* oppressive pain over the lower sternum or spread out over the precordium or anterior chest, lasting at least a half hour, and not relieved by rest or nitrites is enough to make the physician suspect a myocardial infarction patient. Characteristic radiation of the pain to the upper extremities, throat, jaws or interscapular area usually confirms the suspicion.

20. *What is a pulse deficit?*
The difference between the heart rate and the radial pulse rate is known as the pulse deficit.

21. *Can one person take both pulses or beats?*
If you mean at the same time, yes, it can be done but is not recommended.

22. *What is the most accurate way of establishing heart deficit?*
It can be detected by taking an apical-radial pulse. One nurse counts the beats of the heart with the stethoscope placed over the apex, which is the lowest point of the left ventricle. At the same time, the second nurse counts the radial pulse. Both nurses count for one full minute. Before comparing notes, leave the patient's bedside.
23. *Suppose a patient is on digitalis and you are in doubt about which pulse is to be used as indicator?*
The question really is asking: which pulse is supposed to be the "reportable" pulse in deciding whether to withhold digitalis? And the answer, of course, must be that the apical pulse is the most significant.

# 5 CONSIDERATIONS OF STAFFING A CORONARY CARE UNIT

Ordinarily, one would expect an author to present the nursing objectives early in any text discussing a "specialty." However, due to the very nature of the role of anxiety and stress as antecedent factors in the coronary patient, it seems wise to discuss the "type" of nurse who may be best fitted for this particular "type" of patient.

## *Personality of the Coronary Care Nurse*

More and more, the relationship of personality and nursing effectiveness has been considered by a number of investigators. The characteristics cover an almost astronomic spectrum of desirable traits; but this should not be an obstacle to the nurse who truly realizes the need of the characteristics for the particular specialty she desires as long as she has persistence and a true desire to meet those requirements.

Educators and others have been convinced that the successful nurse should have certain personality traits. On the other hand, some studies question the existence of a specific pattern of traits which are characteristic of nurses as a group.

The list of personality traits used most often in attempting to describe nurses in general goes as follows:

| | |
|---|---|
| Adaptable | Loyal |
| Alert | Orderly |
| Broad interests | Performs procedures effectively |
| Cheerful | Physical endurance |
| Cooperative | Plans work |
| Conscientious | Resourceful |
| Courageous | Respect for authority |
| Courteous | Self-controlled |
| Economical | Sense of humor |
| Emotionally mature | Stable |
| Enjoys and appreciates beauty | Sympathetic |
| Enthusiastic | Tactful |
| Frank | Thorough |
| Good attitude toward criticism | Tolerant |
| Good judgment | Trustworthy |
| Independent | Well-groomed |

As you can see, these cover a wide range of behavior. They were presented to a jury of nurse educators who put them into several categories:

Emotional maturity
Relationships with patients and staff
Work habits
Professional attitude
Relationships with co-workers and supervisors
Morale

Those who succeed in particular specialty areas of nursing suggest that these individuals have a greater need for order, for companionship and friendship, for taking care of and nurturing others, and for persisting at tasks in the face of difficulties. They also have less need to be dominating and aggressive or to be concerned with themselves.

## Informal Relationship Develops

Nowhere in the hospital organizational setup is the development of informal relationships seen to arise more quickly than in the coronary care unit. It more than substantiates the social scientist's viewpoints.

In the team plan as characterized in this unit, the informal leader of the group is usually the man or woman who is most fitted to take charge at the moment. Thus, leadership is not a psychologic trait; rather, it is a function of the situation and the nature of the group. For example, the nurse on the spot when cardiac arrest occurs automatically assumes the leadership role and directs activities until the physician arrives. Time is not wasted by notifying the head nurse or supervisor, who might have duties in another part of the unit or hospital. Thus, a person can be a leader in a group at one time and yet be relatively insignificant at another. This explains why the nursing supervisor, in her relationship with the coronary care unit, could be relegated to a mere member of that professional group.

Status is another important characteristic of the informal organization of the group. Status roughly measures the prestige of a person in the group. Hospitals are very status conscious. There is a great status difference between the head nurse on the unit and the maid. The reason behind this status difference is quite simple. Status is based on the degree to which the individual contributes to the purpose of the group. Regardless of the desirability of status, it is very real. Most nurses, for example, would be very indignant if they were asked to do the chores of the maid as a daily diet.

The question has arisen concerning the utilization of nursing auxiliary personnel and where they can be fitted into the pattern of the coronary care unit. Naturally, there are traditional status differences arising from the difference in professional standards that must be taken into consideration. Since at least 30 percent of the professional nurse's time is spent in tasks that do not require professional training as a nurse, the obvious solution would seem to be the introduction of a semiskilled class of worker.

The unit which works together is usually more productive. It is difficult for shirkers to exist in such a situation because everybody can see whether the individual is carrying his share of the load and working to a degree of his potential. Group pressure from the other workers may at times make the supervisor's work that much easier; on the other hand, if the supervisor is inept at handling personal differences, this in itself can disrupt the entire unit's effectiveness.

## Personnel and the Coronary Care Unit

Let us look to the committee on organization and administration of coronary care units as they offer guidelines through the co-chairmen, Hughes Day, M.D., and S. Paul Ehrlich, Jr., M.D.[1]

The first step toward establishing a unit is to assure that the physicians and nurses involved both have the motivation and the knowledge essential to the operation of a successful unit. (A minority of medical opinion holds that if the provisions of such a service were postponed until all personnel were proficient in cardiac care, the patients might suffer. They have suggested that the unit be in operation concurrent with the continuous instruction of all

1. Proceedings of the National Conference on Coronary Care Units, U. S. Government Printing Office, Washington, D.C. 20402.

personnel, thus providing patients the benefits to be derived from monitoring alone.)

The following recommendations were aimed at achieving the most intense surveillance of patients and the most efficient operation of the coronary care unit.

## *Planning Committee*

A broadly based committee must be established, consisting of vitally interested physicians, the nursing director, the proposed supervisor and/or head nurse of the potential unit, and the hospital administrator. (A hospital architect and electrical engineer should be included, also, to meet at appropriate intervals with the committee.)

The planning committee will function as follows:

1. Determine the local needs, available facilities and resources, and, especially, personnel.
2. Establish criteria for admission, length of stay, and discharge. All patients with suspected myocardial infarction should be considered admissible.
3. Define a patient referral system.
4. Determine the specific responsibilities and authority of the staff (physicians, attending physicians, nurses, and all other unit and consulting personnel).
5. Allow for circumstances that will affect the members of all departments, by including them in the plans for the coronary care unit.
6. Develop a written hospital policy covering the role, responsibility, and authority of all medical, nursing, paramedical, and administrative personnel.

It was further suggested:

1. Emergency responsibility be delegated by the attending physician to the unit director and his staff, to ensure maximum benefit to the patient.
2. A record system be devised which will make possible a continual evaluation of the unit. Its efficacy can thus be judged in comparison to other units, and improvements in policy, treatments, etc., can be made.

It was strongly recommended that necessary personnel and equipment never be dispersed to other hospital locations.

*Unit Staffing*

Although the size of the coronary care unit, as well as whether the hospital has a residency and internship program, will dictate the needs in terms of personnel, the following recommendations are made:

- *Medical Director.* A physician with a vital interest in heart disease (preferably a cardiologist) should be appointed unit director by the coronary care committee. He will be responsible for formulating all policy and carrying out overall procedure within the unit. Many hospitals don't have a director for their coronary care unit and are run by a group or committee. Certainly this is less desirable than a single responsible individual.
- *Staff Physicians.* Physician coverage should be based on a 24-hour day, 7 days a week, in larger hospitals, particularly those with house staffs. Staff physicians should be primarily responsible to the unit, and immediately available at all times. Hospitals without a house staff may not be able to provide such physician coverage. In such cases, local policy must be formulated to cover this situation adequately.
- *Staff Nurses.* A regular coronary care unit in a large hospital should have a minimum of two specially trained CCU staff nurses on duty at all times. Nurse-patient ratio should be about 1 nurse for every 2 to 3 patients. If there is a separate intensive coronary care unit for the treatment of patients with serious complications (i.e., acute pulmonary edema and cardiogenic shock), the nurse-patient ratio would be greater—1 nurse for every 1 to 1.5 patients.
- *Selected Staff.* The nurse staffing patterns outlined above may not be feasible in coronary units of small hospitals with less than 100 beds. In such cases, one coronary care nurse should be ever present; a second, trained, experienced individual, such as a licensed vocational nurse, must also be there. Medical technicians may be trained to assist as well.

Ideally, a coronary care unit should be near a general medical ward, a general intensive care unit, an emergency room, or a recovery room. Nurses from these areas with special CCU training may be used in backup and supportive capacities. Small hospitals can ensure an adequate pool of prepared nurses by giving special training to all the nurses on the medical ward, and preferably to all nurses throughout the hospital.

Highly motivated, specially trained *licensed practical/vocational nurses* can be of great value in bedside patient care in the unit. Under the supervision of registered nurses, they provide safe nursing care for selected cases of acute myocardial infarction. The nurses may be of greatest use in small hospitals, where a critical shortage of registered nurses exists, and consideration should be given to this category of nursing personnel, particularly in the intensive care area.

The crucial medical and nursing shortage makes feasible a special training program for interested, responsible, and intelligent individuals, who can then perform cardiopulmonary resuscitation and serve in emergency rooms and coronary care units. It is believed that an untapped source of such personnel consists of former military corpsmen, rescue squad members, firemen, etc. *Nurses' aides* might also assist in CCU's, though in a limited fashion since they have not had the training and experience of licensed vocational nurses.

Use of paramedical personnel should be considered to supplement the staff. The psychologic needs of the CCU patient cannot be met by regular staff members; the medical *social worker* can help a great deal in this area. Although it would be impractical for this member to work full time in the unit, it would be beneficial if an experienced and interested medical social worker were primarily responsible to the unit.

*Inhalation therapists* can be invaluable as CCU staff members. They are essential not only to the cardiac resuscitation team, but to the treatment of cardiorespiratory complications in unit patients.

A full-time *electronic engineer* would be highly desirable in large CCU's or in research units. A technician with interest and training in electronics, who is readily available, would be equally valuable.

*Dietitians* should be consulted about the special food needs of the coronary patients. This member could assume responsibility for explaining the special diet necessities to the patient and the family, especially if the patient is to be discharged on a special diet. Food preparation should be discussed with the member of the family who will have that responsibility in the patient's home.

## *Training Programs for Nurses*

For a nurse to be adequately prepared to function in a leadership position in the coronary care unit, a planned program of instruction and practice is essential (Fig. 1). This program, according to Dorothy V. Wheeler, R.N., and Leonard Scherlis, M.D., who presented the views of the committee on training of nurses and physicians to the conference on coronary care units, should provide the nurse with the opportunity to increase her knowledge and depth of understanding in the following areas:

- The epidemiology of coronary artery disease
- The concept of coronary care units, their purpose, organization, and management

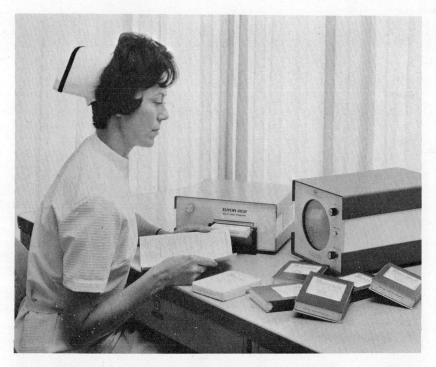

*FIG. 1* Programmed self-instructional machines make it possible for the nursing personnel to study alone and at a pace comfortable to them until arrhythmias can be recognized at a glance.

(Courtesy of Physiological Aid Training Co., San Marino, Calif.)

- The role of the health team in the care of patients treated in these units, with special emphasis on the nurse's role
- The anatomy and physiology of the cardiopulmonary system
- The diagnosis and treatment of coronary artery disease
- Special technology, including:

    1. Proper utilization of electronic monitoring devices for patient observation (Fig. 2)
    2. Interpretation of electrocardiograms
    3. Cardiopulmonary resuscitation
    4. Electrical pacing
    5. Countershock

- Nursing care of patients with coronary artery disease, including the attitudes, knowledge, and skills required for a high quality of comprehensive care during the acute states and for the continuity of this care

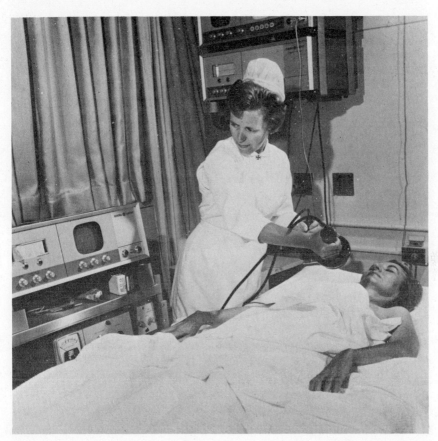

*FIG. 2* In-service programs which bring nursing personnel to the bedside to discuss and simulate action result in better understanding of how to use and handle electronic equipment. Here a cardiovascular nurse specialist discusses care needed in the handling and placement of defibrillator paddles.

This foundation will assist the nurse not only to increase her competence in the more familiar aspects of patient care, but also to master an area of special technology that formerly was not considered within the scope of nursing. Her increased understanding of the therapeutic regimens will enable her to participate in them more effectively. She will be aware of the desired, as well as the undesired, effects of the therapy and will be prepared to take action when necessary. She will be better able to recognize and correctly interpret early and subtle signs of potentially dangerous complications, and will be prepared to participate in the effort to prevent their progression. When

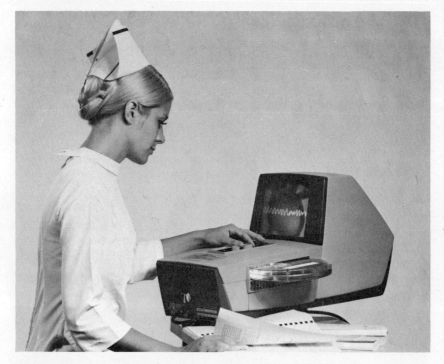

*FIG. 3* Multimedia Instructional System enables nurses to project films and study individually without mechanical know-how.

(Courtesy of ROCOM Division, Hoffmann-La Roche Inc.)

necessary, she will be able to institute lifesaving measures. The attention given to the nurse's role in providing emotional support for the patient and his family will strengthen her appreciation and skill in this area. She will become more effective in assisting the patient to deal with the feelings of fear, unreality, and depersonalization so frequently encountered in coronary care units.

Because of the varied educational and professional backgrounds of the nurses being recruited to work in these units, teaching methods and learning experiences must be varied and carefully planned to insure achievement of the objectives of the program (Figs. 3 and 4). Many of these nurses find the return to the student role trying. They neither tolerate nor benefit from long days of didactic instruction and practice. Lectures, guided clinical experience, clinical conferences, patient-care conferences, review, and, at times, individual tutoring sessions can all be effective. Whenever possible, material presented in class should be related to the clinical situation, with emphasis on the patient's reactions, the required treatment, and subsequent nursing responsibilities.

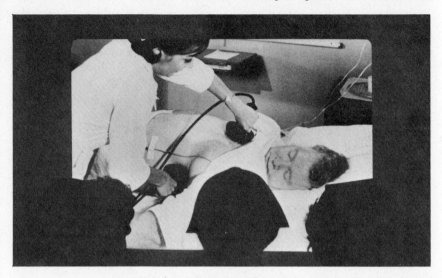

FIG. 4 Nurses training for intensive coronary care through the ROCOM Multimedia Instructional System observe realistic emergency situations on film.
(Courtesy of Hoffmann-La Roche Inc.)

To achieve competence in the area of special technology, the students require guidance and sufficient time to practice these skills in class, in the clinical area, and in the animal laboratory, in addition to experience in the coronary care unit and formal presentations.

The various aids available to teach the interpretation of electrocardiograms should be used to meet the varying needs of the students. These include films, tapes, slides, programmed instruction, and practice strips.

Although the role of the health team and its individual members can be identified and discussed in the classroom, the way in which a team actually functions is best learned in the clinical situation. There the student has an opportunity to observe how effectively team members communicate, how they function in emergency situations, how they plan patient care, and how they provide for evaluation and for continuity of care.

A four- to six-week course allows for adequate time and flexibility in presenting the necessary information and in gaining the experience required. Within this time, provision for independent study can also be made. This unstructured time is necessary for the individual student to assimilate what she is studying and to plan for the responsibilities she will assume in her home situation. This time could also be used in planning a program of continuing study so necessary for the nurse to maintain her competence.

Thus, a four- to six-week program in coronary care unit nursing provides nurses with a comprehensive approach to the care of patients with myocardial infarction. To be successful it should include the opportunity for acquisition of a selected body of knowledge and a change in attitudes, ample time for the development of competence in the technical skills so necessary in this area of specialization, and guided experience to help the nurse incorporate what she has learned into her nursing care, which must be individualized, skilled, and compassionate. These courses are of particular value to community hospitals for the preparation of their key nursing personnel.

## Training Programs for Physicians

It is necessary to prepare a sizable number of physicians to serve as unit directors who, in addition to applying the recent advances in the diagnosis and treatment of acute coronary disease, will disseminate general knowledge to all physicians involved in coronary care. Training of physicians can be divided into three basic categories: (1) at the level of postgraduate and continuing education, (2) at the level of house officer training, and (3) at the level of student training. Coronary care is not an isolated, autonomous entity within the field of cardiology; it incorporates many of the basic principles of diagnosis and therapy that serve as the foundation of sound cardiologic practice everywhere.

In this technical age, a history, physical examination, and routine laboratory investigations are still as important as they ever were; the specific principles which are developing in coronary care are supplements to, rather than replacements for, the fundamentals of medical practice. Therefore, any training program must not be designed merely as a stopgap measure of teaching the physician specialized techniques, but rather must be oriented toward the basic principles of pathophysiology, as well as toward the scientific basis for the use of specialized techniques. The purpose of physician training is to provide knowledge and understanding in depth of the pathophysiology, symptomatology, diagnosis, complications, and management of acute myocardial infarction; to ensure early recognition and prompt treatment of all serious and potentially life-threatening complications; to facilitate preventive measures by early treatment of significant premonitory signs and symptoms which may be forerunners of major complications; and to ensure adequate rehabilitative measures and the prevention of cardiac neurosis.

Such training can be accomplished through short-term courses at university or research centers under the direction of a medical school or in a large medical center. There must be adequate faculty, space, library facilities, and adequate clinical material to allow the necessary depth of exposure and practical experience. The institution should be committed to a program of continuing education for physicians. Two- to three-week courses would adequately meet the needs of most physicians, and should be made available especially to physicians who will serve as unit directors. Specific knowledge and skills to be included in such courses are the principles and practice of electrocardiographic monitoring, closed-chest cardiopulmonary resuscitation, assisted ventilation, electrical pacing, electric countershock, hypothermia, and the principles of hemodynamics and of salt water and electrolyte management.

A second approach, successfully employed by the American Heart Association, the American College of Cardiology, and the American College of Physicians, has been the development of short-term courses lasting from one to five days, usually limited to a particular area of discussion and given at a center where the director is especially knowledgeable. These programs have proved to be immensely successful if the response can be considered a measure of success. They have the advantage of allowing a relatively large number of physicians to be brought up to date in a short period of time. They have the disadvantage of not allowing for practical experience and the development of specific skills.

A third approach to physician training is a program of continuous postgraduate education, covering different aspects of cardiology in weekly periods of two hours or more. Frequent guest speakers are used for these programs, which are based on the total approach to each case, beginning with the history and terminating with sophisticated laboratory investigations. This type of education is again designed primarily to keep the attending physicians abreast of the more recent developments in diagnosis and therapy and does not lend itself to teaching specific skills.

House officer education should be stressed. It has become apparent that to offer a year of broad training in clinical cardiology, which will serve as the basis for subsequent concentrated training in specific areas, it is necessary to provide rotation through the coronary care unit. This gives the house officers an opportunity to study the clinical problems in detail, to learn the indications and techniques of electrical pacing and cardioversion, and to study specific aspects of the problem and become familiar with the experiences of others.

Another group requiring training is the medical students. The acute phase of one of the most serious common American diseases must be emphasized within the medical school program so that the student may learn about the problems of acute myocardial infarction.

In summary, the panel agreed that:

1. Whereas there has been a demonstrated reduction in mortality from myocardial infarction as a result of coronary care units
2. Whereas a successful coronary care unit requires properly trained nurses and physicians knowledgeable in specific techniques and skills

3. Whereas an aggressive team approach is necessary, including medical, nursing, and hospital administration
4. Whereas there is an urgent need for well-trained physicians and nurses for the successful operation of a coronary care unit, the following recommendations are made:

   a. High priority should be given to the training of physicians and nurses in coronary care unit procedures and techniques at an operational level, including in-service training, short-term courses, and other training opportunities. The appropriate Federal agencies, including regional medical programs, National Heart Institute, Heart Disease Control Program, and public health agencies, should provide adequate financial support. There is an urgent need for prompt implementation of this program.
   b. Each coronary care unit should have a director responsible for administering a program of continued training for physicians and nurses, and for maintaining a high quality of patient care. Support from the responsible policy-making group of the hospital *must be provided.*
   c. Instruction in cardiopulmonary resuscitation should be included in the curriculum of schools of nursing and medicine, as well as in hospital programs for house officers, nurses, and staff physicians.
   d. Intensive courses of from four to six weeks should be adequately supported for key nursing personnel of coronary care units.
   e. There is a need for support, study, and evaluation of such additional programs as follows: (1) intensive courses of briefer duration for selected personnel; (2) refresher courses emphasizing newer aspects of coronary care unit nursing; and (3) development of instructional aids for teaching specific techniques and skills.

## Review and Advance

1. *What is considered the correct nurse-patient ratio in the coronary care unit?*
   At best, the optimum effectiveness calls for one nurse to be responsible for two, or at most three, patients. Of necessity, the ratio must remain flexible for it is not unusual for an admission, or a cardiac arrest patient, to become a focal point for many personnel. Therefore, nurses should be available to service the remainder of the patients during such times.
2. *How can a nurse possibly keep up with changes in monitoring or electrical devices?*
   Perhaps we should look to the social scientists for an answer to this question. The modern society is defined as having a dynamic nature, that is, ever-moving, ever-changing. The social institutions of health are no exception.

Since the hospital is essentially dynamic in nature, the nurse must recognize the importance of maintaining a dynamic attitude in her learning experience if she is to keep pace with her work environment. This applies to all nurses, not just the nurses who work in coronary care units. There is no place for set methods in the nursing field. At any given time the facilities and the techniques in use and the general conditions in force are likely to be different from those in use and in force at another time. The skills and knowledge the nurse acquires today may be outdated tomorrow by new skills and knowledge. It is important for the nurse to remember that all the new "monitors" are not to replace her. Rather, they are tools that extend human observation of the physiologic parameters and thereby provide additional measures for lifesaving therapy. The most important element in the success of a coronary care unit is the people that work in it. The architectural design and all the modern equipment certainly are creative and useful elements, but no amount of sophistication of equipment can supplant a well-prepared, competent nursing staff.

3. *Patients being transferred from the coronary care unit sometimes are reluctant to leave and show symptoms of apprehension when being moved to the general medical complex. How can this be "cushioned"?*

The patient-nurse relationship within the coronary care unit develops as one of trust. This is not necessarily because the patient realizes his life is in the nurse's hands in case of an emergency but because he has continuous evidence of the nurse's interest in his welfare through the bedside nursing care she gives. Nurses in the coronary care unit and the other hospital units should be aware of the adjustment that patients must make when they are transferred from the coronary care unit. Some of them, for instance, become attached to the cardiac monitoring equipment and are reluctant to give up the sense of security that it gives to them. Preparation for transfer should begin when the purpose of the unit is explained, and should be continued as part of the patient's education about his illness and care. Transfer will then be accepted as an indication that the special precautions of the equipment of the unit are no longer needed. It is also a good practice for the coronary care nurse to accompany the patient to the unit to which he is transferred, go over the patient's progress record, then accompany the new nurse into the patient's room. Once the patient can identify with "his" nurse, most apprehension will be relieved.

4. *When should the nurses for the new coronary care unit be trained?*

It is always desirable to have nurses adequately prepared for the responsibilities they are to assume. Before such a unit is opened, an in-service educational program should be planned by the nursing service director in conjunction with the coronary care committee. Having determined the goals for patient care and the responsibilities to be assumed by nursing, medical, and other hospital staff, the committee can make immediate and long-range plans for a continuing educational program for all nursing staff working in the unit throughout the 24-hour day.

5. *Why is the nurse turnover so high in the coronary care unit?*

I do not have statistics to prove that the turnover is greater than elsewhere in the hospital. However, if this seems to be a "contagious disease" afflicting a particular hospital, it would do well to examine its method of preparation and continuing education of its personnel. We teach or instruct because we hope that through our instruction those we teach will somehow be different than they were before the instruction. We provide "learning experiences" with the intent that the student—whether undergraduate or registered nurse—will then be a modified person . . . in knowledge, in attitude, in belief, in skill. We teach to influence the capabilities of the learner. In short, we teach because we hope, through our efforts, the learner will know more than he knew before, understand something he did not understand before, develop a skill that was not developed before, feel differently about a subject or specialty than he felt before, or develop an appreciation for something where there was none before.

6.  *Should the educational program be carried on by the supervisor or an in-service instructor?*
    This is not an easy question to answer since it will depend upon what kinds of continuing education programs are in your area on a regional basis, whether courses are offered in local colleges and universities, or whether the entire educational process is in the hands of the nursing director, supervisor, or in-service department. No matter where instruction is carried out, the instructor is far more concerned with influencing how ably the nurse performs after the course is over. Certainly one of the important goals of education is that the influence of an educational experience will extend beyond the period of instruction. This goal is implied in almost every statement of educational objectives.
    There is nothing new about saying we are interested in having the nurses use what has been taught them after instruction has ended. The point may be belabored, but if this goal is worth achieving, it is a goal worth doing more about than just talking. If it is an objective of value, we must act to achieve it and act to learn how well we succeed.

7.  *How do you account for nurses who have taken coronary care courses and have never been assigned to the unit after it opens?*
    This author cannot *account* for it! But this much all instructors should be accountable for: We are supposing that instruction is intended to facilitate performance at some time in the future, after the instruction has taken place. When clinical experiences are an integral part of the course, the instruction has a definite "staying" power. The most important thing the instructor—and it doesn't matter who it is—can convey to the students is that what is being taught is vitally important. If she (or he, for there are many fine male nurse-instructors) goes to the trouble of putting her own thoughts together and organizing effective learning experiences for her students, she will certainly want to avoid hearing a student say, "Boy, I hope I never hear of that subject again!" She would not only have wasted her own talents, but the talents of the student as well.
    In short, whatever else instructors do in the way of influencing the student, the *least* they must strive to achieve is to send him away with a favorable feeling about the subject or activity taught. This might be our minimum, and universal, goal in teaching.
    Thus, it would seem that if a nursing administrator knew her employee had a favorable attitude toward working in the coronary care unit—and whether the student attended a course at her own or the hospital's expense—it would behoove her to place that nurse in a positive environment where

she could prove not only her interest, her skills, and her knowledge, but also her ability and willingness to learn a great deal more about the subject.

8. *What can the director or head nurse of the coronary care unit do to encourage the staff nurse who has just finished a coronary care course?*

If the instructor has fulfilled her function of sending the nurse-student away with tendencies to approach, rather than avoid, the things she wants her to think, feel, and do something about, the director, supervisor, or head nurse of any unit can assist by modeling the very kind of behavior she would like to see displayed by her nurses or nursing personnel and by making certain there are as few aversive conditions present as possible while the new nurse is becoming accustomed to the new unit, e.g., don't force her into the role of being on the unit alone until she feels more sure of her capabilities.

# 6  INTEGRATING OBJECTIVES

At no time in the history of nursing have so many opportunities of knowledge presented themselves to the average professional nurse. The advent of electric monitoring devices represents the most exciting development ever to offer a light on systematized education, as well as increasing emphasis on self-learning and self-regulation of the instructional process. Within the profession of nursing, there is mixed emotion. Leading nursing figures frequently cite the reluctance of nurses to change their habits and traditions of accomplishing high quality nursing care. But nurses have reached for the challenge to be part of the medical and nursing health team who are a vital and necessary aspect of efficient coronary care. Here, in this environment, the combination of grave effort and an imagination can assist the individual nurse to take on new responsibilities because she will know that her success will lie in her own steadfast endeavor to learn as much as she possibly can; she will learn specialized tasks that will show how she will react to emergency situations. By learning and imagining how the goals of the coronary care course can be applied to the clinical situation, she will find that her knowledge and the new skills will fast become integrated into the functioning of the coronary care unit. These are objectives that can be brought to *life*.

## *Objectives*

- To orient nursing personnel to the coronary care unit
- To review basic principles of cardiac and pulmonary physiology
- To develop knowledge and understanding of the underlying principles of coronary heart disease

- To develop better patient care through advanced coronary artery disease
- To develop acuity in professional judgment and observational abilities to interpret visual signs
- To develop a usable knowledge of electrocardiography and an understanding of the principles governing operation of electronic devices
- To develop skills of artificial ventilation and closed-chest cardiac resuscitation
- To develop competency in meeting and instituting emergency measures when the need arises

## Nurse's Role on Admission of Patient

Remembering that approximately 128 per 1,000 persons are admitted to our hospitals each year, the nurse who is well informed regarding current therapy of coronary artery disease and the objectives of nursing care will be able to function intelligently and efficiently.

The goals of therapy and nursing care for the patient with myocardial infarction are expressed in terms of caring for the whole patient and total needs of the illness. This involves more than thoughts concerned only with the survival of the patient; it involves delivering him to his family and the community to continue his life in the most nearly normal manner possible, and keeping the structural, functional, and psychologic effects of the infarction to a minimum. Nursing care must be orderly, well formulated and individualized to fit the patient and his illness. The nurse must be aware of the patient's needs as an individual and not force upon him a stereotyped plan of comprehensive care. Her plan of care should include cooperation with the patient and his physician (Fig. 1). She may need to protect the patient from his families and well-meaning friends. She must provide close supervision for the patient without creating anxiety or emotional disability.

The role of the nurse changes during the care of the patient with myocardial infarction as he progresses through various degrees of the disease. It is important that she know and recognize the usual course of the disease, the complications, and prognosis of a coronary. She must be familiar with the physician's plan of therapy. As the patient progresses from the initial stage, acute stage, through the convalescent stage and into the recuperative stage, the nurse must be prepared to move along with him, change her goals and plan of care as the needs of the patient change.

During the initial stage, the nurse will follow the admitting orders of the physician. Many hospitals have these orders already typed on order sheets which have been prepared by the medical director and/or the coronary care unit committee. An example of such orders is included here. However, it is

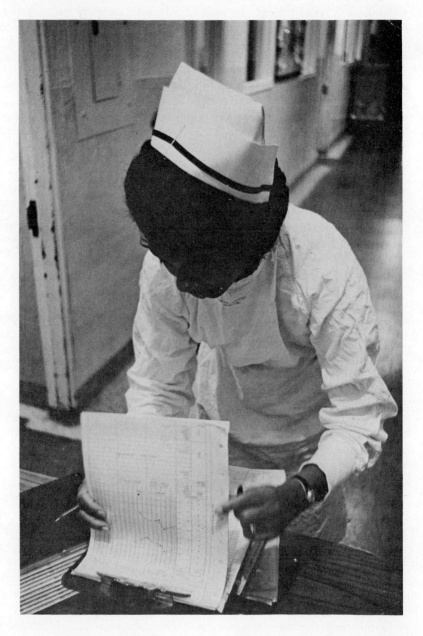

*FIG. 1* The nurse studies the doctor's orders carefully. She will adjust her nursing-care plan accordingly.

(Courtesy of Tufts New England Medical Center, Boston, Mass.)

also good for the nursing staff to have planned nursing orders. The following items should be included in admitting nursing orders:

1. Allay fear!
2. Assess and evaluate physical condition.
3. Evaluate intensity of pain:
    a. By the amount of activity patient does
    b. By the tenseness of shoulders, head and arms
    c. By type and character of respirations
4. Recognize primary symptoms of cardiogenic shock:
    a. Pallor
    b. Clamminess
    c. Perspiring
    d. Mental apathy or dulled response
    e. Hypotension
    f. Arrhythmia
5. Recognize secondary symptoms:
    a. Pallor
    b. Perspiration
    c. Nausea
    d. Vomiting
    e. Faintness
    f. Vertigo
6. Check vital signs:
    a. Pulse—rate, rhythm, and quality
    b. Blood pressure (hypotensive or hypertensive)
    c. Oral temperature if possible (rectal temperature-taking may cause adverse reflex action of the vagus nerve, causing bradycardia and, possibly, ventricular standstill)
7. Institute prompt nursing measures:
    a. Start oxygen per nasal cannula. (Later, the physician may want a tent to be used.)
    b. Place patient in position most comfortable to him:
        1) Elevate head.
        2) Support arms—particularly the left arm. Place arms in position of slight abduction (this is a position of relaxation and may relieve tenseness)
8. One nurse should remain with the patient to give reassurance and explain to him what is taking place, while others assemble necessary equipment.
9. Do not give the impression of frenzy or hurry.

10. Medicate, if order has been left.
11. Maintain flexible nursing care plan geared to the needs of the patient and situation:
    a. Maintain good hygiene and physical comfort through periodic cleansing (patient will not be harmed by unbrushed teeth or unlotioned or unpowdered skin).
    b. Facilitate elimination by assisting patient to use bedpan or commode (if order is left).
    c. Maintain good nutrition. Evaluate nutritional habits.
    d. Maintain body mechanics through periodic turning and moving of extremities without producing fatigue.
    e. Facilitate maintenance of fluid and electrolyte balance by recording and evaluating fluids given and excreted.
    f. Give ordered medications and narcotics as needed, and observe for reactions and adverse side effects.
    g. Record vital signs as often as necessary in accordance with doctor's plan.
12. Be aware of the patient's emotional status:
    a. Communicate by your manner that you accept not just his disease but him as a whole person.
    b. Allow him to communicate his fear, apprehensions, frustrations and bitterness to you.
    c. Explain meaning of "heart attack" to him in lay terms.
    d. Explain reasons why he must be fed, bathed, etc.
    e. Praise him for his patience.
    f. Reassure him as often as necessary.

During the acute stage, it is important that the nurse provide *restful* rest for her patient, i.e., a quiet environment conducive to rest. Although the patient is attached to monitoring leads, laboratory technicians will be in and out of the room often, the attending physician and house staff, and many other individuals will be involved with his care; thus, all of the nurse's care now must be geared to the end of securing the right kind of rest for her patient, both physical and supportive. She will find herself giving less physical care, but providing more and more reassurance as she helps her patient to accept the reality of his attack after the initial stage. She will assume an interpretive role, clarifying for the patient his therapy and progress. When the physician begins to think in terms of moving the patient outside the unit or of discharging him, auxiliary personnel may begin to step in to meet the patient's physical needs, and the professional nurse extends her supportive role through education of the patient and the family, and referral for followup care.

## *Delegation*

The emphasis on the health team influences planning for the nursing care of the coronary patient. The nurse's insight into the special problems of the patient will dictate her decision on whether to assume the care for the patient, or whether she will delegate it to auxiliary personnel. The nurse will evaluate the current status of her patient and identify his presenting needs. During the acute stage, when observations are so important, she will want to assign a professional nurse to the care of the patient. Later, she may assign an auxiliary person to his care. In delegating, she will instruct this person as needed in the principles of cardiac nursing. She will help her plan for spaced periods of rest and activity for the patient. She can help her in modifying routine procedures of morning, afternoon, and sleep care so as to best meet the needs of the patient.

What should the nurse know before making a team assignment? Her approach to the care of the patient must be based upon astute observations of the patient's response to therapy and his acceptance of his illness. Through her solid foundation of knowledge of the usual course and progress of myocardial infarction, she will be especially sensitive to signs of impending complications which may alter or influence the care. The nurse must be aware of the physician's approach to therapy in myocardial infarction. Whether he is aggressive or conservative, she will want to provide the proper atmosphere to support his plans, and further the patient's confidence in his physician.[1]

Above all, the nurse must have learned her responsibilities so well that she will have confidence in her own ability to care adequately for her coronary patient. She cannot expect to feel and put on a constantly cheerful "front"; she must know for a fact that the patient is fearful of impending death, or wracked with worry over how he will meet expenses, or how he can face his family with the burden of respecting an unpotential breadwinner. An apprehensive, insecure nurse can transmit her own fears unknowingly to the patient, thereby complicating his problems. On the other hand, the nurse should not present a carefree or continual jolly attitude either. Her ground must realistically be the middle road, and matching her mood to the patient's mood to offset any negative fears he may present.

Occasionally, the nurse will encounter a patient who just cannot accept the reality of his coronary attack. He looks well, and he feels well. The patient may challenge the nurse's ability and skill in interpreting the need for restricted activity and alternate periods of rest. The nurse may meet the situ-

1. From a paper delivered at the Fifth Annual Cardiac Institute for Nurses by Joan L. Green, March 29, 1961, San Francisco, Calif.

ation where she must help the patient to face certain facts. He is very seriously ill. At the same time, she adopts a positive approach and reassures the patient of the high statistical percentage of patients who *do* return to work after recovery from a coronary.

Included in the core of skill and knowledge, the nurse brings to the bedside of the patient a cheerful and optimistic positive approach, based on a solid foundation of scientific knowledge, and modified according to the individual needs of the patient.

## *Activity*

The objectives of the nursing care are determined by the objectives of therapy. These goals are based upon measures to ensure maximum rest for the heart and circulation. The need for physical and mental rest is present in varying degrees through all stages of the recovery process.

During the emergency stage at the onset of the attack, the nurse must do everything to ensure a minimum of physical activity on the part of the patient. The actual limitations will be established by the physician, depending on the severity of the patient's attack, the presence of complications, and his progress as indicated by the laboratory reports, electrocardiographic readings, and physical findings. At the same time, it is important to avoid establishing a pattern of invalidism, although in certain situations he will be so ill that it is wise not to bathe him at all for a few days.

Nevertheless, the patient on absolute bed rest should not lie absolutely motionless. He will rest better with a change, and real rest is our goal. This is a very important point! What is considered restful to the nurse may not be restful at all to the patient. Most patients will rest better if they are permitted to lie in a position to which they are most accustomed, whether it be on their sides, or on their backs. A patient with myocardial infarction does not necessarily have to be in the high sitting position so often associated with cardiac patients. If the patient has a complication which interferes with his respiration, then he should be rolled up to a position of comfort. Patients who spend the greater part of the day in a sitting position should have a rolled pillow placed below each elbow and forearm for support. The weight of the arm dragging on the shoulder is frequently very exhausting, and may be the forerunner of future complication. Innovative early exercise programs are being started in some experimental units.

The nurse should be aware of the significance of restriction of activity during absolute bed rest, and be able to interpret it to the patient in its proper value: to decrease the body's need for oxygen, thereby decreasing the activity of the heart.

The nurse must learn to feed, bathe, and turn the patient with a minimal amount of physical exertion or mental strain for the patient. Unless she is able to do these things smoothly and efficiently, she may unwittingly be creating more problems for the patient than if he were able to do them for himself. The nurse must be alert to the psychologic effect of such restrictions on the patient. The ego of a virile male may be threatened by what he calls "babying." The nurse should help him to understand that these restrictions are only temporary. If she feels he is still undergoing too much anxiety, then she must call this to the attention of the attending physician, who may decide that there are small things that the patient may do for himself: feed himself if food is cut up, or brush his teeth. However, the nurse is still charged to see that this activity is made as effortless for the patient as possible, by placing things within his reach, uncapping the toothpaste, etc. These can be done quietly and without fuss, so that the patient's attention need not be drawn to the fact.

The nurse should be aware of the psychologic lift that a patient gains from having his hair combed or having a shave. Once again, the nurse can obtain permission from the physician to give the patient a shave when the patient is unable to perform the activity for himself.

Usually the patient may feed himself after forty-eight hours. The nurse must be alert for any evidence of fatigue, shortness of breath, chest pain, or changes in pulse or respiration as a result of the activity. When these occur, the activity is obviously too strenuous for the patient. The same symptoms may occur if the patient indulges in too much conversation during the early part of his illness. Therefore, the nurse watches carefully for the effect of visitors and family. Occasionally, the patient needs the opportunity to express himself and talk over a few things. The nurse must be sensitive to his needs and be practical in the limitations she imposes. Unnecessary restrictions are to be avoided since this only creates frustration or more doubt in his mind regarding his welfare.

Remember, the extent and limitation of activity must be individually prescribed by the physician. Frequently, the nurse may initiate activity by inquiring whether she may encourage deep breathing or flexing the extremities. When a range of motion exercises are done without effort, the patient is then permitted to resume gradually such activities as shaving himself, feeding himself, and other forms of physiotherapy and occupational therapy. Reading a newspaper and using the telephone are frequently restricted in the acute stage of myocardial infarction because of the effort involved in holding up the newspaper, or reaching for the phone. The principles involved in these restrictions are also followed when the nurse sees to it that the signal cord is right where he can reach it without raising his arm. Sometimes nitroglycerin is placed at the bedside so that the patient has to turn over in bed, reach through the side rails, pull open the bedside table drawer to get to it. The professional nurse is alert to such details and makes an effort to assist her auxiliary personnel to become aware of the means to reduce needless, and often harmful, activity by the patient.

After the patient has been free of chest pain for several days, the nurse will anticipate an increase in his activity. He is first permitted to sit on the side of the bed with help, and to dangle his legs for 10 to 15 minutes. This activity is increased to four or five times a day. If this is carried out with no evidence of fatigue or pain, then the patient is permitted to move out of the bed to a chair. After this, he begins to walk within his room and, perhaps, is permitted to walk to the bathroom. This is entirely a separate thing from allowing the patient to use the bedside commode for bowel elimination to avoid exertion.

Throughout this entire program of increasing activity, the nurse continues to observe the effect of such activity and reports any abnormal response. She must be careful to explain the normalcy of such exertion. A certain amount of dizziness, weakness, and rapid heart rate are to be expected after a patient has been on bed rest for three weeks, or even one week. If this is interpreted to the patient his anxiety over the effort is relieved, and the nurse will be better able to evaluate the actual physical response to the activity.

## *Nutrition*

In accord with rest therapy, the patient is offered frequent small feedings of easily digested foods in order to decrease the activity of the heart. During the first week small feedings may be given five times a day with a total caloric intake of not more than 1,200 calories, or regular diet may be prescribed if condition warrants. Calories may be restricted if the patient has an overweight problem. If the patient has renal complications due to cardiac decompensation or failure, he probably will have a definite prescribed sodium restriction in his diet. Nurses must watch the patient carefully during his meals for signs of fatigue. If he does show signs of fatigue, he should be given smaller feedings at more frequent intervals. It is important that the nursing care plan allow a period of rest after each meal.

When the patient is stronger and allowed a variable degree of activity, the caloric intake is generally increased to 1,800 calories. The patient is still taking small intermediate feedings between meals, or five small meals a day. The patient who is overweight or who has had high levels of serum cholesterol may be given a modified fat diet with supplemental polyunsaturates and restricted saturated fat—in other words, approximately 35 percent of his total calories coming from fat. Coffee during this stage of recovery is usually permitted, unless the patient has unfavorable reactions to caffeine.

Usually, fluid intake presents little problem. Fluids should not be forced unless specifically ordered by the physician lest the circulatory system be overloaded with volume. All nursing persons must be aware that extremely hot or cold liquids should never be offered to the patient.

It is sometimes difficult for auxiliary personnel to remember that ice water should not be given to the cardiac patient. If the patient has persistent vomiting or excessive perspiration, the nurse must keep in constant communication with the physician; if fluid intake is greatly hampered due to nausea or vomiting, slow intravenous fluids may be ordered. Even if the patient is feeling well after his severe, acute stage, an adequate intake and output record should be kept.

## *Oxygen Therapy*

Oxygen is used frequently as supportive therapy in myocardial infarction. Many coronary patients are unsaturated because of occult pulmonary edema, and oxygen will push the saturation up, increasing the amount of oxygen carried to the tissues, especially the hypoxic myocardium. It is most important to allay any anxiety that the patient may have regarding its use. If the patient is instructed that oxygen is used frequently as a routine measure in therapy, he will not have the feeling that he is near death's door when it is prescribed. Often oxygen is not used at all unless the patient is in impending failure, or having respiratory difficulty.

In some hospitals, patients are placed in oxygen tents during the summer months simply because there is no air conditioning. Such planning provides for a greater and more constant percentage of oxygen saturation. The nurse must be sure that auxiliary personnel who set up a tent and initiate oxygen therapy are aware that oxygen is heavier than air and will seep through the mattress unless a plastic cover or rubber sheet is placed over the head of the bed, or the mattress is plasti-coated.

Not only does infrequent opening of the oxygen tent maintain a higher level of oxygen saturation, it also provides the patient with the longer periods of undisturbed rest which are so essential to his recovery in the early stages of his attack.

Other practices will also help the patient to accept oxygen therapy. The nurse should check the positioning of the tent so that the plastic canopy is not pushed up against the patient's face. The tent should be large enough to keep the patient from having a feeling of claustrophobia, but not so high that it is difficult to maintain the desired oxygen saturation or that oxygen is needlessly wasted. Frequent mouth care is indicated since oxygen is very drying to the mucous membrane. If the tent is not provided with a funnel which diverts the inflow of oxygen upwards, a light cotton blanket or towel placed around the patient's head and shoulders will keep him from feeling a draft. The nurse can also be sure that the patient is provided with any necessary equipment which he may need inside the tent, such as the hand bell, bottle of nitroglyc-erin tablets, Kleenex tissues, and paper bag in which to dispose of them. Lint should be cleaned from the screen inside the tent frequently so that the air remains at the desired temperature and does not overheat.

The professional nurse should be sure that her auxiliary personnel under-stand the safety precautions regarding the restrictions of smoking and the use of electrical equipment, oil, and other combustible substances in and around oxygen. When oil and alcohol rubs are indicated, auxiliary personnel should be instructed to take the patient out of the oxygen tent and to turn off the inflow valve. The patient can be provided with some other form of oxygen therapy, if nursing care or diagnostic procedures cannot be done while the patient is in the tent. In extreme cases, back care and positioning of the patient may have to be omitted entirely during an acute period when a seriously ill patient cannot do without his oxygen. The professional nurse must assume responsibility for telling the patient's family and relatives that the plastic canopy of the oxygen tent does not interfere with the patient's hearing activity.

Other methods of oxygen therapy include the use of the nasal catheter, nasal cannula, and the face mask. Once again, the nurse must be alert to the effect of such therapy on the patient. It may be necessary to change from one method to another if the patient experiences any anxiety associated with a sense of suffocation when a mask is used. Skin care about the nose and mouth is very important if a patient is getting oxygen continuously per face mask.

When the nasal catheter is the prescribed method, care must be taken that the catheter not be inserted too far. The patient should be asked to swallow after the catheter has been inserted. If he swallows a lump of air, the catheter is down too far, and must be withdrawn slightly. Many cases of severe hiccupping and gastric distention, which complicate a heart attack, are due to the patient swallowing his oxygen rather than breathing it. Another important point is to remove the nasal catheter at least once every six to eight hours. The presence of the catheter in the nose stimulates the secretion of the mucous membranes. Unless the catheter is removed and cleaned, nasal se-cretions may completely obstruct the openings through which the oxygen passes. The catheter should be lubricated with a water-soluble jelly before it is inserted. In the event the patient aspirates the jelly, no harm will be done to the lungs. If preferred, plain water may be used to moisten the catheter for ease of insertion. When possible, reinsert the catheter through the alternate nostril so that the mucous membrane is not continuously traumatized on the one side.

It is important that the nurse be alert to the signs which indicate the need for oxygen. After the first few days of oxygen therapy, the order is generally changed to use oxygen as necessary (p.r.n.) by cannula, catheter, or mask. With skill and experience, the nurse will be able to evaluate the patient's need for oxygen. Restlessness and mild anxiety are often relieved by the use of oxygen. A change of position during the night may permit the gravitation of tissue fluid to the lungs and cause shortness of breath. A disturbing dream may cause a subconscious anxiety reaction and increase the activity of the heart. Once the nurse gets to know the patient, she will be able to decide if it is a medication he needs, or if oxygen is indicated. The judicious, prudent use of the p.r.n. order for oxygen plus reassurance and support from the nurse may eliminate entirely the need for narcotics during the night.[2]

## Pain, Anxiety, and Rest

Relief of pain, distress, and anxiety is a major factor in providing physical and mental rest for the patient. Sufficient sedation is usually ordered by the physician to reduce anxiety and restlessness, but not so much as to produce complete apathy.

A good night's rest can be ensured with a soothing back rub, a warm beverage, the sedative as ordered, and control of the temperature and ventilation of the room.

During the day, the nurse should be alert to those factors which seem to cause stress for the patient. It is important to avoid careless remarks and attitudes which may be misinterpreted. Much apprehension can be allayed by the nurse's confident attitude. If something definite is bothering the patient, he should be permitted the opportunity to get it settled.

Large doses of morphine or other potent analgesics may be given very frequently in order to alleviate the crushing pain of the myocardial infarction. The drug must be given as prescribed in order to reduce the extension of the damaged area of the myocardium. The nurse must be alert, however, for the moment when the patient's pain *suddenly* disappears. There may be an accumulation of morphine in the blood stream, which is not dangerous as long as the patient *is having pain,* but may cause toxic symptoms when the pain is relieved. The nurse should instruct her team members to maintain close watch on the pupils and respirations of any patient receiving morphine in frequent doses.

The nurse can also watch closely for nausea related to morphine injections. Morphine may be the drug of choice for the pain, but the side effect of nausea can result in vomiting, which will increase cardiac output and also increase vagal tone. This may result in bradycardia, but can be managed by use of atropine. When she suspects such toxicity, the nurse can alert the physician to the problem, and perhaps atropine will be given with each injection to relieve the side effects.

2. The section on Oxygen Therapy adapted from a paper delivered at the Fifth Annual Cardiac Institute for Nurses by Joan L. Green, "Care of Acute Cardiac," Santa Clara County Heart Association.

The nurse must never be afraid to give the prescribed narcotic except if pulmonary disease is present and consciousness disturbed. It is essential to relieve the pain as soon as possible in order to prevent further damage to the heart. As long as the nurse is alert for the cumulative effects when the pain is relieved, her patient will be safe.

Milder degrees of chest pain may be relieved through the immediate use of sublingual nitroglycerin. Ambulatory patients observed taking a nitroglycerin tablet should be watched carefully. The vasodilating effect of the drug may cause a severe drop in blood pressure if the patient is sitting up or walking around. Patients should be encouraged to lie down if they have had an episode of chest pain, or if they have felt the need for a nitroglycerin tablet. At the same time, the patient should be instructed to report to the professional nurse any episode of pain. She can then evaluate the situation and, if necessary, provide the patient with a stronger medication.

The nurse should observe carefully for pain which appears to be related to a rapid heart rate, or any increase or decrease in the blood pressure. In these instances, the physician will most likely prefer to treat the cause of the pain by controlling the heart rate and blood pressure, rather than indulging in an excessive use of narcotics.

## Anticoagulant Therapy

The procedure and significance of thrombin and prothrombin time will be discussed fully under laboratory procedures. However, the control of thromboembolism indicates other responsibilities for the nurse. It is important to prevent the development of clots within the vessels which may break off and travel to the lungs. Thromboembolism can be reduced to a minimum through early continued use of anticoagulants and by avoiding stasis in the lower extremities. Changing the patient's position in bed every hour and providing for adequate fluid intake are two nursing measures which will help avoid the formation of clots.

Frequently the physician requests that the patient's lower extremities be wrapped with Ace (elastic) bandages from the toes to above the knees. In some instances, elastic stockings may be used. This measure is directed toward the prevention of stasis in the vessels by providing firm external support to the muscles which support the veins. Many nurses feel that once these bandages are on, they must not be removed. Consequently, the bandages become loose in some areas, and tighten up as a tourniquet in others. This is also a source of general discomfort to the patient. The nurse should remove the Ace bandages at least twice a day, and oftener if necessary. Good skin care can be given to the legs by washing, drying, and powdering carefully. After a brief exposure to the air, the legs can then be rewrapped. The leg should be elevated while the Ace bandage is applied. If the nurse is working alone, she can support the patient's heel on the edge of the bedside table or tray table. The nurse should be careful to avoid a tourniquet effect by wrapping with equal pressure, overlapping the layers equally, and not pulling the bandage too tight. The current trend is to completely encase the toes and the heel so that tissue fluid is not trapped in the foot.

Patients who receive anticoagulants are usually on the therapy for at least two to four weeks. Some patients will go home on the medication. It is important to observe for a smoky urine which will indicate a bleeding condition resulting from an accumulation of the drug. During the bath procedure and other care, the nurse can observe the skin for any signs of petechiae which indicate bleeding through the capillaries. Patients who are taking anticoagulants must be careful to avoid cutting themselves when shaving, and should not be too vigorous with their toothbrush so as to cause bleeding. The nurse has a joint responsibility with the doctor to observe the results of the blood tests which determine the patient's clotting ability.

## Gastrointestinal Problems

Nausea, vomiting, constipation, and distention are complications occurring frequently in myocardial infarction. They not only provide a source of much discomfort to the patient, but also have adverse effects on the heart activity itself. These conditions must be treated promptly, and prevented altogether, if possible, so that the workload of the heart is kept at a minimum.

Carbohydrate beverages may be all that a patient can tolerate by mouth if he has nausea associated with the effect of the heart attack. If the nausea is related to the drug therapy, other measures will be more beneficial. In some instances, the nurse may need to request an order from the physician for a sedative or tranquilizer to control nausea. Fluid intake must be replaced if actual vomiting has occurred so that the patient's electrolytes are kept in balance. Here, too, the nurse may administer drugs which will control vomiting.

The low dietary intake permitted the patient with a heart attack reduces to a certain extent the number of bowel movements which a patient will have. It is important that constipation be avoided. At the same time, patients should not be permitted to attempt to keep bowel activity at a minimum so that there is no strain on the myocardium. Mineral oil, milk of magnesia, or one of the new fecal softening agents such as colace, are administered regularly from the beginning of the heart attack so as to maintain a soft stool which the patient can expel easily when the time does come. Adequate fluid intake will also help. If the patient has been unable to have a bowel movement after several days, in spite of the supportive measures taken, a glycerin suppository may be used. At all times, however, the patient should be encouraged to relax and to avoid undue worry or anxiety over the problem.

It is generally well accepted that the use of a bedpan is far more exerting for the patient than the use of the bedside commode. Consequently, many doctors now permit their patients to use the bedpan on a chair, or to be moved from the bed to the commode. The nurse should be sure that the commode is at the same level as the bed. The patient should be assisted in the transfer from the bed to the commode. In some cases, physicians will order that the patient be lifted.

The nurse should be well aware that the patient permitted this activity is *not* on early ambulation. He is still on absolute bed rest. He is allowed to use the commode only because there is less physiologic stress than to lift and turn to get on and off a bedpan. The implications here are that once again the nurse must see to it that all personnel caring for the patient keep a watchful eye on his personal needs, and decrease the amount of physical activity which he must exert getting in and out of bed to use the commode.

Careful observation of the patient for abdominal distention will initiate treatment for this complication as early as possible. Prevention of constipation and control of nasal oxygen therapy are the two most important means of controlling abdominal distention. Frequently, distention will occur as an indirect result of the heart attack itself. Orders will have to be obtained from the physician for the use of stupes and rectal tubes. If Prostigmin should be used to treat the distention, the nurse must be unusually alert to the heart rate and rhythm. The sensitive and irritable myocardium is especially susceptible to the effects of Prostigmin, and arrhythmias may occur which could result in heart failure.

### Summary

The restrictions placed upon the patient with myocardial infarction have been described throughout this entire chapter. Certainly, they should be reasonable and individualized. The nurse should protect the patient from disturbing visitors, business associates, and relatives during the first several weeks. It is important to exclude or minimize business worries. His access to the telephone may be limited. However, the nurse should be alert to those exceptions that, in the long run, will provide more complete physical and mental rest. Usually tobacco will be restricted during the first four to eight weeks after a heart attack, although recent research investigators stress complete abstinence.

The nursing care given the patient with myocardial infarction is a very important factor in his recovery. Certain fundamental concepts must form the basis of the care plan, but they must be flexible enough to be modified according to the individual patient situation. The professional nurse is charged with the responsibility to use the advantages of team nursing to the best interests of the patient. When auxiliary personnel are involved in the care of the patient with a heart attack, active instruction programs should be developed so that they too are aware of the significance of relating the need for alternate periods of rest and activity to the actual needs of the patient.

As the patient progresses from the acute stage into the convalescent and pre-discharge period, all members of the nursing team must work together in utilizing the teaching opportunities that occur for the patient and his family. Not only are we working for the survival of this patient and his return to full activity in society, we are also hoping to prevent the occurrence of another heart attack.

## Review and Advance

1. *Identify some of the predisposing factors of myocardial infarction.*
   The principal factors associated with "high risk" patients indicate evidence of atheroma of the coronary vessels. Yellowish, fatty material composed largely of cholesterol is gradually deposited along the walls of the arteries causing them to become fibrotic, thick, calcified, and narrow. The resultant reduction in blood supply to the body tissues first affects the myocardium. Other factors that are considered are elevation of blood pressure, obesity, cigarette smoking, emotional stress and anxiety, and possibly heredity. Experimental research continues to struggle with what actually triggers one person to have a "heart attack" when another in the same circumstances does not.

2. *Does atherosclerosis always produce myocardial infarction?*
   If the atherosclerosis develops gradually with progressive narrowing of the coronary arteries but no thrombus formation, a collateral circulation may develop to minimize the amount of anoxia to the myocardium although the blood supply through the coronaries decreases. The collateral circulation is seldom able to circulate enough blood, however, to maintain an adequate supply of oxygen to the heart muscle during excessive exertion. When an acute coronary occlusion occurs, it is thought that some of the cholesterol may break away from the wall of one of the coronary arteries, causing the wall to become ulcerated and a thrombus to form. As this thrombus increases in size, it completely closes off the circulation to a portion of the heart muscle. This is myocardial infarction.

3. *What is the most common cardiac emergency?*
   Acute myocardial infarction is the most common cardiac emergency. The patient typically complains of a sudden, severe, viselike pain in the substernal area. This pain may radiate into the left arm, and sometimes into the right arm, and up the sides of the neck. At other times, it may imitate indigestion or a gallbladder attack, with abdominal pain. The patient is often restless, and may be very apprehensive. He gets up and paces, opens the windows, or has a sudden urge to have a bowel movement. He often has the feeling that he is dying; his skin becomes cold and clammy. He may become dyspneic and cyanotic; he may show signs of shock. The pulse is usually rapid, but it may be barely perceptible; the blood pressure usually falls, and the patient collapses.

4. *Does the electrocardiogram always show muscle damage when the patient has a myocardial infarction?*
It is not unusual for the ECG not to show changes for several days after the attack. The physician relies on many diagnostic aids: the history and physical examination; white blood cell count; sedimentation rate; blood cholesterol; serum tests (SGOT, CPK); temperature .elevation; blood pressure; rate, rhythms or irregularity of pulse; quality and depth of respiration; x-rays; as well as renal output.

5. *What is the main objective in nursing care for the myocardial patient?*
The major objective in caring for the patient who has an acute myocardial infarction is to provide him with physical and mental rest. The damaged heart may be able to maintain basal activity, but additional strain may cause it to fail.

6. *How does healing of the myocardial infarction take place?*
Healing takes place by the substitution of fibrous connective tissue for the injured tissue. When fibrous connective tissue is used in repair, it serves as a patch that preserves or restores the continuity of the tissue. It can do nothing more. It cannot return to its former functional duty. The extent to which the cardiac reserve is diminished will depend on the size of the scar.

7. *Why is it connective tissue that takes over the repair job?*
There are certain circumstances under which repair by the substitution of fibrous connective tissue occurs. Among these are:

- when the conditions in the internal environment are unfavorable to mitosis
- when the quantity of tissue destroyed is too large for it to be replaced by regeneration of the cells in the area
- when highly specialized cells have been destroyed
- when the rate at which parenchymal cells multiply is slow
- when tissues are subjected to repeated injury

Thus, healing by the formation of fibrous tissue restores the continuity after too great a destruction of tissue. It walls off foreign bodies and disease processes, and reinforces weakened structures such as aneurysms of the aorta and other large vessels. There are many other reasons why fibrous tissue is called into action, but it suffices to remember that tissue repair by the formation of scar tissue is beneficial when the process is initiated by an appropriate stimulus and is sufficient to correct the damage caused by the injury. This is one more of the body's homeostatic mechanisms at work.

8. *Many hospitals have standardized procedures for oxygen administration by intermittent positive pressure for coronary patients. How safe is this procedure or practice?*
Oxygen therapy is prescribed by the physician in order to increase the supply of oxygen available to the cells. It should be the physician's responsibility to include in his prescription the method by which it is to be administered, the concentration to be maintained, the duration of the treatment, and whether an inhalant is to be added. Many nurses have worked so long with the same physicians—especially in the coronary care units—that they may well have gained expertise in administering IPPB. However, when inhalation therapists or oxygen technicians are employed, they are usually responsible for keeping the equipment in order, for bringing it to the patient's bedside, and supervising or checking its operation throughout the procedure. This may work

out very well for the general medical unit patients, but the purpose of the coronary care unit is to have all available equipment on hand and limit operations to those nurses or personnel within the unit as a part of patient therapy. Of necessity, she does much more than "hook up" the patient to the respirator. She prepares the patient physically and psychologically for the procedure, applies the appropriate apparatus, supervises the care of the patient so that an effective concentration of oxygen is maintained, and attends to personal, physical, and psychologic problems as they arise. She instructs the patient, his visitors, and personnel in safety precautions and in the essential aspects of treatment. In short, to fulfill her obligations, the nurse should have knowledge of the principles basic to effective and safe inhalation therapy and information about the different methods of administering oxygen, as well as an understanding of the reason why the oxygen was ordered.

9. *How is the adequacy of respiratory function determined?*
   Briefly, respiratory function must be considered in four general types of processes:

   - the movement of air to and from the respiratory membrane
   - its diffusion across the respiratory membrane
   - the transport of oxygen and carbon dioxide to and from the pulmonary circulation and the tissues
   - the utilization of oxygen by the cells

   In years past, tests were limited to measuring vital capacity and to the clinical judgment of the physician, but the advent of thoracic surgery has stimulated the development of many respiratory function tests. Tests include those for determining inspiratory time, inspiratory volume, tidal volume, expiratory reserve volume, residual volume, and total lung capacity.

10. *When vasoconstrictors are used to elevate the blood pressure, does this ensure that the patient has recovered from "shock"?*
    Even when the patient's blood pressure has been restored to normal physiologic levels, the patient may still be in shock. The most sensitive index is urine output. It should be at least 30 cc per hour.

11. *Is there a disagreement about the benefits of having a central venous pressure on all coronary patients?*
    Many physicians are doubtful about the usefulness of the CVP and are hesitant to perform the procedure.

12. *What are the advantages of central venous pressure?*
    The advantage of having a central venous catheter in the right atrium is primarily that the central venous pressure can be monitored. An elevated CVP (greater than 10 cm/water) indicates the inability of the right ventricle to handle the venous return. Serial changes in CVP are a good indicator of myocardial competency and circulating blood volume, and of effective inotropic or fluid volume therapy. In addition, many physicians feel that this provides a stable route for administration of intravenous fluids and medications and a route for phlebotomy is available. Blood for laboratory studies can be withdrawn directly from the CVP catheter without the ordeal of repeated venipuncture; mixed venous blood may be readily obtained from the right atrium for serial determinations of pH, $pCO_2$, and mixed venous oxygen saturation.

13. *What is venous pressure?*
    Venous pressure is simply the pressure exerted by the circulating blood

against the venous walls. The normal venous pressure ranges from 6 to 10 cm of water, although slightly higher rates may be considered normal by many physicians.

14. *When can the venous pressure be expected to be elevated?*
One can expect to find an elevation in the venous pressure in congestive heart failure, acute or chronic constrictive pericarditis, and in venous obstruction caused by a thrombus or external pressure.

15. *Is venous pressure the same in all parts of the body?*
Just as the arterial pressure is not always the same in all parts of the body, so does the venous pressure vary. It is not uncommon to see a physician do an antecubital venipuncture with a needle and a manometer attached to a two-way stopcock. However, central venous pressure, more commonly referred to as CVP, is dependent upon the blood volume, cardiac action, and peripheral resistance or other vascular alterations. If cardiac function or peripheral resistance has been disturbed, a high CVP may be found with a normal or reduced blood volume. On the other hand, if there is a disturbance of cardiac action alone, or in addition to peripheral resistance, a low CVP can be present with a normal or high blood volume. Therefore it cannot be stated as a general rule, but measurements of CVP should be obtained when (1) the blood volume or cardiac action is, unstable, or when large quantities of blood or fluid replacement may be required; (2) the cause of circulatory failure remains obscure and when the condition has failed to respond to previous measures; and (3) problems involve two or more of the major factors which can influence the CVP.[3]

16. *Can electrocardiogram tracings be taken from the CVP?*
Yes, this is an advantage, too. Using the saline bridge technique, intra-atrial electrocardiograph leads are immediately available. With the tip of the CVP catheter in the right atrium, the catheter is filled with *hypertonic* saline solution. The metal cannula at the outside tip of the CVP catheter is connected by an alligator clamp to the chest V-lead of an ECG cable with limb leads on the patient. The intra-atrial ECG is recorded in the V-position.

17. *What are some of the factors which create psychologic problems for the myocardial infarction patient?*
The implications of the diagnosis and the nature of the required treatment alone may result in psychologic complications. As mentioned previously, the highest incidence of coronary disease occurs among men, and they are usually men who are in the prime, productive years of their life, with families dependent upon them for support. Besides the possibility of sudden death, the disease carries the threat of invalidism or, at best, some adjustment in living habits. These factors are all sources of psychologic stress. Bed rest and inactivity are also accompanied by physiologic and metabolic changes which are a part of the total effect. And lastly, the patient may be greatly affected by the attitude of his family and friends.

18. *What are some of the later effects of myocardial infarction?*
As the heart muscle degenerates, rupture of the heart is a possibility. Thrombus formation with release of emboli into the circulatory system is a danger. Venous stasis, congestive heart failure, the shoulder-hand syndrome, develop occasionally.

3. Philip Cooper. *Ward Procedures and Techniques.* New York, Appleton-Century-Crofts, 1967, p. 55.

# 7 LABORATORY IN EVALUATION OF HEART DISEASE

Many substances in the blood have been given recognition as aids to the diagnosis of myocardial infarction. Aside from the routine laboratory procedures which have been established as policy upon admission, there are certain serum proteins, in the form of enzymes, that have assumed increasing diagnostic importance within the past decade. These include polysaccharides, nonenzymatic proteins, inorganic metals, and enzymes. The first two represent secondary, nonspecific responses to injury; the latter two are presumed by researchers to reflect the loss of soluble sarcoplasmic content (semifluid, inter-fibrillary substance of striated muscular fiber) from the injured cell into the circulation.

Enzymes, organic catalysts that are responsible for most of the chemical reactions of the body, are found in all tissues. Some have been identified in the plasma (serum), to which they gain access from injured cells or even perhaps from intact cells. The interest of physicians in serum enzymes began shortly after World War I, with the demonstration of usefulness of alkaline phosphatase levels in the diagnosis of bone and liver disease, of acid phosphatase levels in the diagnosis of carcinoma of the prostate, and amylase and lipase levels for the diagnosis of pancreatic disease. In spite of this clinical demonstration, interest remained relatively dormant until 1953. The demonstration in that year of a transaminase (glutamic-oxalacetic transaminase) in the serum of normals and the subsequent observations that increased levels of this enzyme were helpful in the diagnosis of cardiac and hepatic disease led to a marked intensification of interest in serum "enzymology." Nurses became aware of the importance of enzymes with the initiating of the coronary care units. Although a fully comprehensive discussion is not possible in a text of this type, the usefulness of several serum enzymes used in the diagnosis of the cardiac patient will be discussed.

## Principles of Diagnostic Serum Enzymology

All of the serum enzymes have their origin in cells. Some enzymes are found in many tissues, e.g., lactic dehydrogenase, aldolase, malic dehydrogenase. Other enzymes are, by nature, concentrated in one or two tissues. For example, ornithine carbamyl transferase and sorbitol dehydrogenase are found almost exclusively in the liver; significant amounts of creatine phosphokinase are found only in skeletal muscle, myocardium, and the brain. You can see that an increase in the serum levels of enzymes spread throughout many tissues is a less specific clue to the site of injury. So, in order to concentrate the diagnostic value of enzymes, attention has been directed to the different molecular forms of a given enzyme (isoenzyme) that may be found in different tissues.

Isoenzymes of amylase, alkaline phosphatase, acid phosphatase, glutamic-oxalacetic transaminase, leucine aminopeptidase, lactic dehydrogenase, malic dehydrogenase, isocritic dehydrogenase, creatine phosphokinase and cholinesterase, and other enzymes have been demonstrated in different tissues and are of interest to the physician as well as the physiologist, geneticist, and the clinical researcher. Only the isoenzymes of lactic dehydrogenase and creatine phosphokinase have been of importance clinically.

It must be remembered that the use of serum enzymes as diagnostic aids has been largely empirical, but the values observed in clinical and experimental circumstances permit speculative analysis of the factors that control serum enzyme levels in normal and diseased subjects. The serum levels of a particular enzyme may be increased by diseases that lead to increased rates of release from tissue, increased amount available for release, or decreased rate of disposition. The levels of an enzyme may be decreased in disease that interferes with its production.

Increased rate of release is clearly responsible for the high serum levels of hepatic, pancreatic and myocardial enzymes in diseases that produce necrosis of the respective tissue. The pattern of abnormality of serum enzyme values that results depends on the normal enzyme content of the tissue involved, on the type and extent of necrosis, and on other not yet understood factors. Bearing this in mind, it is understandable that high serum levels of a number of digestive enzymes are found in acute pancreatitis, and a number of enzymes of intermediary metabolism are found in myocardial infarction or acute hepatitis. Although these enzymes are richly concentrated in both liver and myocardium, higher levels are produced in hepatitis than by myocardial infarction presumably because the necrosis and degeneration of hepatitis is diffuse and of infarction, local.

Increased rate of release of enzymes into the circulation may occur without apparent tissue necrosis. Increased permeability of cell membranes seems to account for the elevated serum levels of aldolase, creatine phosphokinase, and other enzymes in progressive muscular dystrophy. The high serum levels of creatine phosphokinase (CPK), glutamic-oxalacetic transaminase (GOT), aldolase, lactate dehydrogenase (LDH) and several others in patients with delirium tremens but without recognizable liver disease also may depend upon increased permeability of skeletal muscle membrane.

An increase in the tissue source of enzymes because of increased rate of production per cell or increase in the number of cells may be responsible for increased serum levels. This seems to be the mechanism for certain enzyme-level increases in patients with peptic ulcer, osteoblastic bone lesions, and prostatic carcinoma.

Impaired disposition or arrangement of serum enzymes has been considered responsible for the increased levels of alkaline phosphatase (AP) and GOT in biliary obstruction and for increased amylase levels in renal failure. Particular attention is given to transaminases, lactic dehydrogenase and its isoenzymes, creatine phosphokinase, and their relevance to clinical use.

## *Transaminases*

Glutamic-oxalacetic transaminase is elevated in diseases involving the tissues that are rich in it. These would include the tissue of heart, liver, skeletal muscle, kidney, brain, pancreas, spleen, lung, and serum. Therefore, cardiac diseases or conditions in which serum GOT is elevated would include myocardial infarction, pericarditis, cardiac arrhythmias, acute rheumatic fever, postcardiac surgery and catheterization, and heart failure. Experimental work with animals suggests that the degree of rise of SGOT is related to the extent of myocardial necrosis (Figs. 1 and 2). This has been difficult to prove in patients.

In patients with electrocardiographic and clinical manifestations of coronary insufficiency rather than myocardial infarction, elevated SGOT levels may occur. It is not clear whether this represents myocardial necrosis or leakage of the enzyme into the serum without myocardial necrosis. Nevertheless, for treatment purposes, these patients are considered to have suffered a myocardial infarction.

Mild elevations of the SGOT levels have been reported in some patients with pulmonary infarction. The incidence of increased values is low, the degree of abnormality slight, and the rise delayed for three to five days after the onset of pain.

Activity

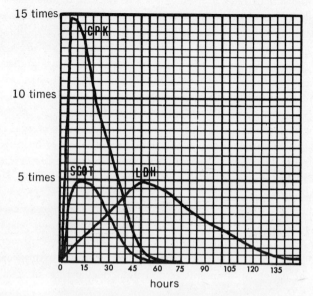

**FIG. 1** During the days following myocardial infarction, CPK is the first to be elevated within 3 to 5 hours after infarction. SGOT rises steeply from 2 to 20 times normal within the first 24 to 36 hours. LDH reaches its peak one or two days later than the SGOT. Between four to ten days the values begin to return to normal.

| Enzyme | Beginning of increase hours | Maximum hours | Return to normal days |
|---|---|---|---|
| CPK | 2 - 4 | 24 - 36 | 3 |
| SGOT | 4 - 6 | 24 - 48 | 5 |
| LDH | 8 - 10 | 48 - 72 | 14 |

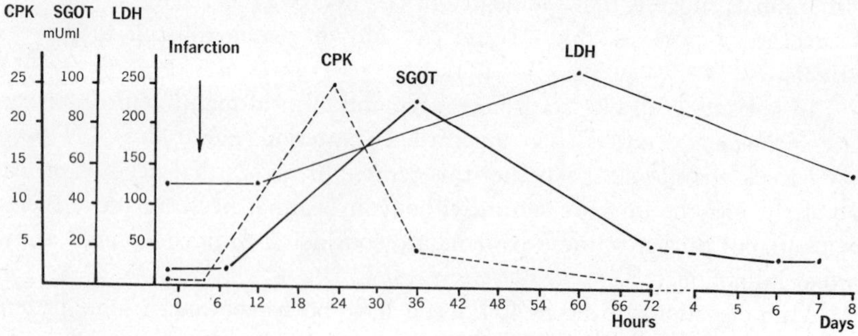

**FIG. 2** The most commonly used enzymatic assessments of myocardial infarction include the evolutionary changes in activity of serum glutamic-oxalacetic transaminase (SCOT), lactic acid dehydrogenase (LDH), and creatine phosphakinase (CPK).

In patients with congestive heart failure and in those with marked tachycardia, mild to moderate degrees of SGOT elevation may occur. These have been attributed to the hepatic necrosis secondary to hepatic congestion. Patients with pericarditis have been reported to have a 50 percent incidence of slightly elevated SGOT. Slight SGOT elevations have been reported after cardiac catheterization and mitral commissurotomy.

SGOT determination is not necessary for the diagnosis of myocardial infarction in most patients with classical clinical symptoms and electrocardiographic evidence of this condition. This determination is of value in patients whose electrocardiographic changes are insufficient to be helpful, e.g., those with left bundle-branch block, Wolff-Parkinson-White syndrome, or those with abnormalities remaining from previous myocardial infarction which obscure acute changes. It is also of value in recognizing the recurrence of an infarction during convalescence. Normal levels obtained at the proper time are of value in ruling out a diagnosis of myocardial infarction.

In patients with myocardial infarction, elevations in the serum levels of serum glutamic-pyruvic transaminase (SGPT) are slight or absent. Heart failure or shock with accompanying hepatic necrosis may lead to elevated SGPT levels.[1] The chief application of determination of this serum enzyme is the diagnosis of hepatobiliary disease.

## *Lactic Dehydrogenase*

This enzyme is widely distributed throughout the cells and body fluids. It catalyzes the reversible oxidation of lactic to pyruvic acid in the presence of other enzymes, and also catalyzes the end reaction of the anaerobic and aerobic pathways of glucose metabolism. The serum and plasma LDH activity are relatively stable at $+4°$ C to $-10°$ C for a few days.[2] LDH is inhibited by the presence of anticoagulants, such as heparin and oxalate; therefore, serum is preferred in testing. There have been five different varieties of isoenzyme forms of LDH isolated.[3]

Serum LDH activity becomes acutely elevated for variable lengths of time for a large variety of conditions: acute injuries of the heart, red cells, kidney, skeletal muscle, skin and liver (Fig. 2). Peculiarly, it is elevated only briefly in severe hepatitis, and only seldom is it increased in chronic liver disease. The serum activity, on the other hand, is persistently elevated in chronic muscle and skin disorders, such as dermatomyositis. It is also per-

1. "Contributions of Serum Enzymes and Isoenzymes to the Diagnosis of M.I. (II)," *Modern Concepts of Cardiovascular Disease*, AHA, Sept. 1967.
2. R. Douglas Collins. *Illustrated Manual of Laboratory Diagnosis: Indications and Interpretations*. Philadelphia, J. B. Lippincott Co., 1968, p. 139.
3. *Ibid.*

sistently elevated in a wide variety of blood disorders or dyscrasias, including the macrocytic anemias associated with folic acid or $B_{12}$ deficiency, in some forms of disseminated neoplasm, and in the proliferative disorder, polycythemia rubra vera.[4] In pulmonary infarction there is frequently a higher incidence of elevated LDH's than SGOT's:

| Infarction | SGOT | LDH | Bilirubin |
|---|---|---|---|
| Pulmonary | Normal | Elevated up to 7 days | Elevated |
| Myocardial | Elevated up to 4-7 days | Elevated up to 7-14 days | Normal |

Cellular injury and necrosis in myocardial infarction leads to the outpouring of intracellular transaminases and dehydrogenases into the blood. As a result, the serum transaminases (SGOT) and lactic dehydrogenases (LDH) rise. There is a high correlation between the size of the infarct and the degree of enzyme elevation. The SGOT rises early (6 to 12 hours after the infarction) and drops to normal within a 4- to 7-day period, whereas the LDH rises later (12 to 24 hours afterward) and falls gradually over a 1- to 2-week period. For some unknown reason, the serum LDH rises in pulmonary infarction, whereas the serum transaminases (SGOT) remain normal unless there is associated congestive heart failure.

The pattern of elevated serum LDH levels in patients with myocardial infarction is quite characteristic. High levels are observed in almost all such patients within a few hours of the apparent onset of infarction. Although the degree of elevation is not so striking as that of SGOT, the elevation persists longer (10 to 14 days). The characteristically prolonged period of elevated LDH values and briefer period of elevated SGOT values provide a pattern that may be useful in the recognition of myocardial infarction.

Most patients with pulmonary infarction have elevated levels of LDH, usually within 24 hours of the onset of pain. The pattern of normal SGOT and elevated LDH levels within one to two days after an episode of chest pain provides suggestive evidence for pulmonary infarction.

The lactic dehydrogenase of human serum has been found to be separable into five different components by electrophoretic techniques. Each of these isoenzymes is distinguishable from the others by serologic, electrophoretic, and various other chemical procedures. The isoenzymes of LDH are designated in ordinary usage according to their electrophoretic mobility. Some American authors have referred to the fraction with the greatest (anodic) mobility as isoenzyme 5 and the fraction with the slowest mobility as isoenzyme 1, with the other three fractions numbered according to relative mobility 2, 3, and 4. European authors have followed the reverse order. They refer to the most anodic fraction as isoenzyme 1 and the least mobile as number 5, and desig-

4. *Ibid.*

nate the other three accordingly. In the United States, the American nomenclature is followed.

The five LDH isoenzymes have the same molecular weight but differ in the charges that they carry. Tissue LDH consists of the five isoenzymes in varying proportions, and the LDH activity of each tissue has a characteristic isoenzyme composition. Thus, the LDH of myocardium erythrocytes and kidney cells consists largely of fast-moving isoenzymes ($LDH_5$ and $LDH_4$). Studies of the isoenzyme composition of the elevated LDH serum levels of various diseases have revealed abnormal patterns that reflect the tissues involved. However, to go into more detail is beyond the scope of this text.

## Creatine Phosphokinase (CPK)

This enzyme, also referred to as a creatine kinase and ATP creatine phospherase, is particularly useful shortly after the myocardial infarction occurs. Its concentration in skeletal muscle and the myocardium is very high; appreciable amounts are found in the brain. Very tiny amounts are found in other tissues. *None* is found in the liver. Many studies have shown that CPK values are high in patients with myocardial infarction, progressive muscular dystrophy, and delirium tremens, but normal in patients with hepatitis and other forms of liver disease. Although CPK is found almost exclusively in myocardium, muscle, and brain, and early reports suggested it to be an almost specific index of injury of myocardium and muscle, more recent reports indicate that inexplicably high serum CPK values can occur in patients with pulmonary infarction and pulmonary edema. Further studies are required to define the degree of specificity of high serum CPK values. At present, it is regarded by clinicians as a useful but not completely specific aid in the diagnosis of myocardial and muscle disease.

## Other Enzymes

The most commonly used enzymatic assessments of myocardial infarction include those of serum glutamic-oxalacetic transaminase (SGOT), lactic acid dehydrogenase (LDH), alpha-hydroxybutyric acid dehydrogenase (HBDH), and creatine phosphokinase (CPK). The less commonly used ones include aldolase (ALD), malic dehydrogenase (MDH), and serum glutamic-pyruvic transaminase (SGPT).

The more common of these have been presented briefly since the nurse should have some understanding of their increasing value. However, if she should wish to expand her knowledge of the research and studies, she is referred to the bibliography.

The nurse should be familiar with the knowledge that other blood and serum and plasma studies also indicate some helpfulness to the diagnosis, but these are not to be discussed here. However, to refresh the memory they will be included in the table of diagnostic laboratory tests at the end of this chapter.[6]

## Summary

Along with the electrocardiogram tracing, the physician depends upon certain other significant laboratory tests. The ECG is discussed elsewhere in the text; the discussion of enzymes has been presented in this chapter because they are not as widely known and understood by nursing personnel.

It must be remembered that increases in serum enzyme activity are non-specific indicators of injury. Such increases do not indicate which organ is injured, nor the etiology of the injury. Also, these tests are rarely done singly since they are most meaningful in combination when assayed daily, for they may provide a pattern suggestive of a specific clinical diagnosis for the physician. The tests, therefore, have relevance only in a clinical context. That is, they either confirm or rule out organ injury that is suspected clinically.

Which of the current enzymatic tests are most useful? Which offers the greatest aid to the physician in diagnosis of myocardial infarction? Evidence has been presented that the simultaneous assay of two enzymes possesses greater value than of one alone. The daily and simultaneous assay of two enzymes, one demonstrating changes of short duration, and one those of longer duration, was found to be superior to reliance on either one alone.[7] The choice of which assays to use routinely is up to the physician. The SGOT and LDH assays probably are more useful, but only because each has been studied extensively, each is simple, and the two cover a major period after the infarction. It seems likely, however, that if the minor technical problems pertinent to CPK assay are resolved, because of its greater specificity it could supplant the SGOT as the assay of choice in the early phase of myocardial infarction.

The great need for means of diagnosing specific organ injury is obvious. Even though anatomically dissimilar, most organs have a number of biochemical features in common, but the diagnosis of specific organ injury by many biochemical means unfortunately is nonspecific. Thus, further study and research based upon these features and directed to identification and assay of unique organ substances which pour into the circulation are continuing in the attempt to resolve and clarify the dilemma.

6. Eugene Coodley. Significance of Serum Enzymes. *American Journal of Nursing,* February 1968, pp. 301–304.
7. *Ibid.*

## *Review and Advance*

1. *In which heart disease does the assay of enzymes in serum have a direct use?*
   Predominantly, in myocardial infarction.
2. *An assay of which enzymes is recommended when a myocardial infarction is suspected?*
   CPK, SGOT, LDH, also SGPT for differential diagnosis and for following progress (liver).
3. *Should enzyme assays be carried out or an ECG be completed first when a myocardial infarction is suspected?*
   Both. Only by a combination of both methods is the maximum information obtained. Enzyme assays are especially useful when there are already one or more ECG tracings showing earlier ECG changes.
4. *Is it important to determine the enzymes at a fixed time in case of a suspected myocardial infarction?*
   Because of the relatively transient nature of the enzyme increases after a myocardial infarction, the time of obtaining a blood sample is of special importance.

| Enzyme | Beginning of Increase (Hours) | Maximum (Hours) | Return to Normal (Days) |
|--------|-------------------------------|-----------------|-------------------------|
| CPK | 2–4 hr | 24–36 | 3 |
| SGOT | 4–6 | 24–48 | 5 |
| LDH | 9–10 | 48–72 | 14 |

5. *Does the extent of the increase in enzyme activity give any indication as to the prognosis?*
   An increase of SGOT over 150 mU/ml and of LDH over 800 mU/ml is unfavorable for the prognosis, as is an increase of CPK lasting longer than the third to fourth day.
6. *Can a second myocardial infarction be recognized by the enzyme levels in serum?*
   Yes, renewed damage to myocardial cells leads again to an increase of enzyme activity.
7. *In myocardial infarction what are the advantages of the assay of SGPT in addition to SGOT of serum?*
   Two main advantages are:
   a. For differential diagnosis: A significantly higher activity of SGOT compared to SGPT from the start is characteristic of myocardial infarction. In pulmonary embolism and acute upper abdominal disease the situation is reversed, with SGPT higher than SGOT.
   b. For following progress: If the activity of SGPT, which is largely liver-specific, increases above that of SGOT, this is an early indication of heart failure with hepatic congestion.
8. *How do the enzyme activities behave in simple angina pectoris?*
   Normal values are found in angina pectoris. If an increase in enzyme activity

is detectable, then in spite of the absence of positive ECG signs, damage to the myocardial muscle cells must be presumed.

9. *Is it worthwhile carrying out enzyme assays in inflammatory heart diseases?*

In inflammatory heart diseases the changes in enzyme activity in serum are usually very small and may be completely absent. However, if an increase in enzyme activity occurs, then, as in the case of angina pectoris, severe cell damage is indicated.

10. *What are the enzyme changes found in heart failure?*

In acute heart failure, increases of SGOT and SGPT are found in serum due to the hepatic congestion, and these rapidly return to normal on successful treatment with digitalis. In chronic heart failure, there are usually no or only slight changes in enzyme activities.

## Cardiovascular Diseases—Diagnostic Laboratory Tests

| Blood Specimen | Normal | Abnormal Indication |
|---|---|---|
| Bleeding Time | 1–5 minutes | |
| Differential count: | | |
| Lymphocytes | 1250–3500/cu mm 25–35% | |
| Monocytes | 200–1000/cu mm 4–10% | |
| Neutrophils | 3000–8000/cu mm 53–80% | Increased in rheumatic fever, acute bacterial endocarditis |
| Eosinophils | 25–400/cu mm 0.5–4% | Decreased in congestive heart failure |
| Basophils | 0–200/cu mm 0–2% | |
| Erythrocytes | 4–5.5 million | Decreased in rheumatic fever, subacute endocarditis. Increased in many forms of chronic heart diseases as in some types of congenital heart diseases and in heart disease with pulmonary complications. |
| Leukocytes | 5–10,000 | Increased in coronary infarction, rheumatic heart disease. |
| Platelets | 200–500,000 | |
| Reticulocytes | 0.5–2.0% red cells females: 37–47% males: 40–54% | Rises considerably in shock |
| Hemoglobin | Females: 12–15 gm/100 ml Males: 14–17 gm/100 ml | See comments for erythrocytes |
| Coagulation Time | 4–12 minutes | |
| Sedimentation Rate | 2–20 mm/hr (depends on method) | Abnormal always higher. Useful in following the course of acute rheumatic fever and myocardial infarction |
| Blood urea nitrogen | 10–20 mg/100 ml | Elevated when heart disease disturbs renal circulation |

| Blood Specimen | Normal | Abnormal Indication |
|---|---|---|
| Nonprotein nitrogen | 15–35 mg/100 ml | |
| Blood Sugar | 70–100 mg/100 ml | Used because of susceptibility of diabetic to arteriosclerosis |
| Blood serum protein | 6–8 gm/100 ml | Measured because edema sometimes results when protein content is low |
| Blood cholesterol | 160–270 mg/100 ml | High in arteriosclerosis |
| Serological test for syphilis | | Used because of aortic aneurysm resulting from syphilis |
| Prothrombin time Prothrombin index | 14–18 seconds 70–100% | Measured frequently because of anticoagulants in treatment and prevention of embolism |
| Blood cultures | Negative | Positive in bacterial endocarditis |
| Antistreptolysin titer | | 400 units is consistent with, but not diagnostic of, rheumatic fever |
| C-reactive protein | Negative | A protein substance, not normally present, is found in active rheumatic fever, myocardial infarction and pulmonary infarction |
| Transaminase (SGOT, SGPT) glutamic-oxalacetic glutamic-pyruvic | 5–40 units/100 ml 8–40 5–35 | Increased in myocardial infarction SGOT—briefly within first 2 days, then drops abruptly SGPT—lags considerably—not helpful to diagnosis of M.I. |
| Lactic acid dehydrogenase (LDH) | 50–400 units/100 ml | Reaches peak in 1–2 days, gradually declines |
| Creatine phosphokinase (CPK) | | Dramatic early and short-lived increase—Marked elevation 3–4 hours post M.I. |
| Calcium | 9–11 mg/100 ml | All of these from this point are important in fluid retention and electrolyte balance |
| Chlorides (E) | 340–380 mg/100 ml | |
| Phosphorus | 3–4.5 | |
| Potassium (E) | 13.5–19.5 | |
| Sodium (E) | 310–335 | |
| Magnesium | 1.25–2.5 | |
| Hydrogen Ion Concentration pH | 7.33–7.39 | Gives a clearer picture of shifting of body metabolism in serial assay |
| $CO_2$ Combining Power (E) | 53–77 cc $CO_2$/100 cc plasma | |

# 8 ELECTROLYTE DISTURBANCES

## *What Electrolytes Are*

Water and electrolyte "metabolism" is an integral part of every branch of medicine and biology. Living organisms cannot exist without them. Water in the body serves as the universal solvent of various solutes. These solutes may be electrolytes such as sodium chloride, calcium sulfate, or potassium phosphate, or nonelectrolytes such as glucose and urea.

Electrolytes are substances whose molecules dissociate or split into ions when placed in water. Some develop a positive charge, some a negative charge. Ions with a positive charge are *cations* (+). They migrate to the *negative* pole (the cathode) when an electric current is passed through the solution. Sodium ($Na^+$) is an example.

Ions with a negative (−) charge are *anions*. They migrate to the positive pole (the anode) under influence of an electric current. Chloride ($Cl^-$) is an example.

With the milliequivalent system, electrolytes are expressed as milliequivalents per liter and electrolyte balance of anions and cations has a clear-cut meaning. A milliequivalent is 1/1,000 equivalent weight of a molecule which is related to the molecular weight of a substance and its valence or charge. Equivalence or milligram contain the same number of molecules so they can be compared.

Total cations always equal total anions. They balance each other. This equality *does not exist* when expressed as milligrams per 100 millimeters. With the milliequivalent system, both the reacting capacity (number of ionic charges) and osmotic activity (number of solute particles) of a solution are known. Thus calculations are greatly simplified; electrolyte imbalances are easier to evaluate; electrolyte shifts are virtually impossible to follow unless expressed as mEq per liter.

## Plasma Electrolytes Expressed As Milliequivalents Per Liter

| Cations | mEq/L | Anions | mEq/L |
|---------|-------|--------|-------|
| $Na^+$ | 142 | $HCO_3^-$ | 24 |
| $K^+$ | 5 | $Cl^=$ | 105 |
| $Ca^{++}$ | 5 | $HPO_4^=$ | 2 |
| $Mg^{++}$ | 2 | $SO_4^=$ | 1 |
| | | Org. Acid$^-$ | 6 |
| | | Protein$^-$ | 16 |
| | 154 | | 154 |

A basic understanding of electrolytes must be viewed first from an understanding of the movement of water from one body compartment to another. Osmosis causes water to be drawn from regions with low concentration into the solution of high concentration.

The force causing this movement through a semipermeable membrane is osmotic pressure or "pull." Exertion is in direct proportion to the concentration of particles in the solution. Thus it is "osmolality" or particle concentration that is essential to maintain constancy of fluid volume in each body compartment. In the living animal it is the proteins which exert the effective osmotic gradient resulting in most physiologic fluid shifts.

For example, if the concentration of extracellular sodium is above normal (hypertonic) water will be withdrawn from the tissue cells. The cells will shrink in size (Gibbs-Donnan Equilibrium Theory). The prominent cation in extracellular fluid is sodium. It constitutes more than 90 percent of the total cations at a concentration of 142 mEq per liter.

If the extracellular fluid is hypotonic (concentration of sodium below normal) the tissue cells will take up water and swell, just as the red blood cells do in a hypotonic salt solution. With hypotonicity, ADH (antidiuretic hormone) is inhibited and diuresis can result (loss of extracellular fluid).

Solutions are considered isotonic or isosmotic if they have the same osmotic pressure (particle concentration) as body fluids. An isotonic solution when given intravenously will neither increase or decrease the size of the red blood cells. Sodium, or isotonic saline, is the chief electrolyte in regard to normal balance and distribution of water.

## The Cation Sodium

As stated previously, sodium is the most prevalent of the extracellular electrolytes. It comprises more than 90 percent of the total cations at its normal concentration of 142 mEq per liter of plasma. Because of its dominance in quantity, appreciable change in total cations represents a change in sodium.

This, plus the fact that sodium does not easily cross the cell membrane, gives it the primary role in controlling the distribution of water throughout the body. It is this function of sodium that makes it so important in fluid balance. A decrease in serum sodium concentration will prevent water retention (ADH inhibited) in an effort to reestablish the normal concentration of sodium. An increase in serum sodium concentration stimulates water retention (ADH release), diluting sodium back to its normal level.

When sodium is lost or retained, it is accompanied by water. Water accounts for 45 to 70 percent of body weight. The percentage is higher in thin than in obese persons, in infants than in adults, and in males than in females. Total water in the body constitutes 60 percent of the average adult weight and remains remarkably stable (within 1 to 2 percent) for a given individual. Approximately two-thirds of body water is intracellular (ICF) and one-third extracellular (ECF). Approximately three-fourths of the extracellular fluid is interstitial (IF) and one-fourth intravascular (plasma).

Alterations in the sodium concentration can produce profound clinical effects in markedly influencing blood volume. With severe sodium depletion, the loss of water continues and results in dehydration. This leads to periphery circulatory failure and then to impaired renal function, reduced renal flow, and glomerular filtration. With reduced glomerular filtration the serum urea nitrogen will rise and the excretion of water and salts is delayed.

Sodium bicarbonate varies directly with intracellular sodium. Sodium enters the cells when there has been a loss of intracellular potassium. Normal intracellular sodium has been reported as being equal to about one-sixth to one-ninth of the total extracellular sodium.

The exact daily requirement of sodium for man is not known. Dietary sodium is usually obtained as sodium chloride. The amount ingested varies largely with the taste of the individual. The National Dietetic Society suggests the following:

### Dietary Intake of Sodium Chloride in Normal Individuals

In adults: 104 to 260 mEq in 24 hours, or 6 to 15 g of sodium chloride in 24 hours.
In children: 52 mEq in 24 hours, or 3 g in 24 hours.
In infants: 17 mEq in 24 hours, or 1 g in 24 hours.

The average daily requirement of sodium chloride for adults is approximately 6 grams.

Daily excretion of sodium as sodium is approximately 111 mEq in 24 hours; and as sodium chloride, 111 mEq, or 6.49 g in 24 hours or 2.55 g. The body has remarkable ability to retain sodium and urinary sodium concentration approaches zero in terms of deprivation; thus, excretion is directly related to intake in the healthy individual in more usual environments.

## *The Cation Potassium*

The unique feature of potassium is that it can be life-supporting or extremely toxic depending upon circumstances. The kidneys are less able to conserve potassium than sodium, and potassium may be flushed out by diuresis even in the presence of a body deficit. On the other hand, if the kidneys fail to excrete it normally from the body, toxic levels can prevail.

Most of the potassium is in the cells. It is the principal cation of cellular fluid with a normal concentration of about 150 mEq per kilogram of water. Plasma concentration is only about 5 mEq per liter. Variations from either of these levels can produce profound clinical effects.

The plasma level of potassium reflects only the concentration in the extracellular fluid. It does not necessarily reflect its concentration intracellularly. A deficit in potassium therefore may exist in either plasma or cellular fluid or both. A potassium deficit in cellular fluid may coexist with an excess of potassium in plasma. Entrance of potassium into the cells depends upon normal metabolism and glucose utilization.

There seems to be a reciprocal relationship between sodium and potassium. Sodium enters the cells where there is a loss of cellular potassium. An intake of large amounts of sodium results in an increased loss of potassium and vice versa.

Deficit of potassium is a more prevalent condition than is commonly appreciated. Early symptoms are vague and confusing. Anyone who stops eating food and drinking liquid containing potassium can develop a severe deficit within days. If an adult is fasting or on a diet adequate in calories but potassium-free, the loss of potassium from the body still goes on; 40–50 mEq or 1.56–95 g are lost daily in the urine. The obligatory urinary loss of potassium in the healthy individual is 10–20 milliequivalents per day, but is higher in stressful situations and with illness. Potassium concentration is quite high in the succus entericus (alkaline intestinal secretions) and vomiting and diarrhea may result in marked depletion. The magnitude of potassium depletion cannot be estimated from the value of the serum potassium concentration alone. With moderate potassium deficits, for example, the serum potassium level may be increased if the patient is acidotic and minimally or moderately or markedly decreased if the patient is alkalotic.

The normal diet contains 50–100 mEq potassium per day. Only about 10 mEq are excreted in the stool and sweat; the remainder is excreted in the urine. The kidney can greatly increase excretion to adjust to high potassium intake but is less capable of adjusting to a very low potassium intake. In fact, in the absence of potassium, the kidney is unable to maintain potassium balance.

*Hypokalemia* is the name given to the condition when there is a decrease of potassium in the blood plasma. It results either from loss of potassium from the body or from a shift of potassium into the cells. Losses may be gastrointestinal or urinary. The condition rarely develops before the serum concentration has fallen below 3.0 mEq/L unless the rate of fall has been rapid. Signs and symptoms include neuromuscular disturbances (weakness, flaccid paralysis, or tetany) and cardiac abnormalities (arrhythmias, increased sensitivity to digitalis, and ECG changes). The ECG abnormalities occur sequentially and include flat or inverted T waves, prominent U waves, depressed S-T segments; at times a prolonged P-R interval is visualized, with tall P waves, and possibly widening of the QRS complexes, since the U wave frequently is superimposed upon the T wave thereby producing an appearance of a prolonged Q-T. Metabolic alkalosis and hypokalemia are often associated. The ECG serves as a reasonably satisfactory guide to serum potassium levels when actual determination of the serum potassium is not available.

Patients treated with diuretics or corticosteroids are susceptible to potassium depletion and should be advised to take adequate dietary potassium, particularly supplemental fruit or fruit juices. Cranberry juice has been found to be a high source of potassium. The serum potassium should be measured at intervals if therapy is prolonged, and potassium supplements should be supplied if indicated. Particular care to prevent potassium depletion is necessary in patients taking digitalis, since severe cardiac arrhythmias may otherwise develop. Patients receiving only parenteral fluids should be given 40 mEq potassium daily unless oliguria or other contraindications exists. Lethal hypokalemia may occur during the treatment of diabetic ketoacidosis.

*Hyperkalemia* is the increase of potassium in the blood serum. It may result from decreased renal excretion of potassium, rapid release of potassium from the cells, or administration of potassium.

Decreased excretion is common in acute renal failure and adrenal insufficiency. Rapid release from cells results from severe acidosis or increased tissue breakdown (e.g., following surgery, crush injury, extensive infection, massive hemolysis); these conditions may also be associated with impaired renal excretion of potassium.

In patients with significant elevation of the platelet count, or in situations in which the *tourniquet has been left in place* for a prolonged period of time before venipuncture, the blood sample hemolyzed or refrigerated, or separation of red blood cells from the plasma delayed, the potassium value in the serum sample may be high although the patient's true potassium concentration is normal.

Manifestations are usually absent; if they appear, they may resemble those of hypokalemia. *Cardiac manifestations* are frequent when the serum potassium level exceeds 8.0 mEq/L (uncommon at concentrations of less than 7.0 mEq/L) and include bradycardia, hypotension, ventricular fibrillation, and cardiac arrest. The sequential ECG manifestations are tall peaked T waves, depressed S-T segments, decreased amplitude of R waves, prolonged P-R interval, diminished to absent P waves, and widening of the QRS complexes with prolongation of the Q-T interval, resulting in a sine-wave pattern.

Hyperkalemia may be treated with measures that antagonize the effects of potassium, force cellular entry of potassium, or actually remove potassium from the body. Which measures should be used depends upon the degree of hyperkalemia and the severity of the manifestations. Urgency is assessed on the basis of both the serum potassium concentration and the ECG changes; the situation is urgent if the serum potassium level is greater than 8.0 mEq/L or the ECG reveals absent P waves or a broad QRS complex.

The following tabulation lists the time of onset and duration of effect of the measures commonly employed in the treatment of hyperkalemia.[1]

|  | Onset of Effect | Duration |
|---|---|---|
| Calcium gluconate, IV | 1–5 min | ½–2 hours |
| Sodium bicarbonate, IV | 5–10 min | 2+ hours |
| Glucose-insulin, IV | ½–1 hour | 6–24 hours |
| Resins, orally or rectally | ½–2 hours | As long as continued |
| Dialysis | 0–2+ hours | As long as continued |

Calcium antagonizes the cardiac toxicity of hyperkalemia, particularly if hypocalcemia is also present. If the patient is receiving digitalis, however, calcium administration is sufficiently hazardous that calcium cannot be given.

## The Cation Calcium

The uniqueness of calcium is its versatility. Calcium not only provides the framework of the bones and teeth but is also involved as ionized calcium in normal clotting of the blood and in neuromuscular irritability and in myocardial contraction. Calcium also exerts a sedative effect on the cells of the nervous system. When the concentration is low, excessive irritability, even convulsion, occur.

The absorption of dietary calcium is stimulated by vitamin D. Unless there is adequate protein in the diet, the body is unable to use calcium.

1. Robert C. Packman, ed. *Manual of Medical Therapeutics.* Boston, Little, Brown and Company, 1962, p. 53.

Digestive juices secreted into the intestinal tract contain 5 to 10 mg of calcium per 100 ml, or about 8 mg average. In other words, 500 mg of calcium are secreted into the gastrointestinal tract daily and are reabsorbed. Calcium is never completely absorbed from the gastrointestinal tract. If the gastrointestinal tract conditions do not favor absorption, a negative calcium balance can exist, especially if calcium intake is low.

Calcium deficit is seen quite frequently in diseases in which calcium of the extracellular fluid is trapped in diseased tissues, in extensive infections on the body skin, in burns and in diarrhea. Calcium may be trapped in the form of calcium "soaps" in patients with malabsorption syndromes.

The patient suffering from calcium deficit will have muscle tremors. He may have cramps. If the deficit persists, calcium will be removed from his bones. Fractures may occur. In·calcium deficit the level of calcium in the extracellular fluid is usually below its normal plasma level of about 5 mEq per liter. If the deficit is acute, intravenous calcium usually is indicated.

The parathyroid hormone secreted by the parathyroid glands located within the thyroid gland is responsible for the handling of calcium and phosphorus by bone, intestine, and mammary gland.

The concentration of the ionized calcium is the important physiologic fraction. It aids in regulation of neuromuscular irritability. In bicarbonate excess (e.g., metabolic alkalosis), ionization of calcium is depressed and tetany may result.

Calcium requirements for normal adults vary widely, even in the same individual at different times. The body content of calcium in adults is 20.1 g per kg, in infants, 9.2 g per kg. In adults, practically 20 percent is excreted in the urine.

### The Cation Magnesium

The last of the four most important cations is magnesium. Its unique feature is its role in enzyme activity. It is an important "coenzyme" in the metabolism of both carbohydrates and protein. Magnesium is also involved in neuromuscular activity.

The serum concentration of magnesium is 1.7 to 2.3 mEq per liter, or 2.0 to 2.7 mg per 100 ml. About 35 percent of the serum magnesium is bound to protein.

Magnesium proteinate in serum acts as a dissociated salt according to the mass law relationship, and diffusible magnesium is practically all in ionic form. It is the only cation that is higher in concentration in the cerebrospinal fluid than in the serum. The average value in spinal fluid ranges from 2.4 to 3.0 mEq per liter. This cannot be considered ultrafiltrate of plasma.

The intermediary metabolism of magnesium resembles that of phosphorus. Both are present in bone and within tissue cells. It is probable that the same factors that control calcium absorption also govern absorption of magnesium, and have the same influence on the deposition of protein as potassium.

The exchange of magnesium in the tissues is accelerated when insulin and dextrose are given parenterally. It has been reported to slow the rate of experimental atrial flutter, to restore normal sinus rhythm, and to abolish toxic rhythm produced by digitalis. Clinical studies of altered magnesium levels are not too prevalent because magnesium determinations have been difficult.

The normal dietary intake of magnesium for adults is about 250 mg in 24 hours, in infants about 150 mg in 24 hours, and in pregnancy and lactation 400 mg daily. The average adult daily intake is about 300 mg. In adults, the daily excretion of magnesium is about 60 percent of the dietary intake via the feces and about 40 percent via the urine. In normal man, probably no more than 8 to 10 percent of the filtered load of ionized magnesium is excreted in the urine in 24 hours.

## The Anion Bicarbonate

Metabolic acidosis and metabolic alkalosis acid-base balance is largely determined by the concentration of the bicarbonate ion. The bicarbonate concentration depends upon kidney and pulmonary function which regulates the amount of cations available to combine with bicarbonate (Table 1). Very little bicarbonate is excreted in acid urine but primarily in alkaline urine.

| | NORMAL | METABOLIC IMBALANCES | | RESPIRATORY IMBALANCES | |
|---|---|---|---|---|---|
| RATIO of bicarbonate to carbonic acid is 20 to 1 | Carbonic acid 1.2 mmol/L | Carbonic acid 1.2 mmol/L | Carbonic acid 1.2 mmol/L | Carbonic acid 1.84 mmol/L | Carbonic acid 0.6 mmol/L |
| | $HCO_3^-$ 24 mEq/L | $HCO_3^-$ 12 mEq/L | $HCO_3^-$ 36 mEq/L | $HCO_3^-$ 24 mEq/L | $HCO_3^-$ 24 mEq/L |
| pH = 7.40 | | $Na^+$ 142 Cations / $Cl^-$ 116 Anions | $Na^+$ 142 Cations / $Cl^-$ 90 Anions | $Na^+$ 142 Cations / $Cl^-$ 105 Anions | $Na^+$ 142 Cations / $Cl^-$ 105 Anions |
| | $Na^+$ 142 / $Cl^-$ 105 | METABOLIC ACIDOSIS | METABOLIC ALKALOSIS | RESPIRATORY ACIDOSIS | RESPIRATORY ALKALOSIS |
| | $R_{c+}$ 12 / $R_{a-}$ 25 | The concentration of the bicarbonate ion is determined by renal function. | | The concentration of carbonic acid is determined by respiratory function. | |

Courtesy of Travenol Laboratories, Inc., Morton Grove, Illinois

## Electrolyte Balance and Imbalance Picture

METABOLIC ACIDOSIS
> The primary alteration is a deficit of bicarbonate. Ex: Ratio of bicarbonate (12 mEq/L) to carbonic acid (1.2 mmol/L) is decreased to 10 to 1. Normal ratio is 20 to 1. pH is also decreased from 7.40 (normal) to 7.10 (acidosis).

METABOLIC ALKALOSIS
> The primary alteration is an excess of bicarbonate. Ex: Ratio of bicarbonate (36 mEq/L) to carbonic acid (1.2 mmol/L) is increased to 30 to 1. Normal ratio is 20 to 1. pH is also increased from 7.40 (normal) to 7.58 (alkalosis).

The concentration of the bicarbonate ion is determined by renal function in metabolic acidosis and metabolic alkalosis.

RESPIRATORY ACIDOSIS
> The primary alteration is an excess of carbonic acid. Ex: Ratio of bicarbonate (24 mEq/L) to carbonic acid (1.84 mmol/L) is decreased to 13 to 1. Normal ratio is 20 to 1. pH is also decreased from 7.40 (normal) to 7.21 (acidosis).

RESPIRATORY ALKALOSIS
> The primary alteration is a deficit of carbonic acid. Ex: Ratio of bicarbonate (24 mEq/L) to carbonic acid (0.6 mmol/L) is increased to 40 to 1. Normal ratio is 20 to 1. pH is also increased from 7.40 (normal) to 7.70 (alkalosis).

The concentration of carbonic acid is determined by respiratory function in respiratory acidosis and respiratory alkalosis.

Courtesy of Travenol Laboratories, Inc.,
Morton Grove, Illinois

The bicarbonate concentration is 22 to 26 mEq per liter in arterial and 24 to 28 mEq per liter in venous blood. There is a significant lower serum bicarbonate in women of about 2.5 mEq per liter in opposition to their higher serum chloride concentration.

Under normal circumstances, a supply of bicarbonate is always present as a result of the production of carbon dioxide as an end product of metabolism. A primary alteration of bicarbonate concentration reflects metabolic acidosis or alkalosis, i.e., low serum bicarbonate as seen in metabolic acidosis and excess serum bicarbonate in metabolic alkalosis. In metabolic alkalosis, there is an increased urinary excretion of potassium. In metabolic acidosis, there is a decreased urinary excretion of potassium. With an *increased plasma* bicarbonate, there is a decrease in cellular potassium, and an increase in intracellular sodium. Potassium leaves the cells as sodium enters. Serum bicarbonate varies indirectly with intracellular potassium.

In respiratory acidosis and alkalosis, opposite bicarbonate levels prevail in response to variable elimination of carbon dioxide from the lung. In respiratory acidosis, carbonic acid is in excess. The patient has a high alveolar carbon dioxide concentration because of hypoventilation. Plasma bicarbonate is above normal. In respiratory alkalosis, there is a deficit of carbonic acid. The patient has a low alveolar carbon dioxide concentration because of hyperventilation. Plasma dicarbonate is slightly below normal. There will be more about this later.

### The Anion Chloride

Even though the intracellular chloride is very small, it is obvious that chloride is found in certain specialized cells. The bulk of chloride is present in the interstitial and lymph fluid compartments.

Normal venous serum or plasma chloride is 100 to 106 mEq per liter. Women have plasma chloride levels about 2.5 mEq higher than men. The amount of chloride found within the cells is only about 1 mEq per kilogram of cell water.

Chloride is unique in several ways since its presence influences the shifts of other electrolytes in the body. For instance, a deficiency of either chloride or potassium will lead to a deficit of the other. Usually chloride losses follow those of sodium; however, the proportion will differ since a loss of chloride can be compensated for an increase in bicarbonate. This reciprocal compensation tends to preserve the osmotic pressure and water balance of the body.

Changes in acid-base balance due to altered bicarbonate are reflected by changes in chloride concentration. Chloride also plays an integral part in buffering action when oxygen and carbon dioxide are exchanged in the red blood cells. When blood is oxygenated, chloride travels from the red blood cells to the plasma, whereas bicarbonate leaves the plasma. This exchange is known as "the chloride shift." This same type of shift in the ratio of cell chloride also occurs when the blood becomes more alkaline. As a result (chloride leaving the cells and going to plasma), venous blood will have a lower concentration of plasma chloride than oxygenated arterial blood. Since water travels the same direction as chloride, the red cells become relatively dehydrated when blood is oxygenated.

The normal chloride requirement, although not known precisely, is expressed as sodium chloride; in adults, the range is 104 to 260 mEq in 24 hours or 6 to 15 g of sodium chloride in 24 hours. In children, the normal dietary intake is 52 mEq or 3 g of sodium chloride in 24 hours; and, in infants, 17 mEq or 1 g of sodium chloride in 24 hours. The daily urinary excretion in adults, as sodium chloride, is 119 mEq or 6.96 g in 24 hours.

### Acid-Base Disturbances

The most important cations and anions have been briefly presented; others that might have been included are the phosphates, sulfates, the organic acid anions (pyruvate, acetoacetate, citrate), and the anion proteinate. However, it is not the author's intent to burden the reader with excessive depth information, but to provide that bit of knowledge that will enable her to be aware of major changes in the electrolyte and acid-base reactions within the body.

We have now shown that the electrolytes are related to at least *four fundamental physiologic processes:* 1) water distribution, 2) osmotic pressure, 3) neuromuscular irritability, and 4) acid-base balance. It is necessary now to take a closer look at this last process.

A word of caution is necessary to remind the reader to remember some of her or his basic chemistry. Acids are hydrogen ion (proton) donors; bases are proton acceptors. These terms are *not* synonymous with the terms anion and cation, for the cations sodium ($Na^+$) and potassium ($K^+$) are neither bases nor acids, the cation $NH_4^+$ is a weak acid, the anions chloride and sulfate are weak bases, and at normal blood pH the anion bicarbonate ($HCO_3^-$) is a weak base and the anion phosphate ($H_2PO_4^-$) a weak acid. The reaction or acidity of biologic fluids may be expressed as hydrogenions in concentration or as *pH*, the *negative logarithm* of $H^+$. The normal pH of venous blood 7.35–7.40 represents 35–40 millimicroequivalents $H^+$ per liter.

Metabolism both produces and uses up acid. Natural carbohydrate and fat, when incompletely oxidized, release protons, even though this release is only transient because complete combustion yields carbon dioxide and water. The carbon dioxide ($CO_2$) is a potential acid because, when hydrated, it forms carbonic acid. These reactions are reversible, however, and the 22,000 mEq of carbon dioxide produced each day by metabolism are excreted by the lungs. If ventilation is not disturbed, the production and elimination of this end-product acid has no net effect on pH. Metabolism also results in the production of nonvolatile, or fixed, acid that does require renal excretion. Thus, the lungs and kidneys, and buffers provide a defense against acid-base disturbances. Chemical buffers ($HCO_3^-$, $PO_4^-$, proteinate, hemoglobin, and bone carbonate) react immediately with acid or alkali to minimize changes in pH, but are thereby used up, or consumed, leaving the individual less able to withstand further stress on neutrality. Respiratory adjustments, which also occur promptly, minimize pH changes by increasing or decreasing the excretion of the end product ($CO_2$), but such adjustments in ventilation are also limited. The *ultimate* correction of acid-base disturbances and restoration of buffer, then, are dependent upon the kidney, even though renal excretion of acid and, to a lesser extent, alkali occurs slowly. The role of the kidney in *the acid-base regulation is to restore bicarbonate to the blood* and excrete $H^+$.

To summarize up to this point, then, the simple disturbances of acid-base equilibrium are metabolic and respiratory acidosis and alkalosis. Each of these four disturbances evokes compensatory responses that tend to minimize the changes in pH, but overcompensation does not occur.

In *metabolic acidosis,* the primary mechanism is retention of fixed acid or loss of alkali (i.e., a decrease in $HCO_3^-$ or ketoacidosis of diabetes mellitus); the compensatory response is hyperventilation and resultant fall in $pCO_2$. In *respiratory acidosis,* the primary mechanism is pulmonary retention of $CO_2$

(i.e., increase in $pCO_2$) resulting in a small increase in total $CO_2$. The large significant increase in total $CO_2$ is due to the compensatory renal regeneration of $HCO_3^-$, the equivalent to renal excretion of acid.

In *metabolic alkalosis*, the primary mechanism is loss of fixed acid or gain of alkali (i.e., an increase in $HCO_3^-$ or total $CO_2$); the cause is almost invariably ingestion of alkali or inability of the kidney to do its job, usually from potassium loss. Thus, compensatory mechanisms are inoperable. In respiratory alkalosis, the primary mechanism is hyperventilation and a resultant fall in $pCO_2$; the compensatory response is a decrease in $HCO_3^-$ or total $CO_2$ due to increased endogenous acid production and decreased renal acid excretion.

Although there is still some controversy on whether or not arterial blood is necessary for pH determination, there seems to be a feeling that arterial blood samples are *not* necessary for determination of acid-base status. Venous blood is quite adequate, say some observers, if samples are properly collected, if peripheral circulation is not impaired, and if the difference between arterial blood and venous blood values is appreciated. Normal values are listed. (For $pCO_2$ measurements, however, arterial blood is needed.)

|  | pH | $pCO_2$ | Total $CO_2$ |
|---|---|---|---|
| Arterial blood | 7.38–7.43 | 35–45 mm Hg | 24–29 mEq/L |
| Venous blood | 7.35–7.40 | 40–50 mm Hg | 26–32 mEq/L |

The syringe should be coated with heparin (1,000 units/ml) to serve as anticoagulant and to seal the barrel against air leaks. Venipuncture should be performed without a tourniquet if possible; if not possible, the blood sample should be drawn before the tourniquet is released. Air bubbles should be expressed from the syringe and the syringe then capped, or the attached needle inserted into a sponge or cork. If pH and total $CO_2$ cannot be measured promptly, the capped syringe may be stored in ice water for as long as two to three hours.

Although the most reliable evaluation of acid-base status is afforded by measurement of pH or $pCO_2$ in addition to total $CO_2$ content, the latter value alone usually permits the most significant knowledge to the physician in his clinical diagnosis. In certain circumstances, however, diagnosis may require measurement of pH and/or $pCO_2$, such as in the hyperventilating patient with either respiratory alkalosis or metabolic acidosis.

## *Summary*

Body fluid equilibrium in health is based on intake-output records—the amount of fluid taken in and the volume excreted. A person who is eating a normal diet will satisfy his needs for various electrolytes. It is the sick patient who suffers the greatest losses since ingestion of water and food diminishes or ceases entirely. Under such conditions, the patient may become seriously ill by loss of body fluids and electrolytes in a matter of days and in some instances, even hours. In understanding the concept of body fluid balance—that is, how it is supposed to work—the nurse will be better prepared to assist the physician in his plan of medical care, as well as to take an active part in the education of her subordinate and team members, the patient, and his family.

## *Review and Advance*

1. *What are the divisions of fluids in the body?*
   Briefly, the divisions of fluids in the body are two: extracellular and intracellular.
2. *Is the extracellular broken down into other classifications?*
   It has been said that the extracellular fluid compartment is that fluid where the tissue cells safely graze. The extracellular fluid compartment is further divided into two parts: the intravascular portion, which consists of those fluids in the arteries, veins and lymphatics; and the extravascular compartment, which is outside the vessels and is divided into (1) interstitial spaces, (2) the fluid of connective tissue and cartilage, (3) the fluids in bone, and (4) a transcellular fluid which is a secretion from cells into the gastrointestinal tract and into the subarachnoid space. This last one is very seldom mentioned.
3. *How does the change of ions take place?*
   This is an important point. The *interchange* of ions and small molecules between plasma and interstitial fluids is extremely rapid. This makes them almost continuous with respect to their electrolyte composition and balance. Further, the electrolytes in the extracellular fluid compartment can be studied with much more accuracy than the intracellular compartment. In fact, because of the nature of the intracellular fluid compartment, there are probably no studies made that the mixture of some extracellular fluid does not take place. The one possible exception would be in the study of washed hemocytes. However, these studies do not represent accurately the composition of the body fluids and electrolytes in a general way.
4. *What are electrolytes?*
   Electrolytes are acids, bases, salts, and aqueous solutions which have dissociated into ions, i.e., electrically charged particles. There are substances in the body, in the circulation, such as urea and glucose, which do exist as molecules but are not electrolytes. The normal concentration of body electrolytes which is usually expressed in milliequivalents per liter varies depending upon whether they are in the extracellular or intracellular fluid. These electrolytes can be both cations or minerals or anions. Any good text on fluid and electrolytes, or any medical text, will give a further breakdown than is presented in this chapter for those who wish further information. However, remember that sodium is the largest and most important extracellular cation. Of the intracellular fluid, potassium is by far the most important cation. In order for a human being to remain alive, all these fluids and all

these minerals, the electrolytes as we have called them, must remain in fine balance.

5. *How does the body keep this fine balance?*

The body has acids and ingests acids. It has bases, and also ingests bases. A base is a hydrogen ion *acceptor*. An acid is a hydrogen ion *donor*. How does the body keep this fine balance? The body must maintain a pH between 7.38 and 7.44. Any deviation below or above these figures can be very serious. Very briefly, the pH is maintained by several methods. First of all, there are the blood buffering actions. These are brought about by the phosphates, the bicarbonates, the protein buffers, and hemoglobin buffers which are intracellular. Very often one hears of the *alkaline reserve*. This is usually referred to as the blood bicarbonate level because this is really the largest and most effective of the buffering systems. Actually, though, it is the sum total of all basic ions, but mainly the bicarbonates. These blood buffering systems, however, do need some help. A big help is given by the respiratory system throwing off carbon dioxide. This is very, very beneficial in helping maintain a good system. If carbon dioxide is retained by the lungs, there is respiratory *acidosis*. If it is increased by an increased respiration, therefore lost at a greater rate, there is respiratory *alkalosis*. This system works rapidly and keeps a keen equilibrium.

There is still another way to maintain a good buffering action: excretion. This is not as rapid as the respiratory mechanism, but it is as good. It is the function of the kidneys. The kidneys can conserve bicarbonate if the need for bicarbonate becomes necessary, or they can excrete bicarbonate if it becomes low. Most bicarbonate is reabsorbed in the kidney tubules. This is done mostly by the proximal tubules but partly by the collecting tubules.

6. *Are all of the fluid compartments composed of water?*

This leads us into "water balance." To say specifically that the fluid compartments of the body are composed of water is somewhat misleading Actually, these compartments are filled with salt water, which resembles sea water somewhat but is of considerably less salinity, especially the fluid in the intracellular fluid compartment. In a healthy individual, one who is able to eat and drink normally, water for the body is gained by ingestion of fluids, solid foods, and by the oxidation processes within the cells. Water loss in a healthy man is by three routes: urine, stool, and insensible water loss which is in the form of water vapor from the skin and lungs. This balance is again keen. When the volume of water in the body relative to the body's solids, that is, the electrolyte volume, increases, the oral gain diminishes and the renal loss increases. Conversely, when the water volume relative to the solid volume decreases, the oral gain increases and renal loss diminishes. The kidney is responsible for removing any excess of body fluids and, on the other hand, conserving such vitally important ions as sodium and chloride when they are being depleted through some abnormal route. The kidney can throw off 35 g of solid per day. It can concentrate the urine to a specific gravity of 1.032 if 35 g of solid are excreted in 500 cc's urine; but, if the concentration of the kidney is only at best 1.010, it will require 1,400 cc's of water for the excretion of those 35 g of solids. It becomes very important to know the specific gravity of urine rather than urine volume. All this makes it very obvious that one can encounter a varying amount of clinical conditions relative to the fluids and the electrolytes in the body. (For example, sweat is hypotonic.)

7. *What is a hypotonic solution?*

    An isotonic solution, sometimes called a physiologic solution, is a solution of equal osmotic pressure to that found in the body. In other words, it is a solution containing just enough salt to prevent the red blood cells from being destroyed when added to the blood. Therefore, a *hypotonic* solution is simply that type of solution that does not equal the osmotic pressure in the system; it is lower. The solids, the electrolytes, are lower. A *hypertonic* solution is one that contains more concentrated amounts of solids and, therefore, the osmotic pressure is higher. For example, if a patient is perspiring profusely and has not taken in sufficient amounts of fluids, because the perspiration— or sweat—is very hypotonic, he will lose more fluid than minerals. This individual will really need more fluid replacement relative to electrolyte replacement. Therefore, it would be logical to use a hypotonic solution giving more fluid and less electrolytes. During the summer, in a room without air conditioning, the patient loses about 600 cc's of water per hour as perspiration; in an air-conditioned room, this amount rarely exceeds 200 cc's per hour. Replacement of fluids involves keen clinical judgment. Today, it is the judgment of the physician, or of the clinician. Tomorrow, it might very well be the judgment of the nurse-clinician.

8. *What are some of the isotonic solutions most commonly used?*

    Sodium chloride, 0.9 percent, bicarbonate solution, 1.3 percent, sodium citrate solution, 2.5 percent, and dextrose solution, 5 percent.

9. *Can vomiting cause a serious electrolyte imbalance?*

    If a patient is vomiting, or undergoing gastric suction, the electrolyte losses will be largely on the cation side, particularly chloride. There will be some potassium loss also. Upper small bowel losses will usually be in equal amounts of both anions and cations, particularly sodium and chlorides and bicarbonate. This is through the bile, pancreatic, and jejunal secretions. Ileal and colonic losses are predominantly basic cations, such as sodium, potassium, and magnesium.

10. *Is the intravenous route of fluid always desirable?*

    The oral route is always preferrable for fluid replacement. Theoretically, the rectal, subcutaneous, and intramuscular methods are next in order of preference mainly because of the opportunity for selective absorption and venous pressure regulations and consequent avoidance of any pulmonary or cardiorenal complications. Practically, however, especially in the presence of peripheral circulatory failure, the intravenous route is usually the method of choice when the patient is unable to eat or drink. Again, remember that the replacement of water and electrolytes is a matter that requires the best clinical judgment.

# 9 THE NUTRITIONAL NEEDS
## OF THE CORONARY PATIENT

The nurse can be an invaluable aid to the patient with heart disease. Patients with long-established eating habits find they have much difficulty in adjusting to changes, and even relatively uncomplicated instructions may be confusing to some patients. The nurse can further interpret the dietary instructions provided by the physician and the dietitian; she should encourage the patient to follow his diet and answer any questions he may have about it. Later, follow-through by the public health nurse may be advisable, and her encouragement of the patient to remain on his diet may contribute greatly to his cooperation.

### Cardiac Dysfunction and Compensatory Mechanisms

The role of the heart may seem to need little explanation. Briefly, in review, the heart is the pump or driving force that pumps the blood throughout the body on its mission of supplying nutrients to various parts and collecting metabolic wastes for disposal. The heart may not be functioning normally. There may be changes in the arteries and veins. Kidney perfusion may be reduced, resulting in less removal of the products intended for urinary excretion. The interrelation may seem obvious and simple: complications in any one system may result in impairment of the others.

The heart itself may suffer functionally or organically and various parts may be affected. The stage in which the dysfunction exists is also of importance. In the first stage, circulation usually is maintained although the heart may enlarge and beat more rapidly in an effort to compensate.

**129**

The initial physiologic finding is usually the elevation of the filling pressure, or "end diastolic" volume. The heart is on a new "Starling curve." The elevated filling pressure may result in accumulation of edema "behind the heart"—that is, in the lungs or peripheral vessels—depending on whether cardiac failure involves the left side of the heart, the lesser circulation, or is biventricular. As the situation worsens, the compensatory mechanisms of the autonomic nervous system fail, and the cardiac output begins to suffer.

When cardiac output declines, renal compensatory mechanisms come into play with increased reabsorption of salt and water. The antidiuretic hormone is secreted, resulting in water conservation. The renal-adrenal axis is activated as renin is secreted by the juxtaglomerular apparatus converting angiotensinogen to angiotensin, which results in aldosterone secretion by the adrenal cortex. Aldosterone is a very potent salt-retaining corticosteroid. *Our dietary efforts are pointed at these events.*

The logic of dietary adjustment instituted to relieve cardiac strain must be understood. The work of the heart must be saved as far as is compatible with good nutrition. As obesity may be a problem, it should receive attention in planning the diet.

## *Obesity Factors*

Certain clinical features of cardiac failure deserve emphasis briefly. Although the mechanisms leading to enlargement of the cardiac myocardium in the very obese patient are not well defined, the appreciable increase in the work of the heart must play a significant role. Some researchers indicate circumstances accompanying gross obesity may be similar to those under experimental conditions of prolonged or continual physical exercise. However, development of congestive heart failure secondary to prolonged physical exertion in otherwise healthy individuals or in experimental animals has not been reported.

A current hypothesis regarding the pathogenesis of heart failure in very obese individuals is that initially myocardial enlargement (hypertrophy) and reduced ventricular contraction result largely from the increased workload on the heart, with resulting rise in left ventricular filling pressure and pulmonary hypertension at rest or during exercise. Later, as progressive hypertrophy itself hinders myocardial contractility, and the work of the heart remains the same, cardiac failure develops.

Edema of the lower extremities is common in patients with extreme obesity and it is not clearly related to the amount of excess weight. Since the presence of edema in these patients is often unassociated with elevation of the central venous pressure or cardiac failure, other factors must account for its development in at least half the patients. Many large varicose veins are often found in the legs of these patients, which could play a role in edema formation. In addition, the presence of high intra-abdominal pressure may cause compression of the inferior vena cava and pelvic veins, resulting in obstruction to venous return to the heart.

Although more could be said of obesity and its many augmented factors, it is enough here for the nurse to see that there are disadvantages: lack of balance between the body mass and heart strength, an undesirable condition even when the integrity of the heart is unimpaired; return venous flow impairment may result in edema; arteriosclerosis and atherosclerosis may involve the coronary arteries which supply the blood to the myocardium.

## Principles of Diet

During illness, foods that under normal conditions would be completely digested and absorbed may be digested very incompletely and, even if digested, may be poorly absorbed into the blood. Therefore, with the exception of the restriction of salt, the dietary regime has two main elements or principles: (1) low caloric intake if the patient is overweight, and (2) small, frequent feedings. Otherwise, the general rules of dietetics are followed. However, often the diet is modified by associated conditions such as fever, obesity or malnutrition, peptic ulcer, irritable spastic colon, vitamin deficiency, anemia, or diabetes. The benefits of a low-caloric diet result from the reduction of the work of the heart. In short, further guidelines from such a diet may be listed under four main headings:

1. Foods are chosen that require little digestion or which are partly predigested, such as milk in the form of junket, toast in which starch is already partially changed to dextrin, and fruit juices containing glucose and fructose which can pass directly into the blood without being broken down by enzymes.
2. As the patient may feel too ill to chew his food thoroughly, foods are allowed in such small particles that enzymes can surround them and thus digest them more completely than large pieces. Liquids are given first place (unless restricted) because much of the food they contain is already dissolved and is therefore in small particles. Any solid food which does not readily break into small particles (as dry toast) or melt (as oils and some fats) should be pureed or mashed.
3. Only small meals shall or should be given because they can be more completely digested than can large meals by the limited amount of juices, the number of enzymes, and the muscular contractions.

4. Frequent feedings are essential, not only to replenish the glucose supply but also to enable the diet to meet the protein, vitamin, and mineral requirements.

Other indications for low-caloric diet in patients with hypertensive and coronary heart disease, other than obesity, take into consideration whether or not the patient is entirely confined to bed by symptoms of heart failure. On the other hand, children suffering from heart failure and rheumatic fever with carditis are usually undernourished, as are many patients with cardiac failure secondary to vitamin deficiency and those with right-sided heart failure. In these cases, as well as those due to constrictive pericarditis, hypoproteinemia may be quite severe and rigid dietary restrictions may be unwarranted. Thus, the physician usually orders a high protein diet in such cases. There are other factors, such as the patient with diabetes and coronary heart disease who is on insulin therapy and must receive an adequate carbohydrate allowance in order to ward off anginal pain due to hypoglycemia (insulin shock).

The vitamin content of the diet is usually supplemented by vitamin concentrates, particularly vitamin B in the form of thiamine chloride, 5 to 10 mg daily in divided doses. Occasionally, when there is reason to suspect a severe vitamin $B_1$ deficiency, it may be given parenterally. Protein must be adequate to spare tissue protein. Low serum protein is not uncommon in the later stages of cardiac dysfunction.

The diet is planned to prevent digestive upset and flatulence; therefore readily digested foods are most desirable.

To prevent edema, which would put added strain on the heart, a moderate intake of water and sodium chloride is indicated, or in more cases than not, the physician will specify a certain "sodium" diet which the dietitian is instructed to follow implicitly.

In coronary occlusion, water, fruit juice, and milk should be the only food offered during the acute stage. After this has passed, there may be a gradual return to a more normal diet. However, if the physician has evaluated the patient's condition and allows the patient more than liquids during the acute stage, he will usually suggest small feedings of bland, low-sodium, low-caloric, low-residue meals, along with vitamin supplements. Evaluation of the previous intake of sodium will provide a base line upon which to gauge the degree of restriction required. Before drastic sodium restriction is instituted, the renal function is usually evaluated to determine if the kidneys can conserve sodium. In an occasional case, 350 mg or less of sodium may be the maximum tolerance without development of edema, although such extreme restriction is usually necessary only when failure is first treated. Again, vitamin supplements may be indicated. Restricted diets and anorexia may lead to malnutrition and avitaminosis, with a superimposed type of failure.

## Counseling the Patient

Standard printed guides for patients on sodium restricted diets are geared to the problem of the average patient. Because patients have their own individual problems that may be due to limited education, insufficient income, or lack of interest, they should have additional help from the physician, the nurse, or the dietitian. Many times, it is up to the nurse to suggest a visit by the dietitian but, where this is not possible, she should have some ready knowledge of the purposes and principles of sodium restriction diets. Generalizations must be kept at a minimum when instructing the patient. She should know detailed differences between the types of sodium restricted diets, the correct terminology to use, the relation of sodium to food and other dietary products, and how to select and prepare food according to the specific restriction prescribed.

It is helpful if the nurse can explain some of the fundamentals of sodium restriction. For example, we cannot expect all people to know and understand the difference between salt and sodium. Sodium is not salt, but salt contains a good deal of sodium.

Many foods contain some sodium, either because it is present naturally or else because it has been added. Normally, fruits contain little natural sodium, whereas meat, poultry, fish, eggs and milk have a relatively large amount. Vegetables vary from those having very little natural sodium to those having a large amount.

Sodium is frequently added to foods when they are processed, and this fact is indicated on the label according to the national food laws. Sodium compounds most frequently used in food processing commercially include disodium phosphate, present in some quick-cooking cereals and processed cheeses; monosodium glutamate (although there is some indication it may be withdrawn from the market); sodium sulfite, used as a preservative in some dried fruits; baking powder, used to leaven bread and cakes; baking soda, also used to leaven bread, muffins and cakes, and sometimes added to vegetables in precooking of frozen foods; and table salt, often used in canning, processing, and cooking foods.

It is good for the patient to know how sodium is measured—in milligrams —and how important it is to stick to the exact amount of milligrams prescribed by his physician, since it only takes such a small amount to run over his limit. For instance, one bouillon cube contains approximately 1,000 mg of sodium; a slice of bread contains approximately 200 mg; a small pat of butter, 50 mg; one level teaspoon of salt weighing 5.8 g contains about 2,300 mg of sodium and one level teaspoon of baking soda, 1,000 mg.

A sodium diet must do much more than restrict sodium. It must provide a variety of foods the patient needs, in the correct number of calories. Sample menus are available at local heart associations. These menus have been worked out so that each one provides a balanced diet, providing proteins, fats, carbohydrates, minerals, and vitamins. Sometimes, the physician may prescribe additional vitamin supplements of vitamin A, $B_1$ or B complex and protein.

Other information valuable to the nurse who is acting as a diet counselor includes knowing about the two types of salt substitutes, and the two labeling regulations that pertain to sodium-restricted diets; one applies to special diet foods, and the other relates to regular frozen vegetables. In addition to being familiar with the sources of special food products and when they are required by the patient's diet prescription, she also knows when they are not indicated. Since new foods appear on the market every day, the nurse needs to keep abreast of these to be able to keep the patient informed. It is a good practice in hospitals who have regular dietitians on duty to request in-service educations periodically to refresh and keep nursing personnel abreast of new information. Smaller hospitals with no registered dietitian on duty full time are encouraged to request aid and in-service programs from the dietitian consultant either from the local heart association or county health department.

When the patient is discharged from the hospital, or if the patient is ambulant and able to lead a fairly normal life, he should still have available to him, by referral to a community public health or counseling nurse, help in measuring and determining sodium content and adjusting recipes to the newly imposed regulations and restrictions. Individual counseling is most necessary at this point. The successful nurse-counselor instructs patients in such a way that they develop confidence in carrying out their instructions and feel free to ask for additional help.[1]

## Low Cholesterol

The correlation between the elevation of the blood cholesterol and formation of the atheroma has been the subject of many investigations for the past decade. Cholesterol is found in animal tissue, transported by the blood, stored in the liver, and excreted by the bile. An excess of fat in the diet increases the synthesis of cholesterol beyond that amount that can be stored in the liver. Thus an excess is left circulating in the blood. It is this free cholesterol that joins with lipids and protein to form a complex compound which is not easily eliminated from the body. The deposit of these large particles in the arterial wall is a phase in the pathologic condition of atherosclerosis. More

1. Beth Heap. Sodium-Restricted Diets. *American Journal of Nursing*, Vol. 60, February 1960, Reprinted by Public Health Service, Washington, D.C.

studies have shown that an increase or decrease in calories, mainly or entirely through carbohydrates, can increase or decrease some of the lipoproteins in the blood. Still other researchers feel there must be something about the chemical nature of cholesterol that needs more studying; that it is not the deposits that cause the trouble, but how cholesterol combines chemically with other substances in the blood so that these large molecules find their way into the inner lining of the vessels.[2]

One of the outstanding advances of clinical investigation in recent years has been that the hyperlipidemias are responsive to therapy of diet control. At present, extensive findings have been reported from five major studies: the Chicago Coronary Prevention Evaluation Program, the Los Angeles Veterans Administration Domiciliary Study, the New York Anti-Coronary Club, the National Diet-Heart Study, and the Oslo Study. The nurse interested in detailed findings of these reports is referred to the American Heart Association for copies of their bulletins in diet and coronary heart disease, or to the Chicago Health Research Foundation, Chicago, Illinois.

These investigations recruited large numbers of middle-aged male volunteers, largely from the ranks of the general public, with or without clinical coronary heart disease. Diets used for correction of hyperlipidemia were essentially similar in all studies. They were based on evidence demonstrating that the cornerstone of nutritional management of moderately severe hypercholesterolemia is sizable reduction in saturated fat and cholesterol intake, assisted by increased intake of polyunsaturated fats, in an overall diet moderate in total calories, fats, carbohydrates, alcohol, and high in proteins.

Experiences of the National Diet-Heart Study were especially valuable, since both free-living volunteers and an institutionalized population sample were studied on the same fat-modified diet plans.[3] Since the nutritional control was tighter in the institutionalized population, a more precise measure was afforded of the potential of diet to correct hyperlipidemia, and the influence of degree of adherence. It was of interest that the largest drop in serum cholesterol was experienced by men with the largest decreases in weight and the highest initial cholesterol levels. Along with decrease in serum cholesterol and body weight, the diastolic pressure was observed to fall. Serum triglycerides, particularly in men with elevated base-line levels, were lowered by the hypocholesterolemic diets. About 20 percent of smokers quit cigarettes while in the study.

These studies conform or correspond closely to other studies. Thus, precedented experience in thousands of men clearly demonstrates the key role

2. Walter Modell et al. *Handbook of Cardiology for Nurses,* 5th ed. New York, Springer Publishing Co., 1966, pp. 76–77.
3. National Diet-Heart Study Research Groups: National Diet-Heart Study Final report. Circulation 37 (suppl. I): 1968. National Heart Assoc.

of dietary fat-cholesterol modification, together with caloric control, for the correction of moderately severe high cholesterol and lipid content common in our middle-aged population. The key alterations in nutrition, in most cases, are sizable reductions in saturated fat and cholesterol intake, correction of overeating and obesity, moderation in intake of total carbohydrate, sugar and alcohol, as well as total fat. This is especially important in a relatively common type of hyperlipoproteinemia that is induced by carbohydrates rather than fat. These individuals are usually prediabetic and their triglycerides may be markedly elevated.

## *Practical Application*

Sustained motivation and detailed indoctrination of the patient and the person preparing his food are absolutely essential for successful nutritional therapy. It is important that a permanent change in the patient's food habits be accomplished. This often takes considerable time since the patient needs "deconditioning" and "reconditioning." Control of saturated fat and cholesterol intake requires simultaneous attention to all five major sources of these nutrients in the usual American diet: high-fat meats, high-fat dairy products, commercial baked goods, spreads (butter, margarine, shortening), and egg yolks. Therefore, the pattern emphasizes moderate quantities of lean meats and poultry (round steak, veal, game, chicken, turkey), fish and seafood, skim or nonfat milk, cottage cheese, whole grain or enriched flour products, fruits (including citrus), vegetables (including dark green and yellow), vegetable oils, and the new soft margarines in modest quantities during the months of weight reduction. To be de-emphasized are fat cuts of meat, table spreads, solid cooking fats (butter, "older" margarines, suet, lard, hydrogenated vegetable fats, bacon, salt pork), and cooking methods that add solid fat rather than remove it.

When nutritional management does not accomplish satisfactory control, the physician considers supplementary drug treatment for lipidemia, hypertension, and/or diabetes. And the effort to control other coronary risk factors, e.g., cigarette smoking, lack of exercise, is also attempted.

## *Summary*

The importance of adequate education for patients cannot be overemphasized, since it is the patient himself who is responsible for the daily task of carrying out his diet prescription. But it is the nurse, acting as liaison between physician, dietitian, and patient more often than not, who enables him to do this. Her assurance and encouragement inspire him to accept his diet, to learn to follow it, and to persevere in carrying out instructions. This chapter has included some of the homeostasis mechanisms which come into play in an attempt to assist the body to maintain its functioning equilibrium. It is necessary that the nurse become familiar with these changes—sometimes referred to as inotropic and chronotropic mechanisms—which can modify action and reaction in the body.

### DIET INFORMATION

If the diet is also to be low in cholesterol, then the following foods must be omitted in addition to those on the controlled fat diet:

1. Glandular organs such as liver, brains, kidney, sweetbreads
2. Oysters, shrimp

If the diet is also to be high in unsaturated fat it should include liberal amounts of the following:

1. Oils that can be incorporated in salad dressings, or added to soups, to non-fat milk, to cereal, to vegetables
2. Walnuts, almonds, Brazil nuts, filberts, pecans
3. Extra margarine in or on foods

### COOKING TIPS FOR MEATS

Meat, fish and poultry may be prepared in almost all the familiar ways. The only exception is deep frying, which is not allowed because the amount of fat cannot be measured. The meat must be lean, of course. But the fat can be further reduced by a few simple rules:

1. Use a rack when boiling, roasting or baking so that the fat can drain off. If possible, do not baste, since basting returns some of the fat to the food.
2. When making stews, boiled meat, soup stock, or other dishes in which fat cooks out into the liquid, do the cooking a day ahead of time. After the food has been refrigerated, the hardened fat can be removed easily from the top.
3. Make gravy for meat and poultry after the fat has hardened and been removed from the liquid.
4. Avoid pan-frying meats such as loin pork chops.

### SHOPPING POINTERS

Labels on packaged foods give very little information as to fat content—either the type or amount. If and when in doubt, the safest course is: Don't buy.

The following pointers may be helpful as a general shopping guide:

1. Any kind of packaged or prepared food that contains no fat at all and is otherwise allowed on your diet is all right to buy. Examples are vegetarian beans (baked) and angel food cake.
2. Packaged or prepared foods with fat may be used only if fat is one allowed on your diet. For example, you may use sardines packed in cottonseed or soybean oil. Avoid packaged popcorn, potato chips, French fried potatoes.
3. Do not buy frozen dinners or other ready-to-eat canned or frozen-food mixtures which contain fat, since you usually cannot tell what kind of fat was used, or how much.
4. Dehydrated foods, such as potatoes, pancake mixes, or other mixes to which you add the fat yourself, are usually all right; but, if in doubt, check with your physician. Read the label to be sure they do not contain any fat.

## Controlled Fat Diet

| Foods Allowed | Foods Not Allowed |
|---|---|
| **Soups:** | |
| Bouillon cubes, vegetable soups, and broths from which fat has been removed. Cream soups made with non-fat milk. | Meat soups, commercial cream soups, and cream soup made with whole milk or cream. |
| **Meat, Fish, Poultry:** | |
| Only one or two servings daily (not to exceed a total of 4 ounces) lean muscle meat, broiled or roasted. Beef, veal, lamb, pork, chicken, turkey, lean ham, organ meats. All visible fat should be trimmed from meat. All fish and shell fish. | Bacon, pork sausage, luncheon meat, dried meat, and all fatty cuts of meat. Weiners, fish roe, duck, goose, skin of poultry, and TV dinners. |
| **Milk and Milk Products:** | |
| At least one pint non-fat milk or non-fat buttermilk daily. Non-fat cottage cheese. Sapsago cheese. | Whole milk or cream. All cheeses (except that containing safflower oil), ice milk, sour cream, commercial yogurt. |
| **Eggs:** | |
| Egg whites only | Egg yolks. |
| **Vegetables:** | |
| All raw or cooked as tolerated. Leafy green and yellow vegetables are good sources of vitamin A. | No restrictions. |
| **Fruits:** | |
| All raw, cooked, dried, frozen, or canned. Use citrus or tomato daily. Fruit juices. | Avocado and olives. |
| **Salads:** | |
| Any fruit, vegetable, and gelatin in salad. | |

Cereals:
All cooked and dry cereals. Serve with non-fat milk or fruit. Macaroni, noodles, spaghetti, and rice.

Breads:
Whole wheat, rye, enriched white, French bread, English muffins, graham crackers, saltine crackers.

Commercial pancakes, waffles, coffee cakes, muffins, doughnuts, and all other quick breads made with whole milk and fat. Biscuit mixes and other commercial mixes, cheese crackers, and pretzels.

Concentrated Fats:
Corn oil, soybean oil, cottonseed oil, sesame oil, safflower oil, sunflower oil. Walnuts and other nuts except cashew and those fried or roasted.
Margarine made from above oils, such as Award, Mazola, Emdee, Fleischmann's, and Kraft Corn Oil.
Commercial French and Italian salad dressing if not made with olive oil.
Gravy may be made from bouillon cubes, or fat-free meat stock thickened with flour and added oil if desired.
Freshly ground or old-fashioned peanut butter.

Butter, chocolate, coconut oil, hydrogenated fats and shortenings, cashew nuts. Mineral oil, olive oil, margarine, except as specified.

Commercial salad dressings, except as listed.

Gravy, except as specified.

Hydrogenated peanut butter

Desserts:
Fruits, tapioca, cornstarch, rice, junket puddings—all made with non-fat milk and without egg yolks. Fruit whips made with egg whites, gelatin desserts, angel food cake, sherbet, water cubes and ices, and special imitation ice cream containing vegetable safflower oil. Cake and cookies made with non-fat milk, oil, and egg white. Fruit pie (pastry made with oil).

Omit desserts and candy made with whole milk, cream, egg yolk, chocolate, cococa butter, coconut, hydrogenated shortenings, butter, and other animal fats.

Sweets:
Jelly, jam, honey, hard candy, and sugar.

Beverages:
Tea, coffee, or coffee substitutes. Tomato juice, fruit juice, cocoa prepared with non-fat milk.

Beverages containing chocolate, ice cream, ice milk, eggs, whole milk or cream.

## *Review and Advance*

1. *Are salt and fats always restricted in the cardiac diet?*
   If warranted, the patient may be placed on a modified fat diet with supplemental polyunsaturated and restricted saturated fats. A 1,200-calorie, full liquid, 1,000 to 2,000 mg sodium diet is usually adequate for the acutely ill patient. As pain and nausea clear, a 1,500- to 1,800-calorie soft diet with no added salt can be given. Salt substitutes should be offered. Dietary reeducation must be started while the patient is still in the hospital.
2. *Can diet and anticoagulants get rid of atherosclerotic plaques?*
   No, once fully formed, atherosclerotic plaques are irreversible and the scars remain until death.

3. *If atherosclerosis cannot be found in the small arteries and capillaries, what causes peripheral artery disease?*
Peripheral artery disease is referred to as arteriosclerosis obliterans, and commonly involves the bifurcation of the aorta, the iliac, femoral, popliteal, anterior tibial, and posterior tibial arteries. Less frequently, it may also involve the radial and ulnar arteries. The lesion present is usually atherosclerosis combined with medial arteriosclerosis and a thrombus.

4. *What is intermittent claudication?*
This term refers to pain in the legs when walking. It is an early sign of ischemia of the muscles. Pain may involve the back, hip, thigh, calf, or foot depending upon the site of the lesion. The pain is relieved sometimes by sitting up with the feet elevated. These lesions may be visualized on arteriograms.

5. *What dietary measures can help cut down the amount of cholesterol in the blood?*
Several methods have been suggested as ways to reduce the blood cholesterol concentration. First, eat less foods containing cholesterol: egg yolk, liver, kidney, brains, sweetbreads, fish roe—all are high in cholesterol. Lesser amounts are found in whole milk, cheese, cream, ice cream, and meat. Second, reduce the total caloric intake by decreasing the amount of ordinary fat in the diet. This also helps the overweight problem many cardiac patients have. Fat is usually restricted to 25 percent of total calories. Such a diet is called a "fat-restricted diet."

6. *Where can the average layman acquire information on diet and heart disease?*
Every major city in the United States has a local city or county heart association that offers dietary advice in the form of literature and consultative services. Many of their diets list helpful information on how dietary control may contribute to retardation or prevention of coronary disease. These booklets are also available from the American Heart Association, 44 East 23rd St., New York, N.Y. 10010.

7. *What are the principles of dietary treatment for cardiac disorders?*
These will vary with the severity of the illness. In the acute stage, minimal nutritional requirements may be sustained for short periods, followed by necessary diet adjustments to meet all needs. The diet may be advanced from liquid to soft to light, depending upon severity.

8. *Then dietary changes can be adapted to meet the patient's needs, if he progresses to a stage and remains at a plateau?*
In referring to the patient who has reached the chronic stage, either by compensation or by slow progression, we usually assume that normal circulation is maintained by an enlarged heart and an increased pulse rate. The patient may have a normal diet with the following adjustments:
   a. Low calories—if the patient is inactive and slightly obese—to lessen the burden on the heart.
   b. Use carbohydrates to furnish the bulk of calories.
   c. Five or six small meals rather than three large ones.
   d. Cut out all gas-forming, indigestible, or bulky foods to prevent pressure on the heart.
   e. Limit stimulating drinks, such as tea and coffee.
   f. Careful choice of foods to prevent constipation.
   g. Possible salt restriction if edema is present or a possibility.
   h. Vitamins and minerals may be ordered in concentrated form.

9. *What about dietary regime in the decompensated heart patient?*
   In the chronic decompensated patient, the heart is unable to maintain normal circulation; that is, the heart is no longer able to adequately carry oxygen and nutrients to the tissues throughout the body and unable to gather waste products from the tissues and route them toward excretion. Edema may be present as sodium and water are literally held in the tissues. Thus, there must be a much more rigid diet to prevent strain and further damage to the heart. Again, calories play an important part and must be maintained so that the weight of the patient may be kept at normal or slightly below normal. In addition
   a. Carbohydrates are used as the chief source of calories because they are digested and leave the stomach quickly.
   b. Protein normal—1 gram per kilogram of body weight.
   c. No bulky or gas-forming foods.
   d. Vitamin and mineral supplements may be ordered.
   e. Small meals to prevent pressure on the heart.
   f. Salt and fluid restriction is adjusted to the individual patient according to the amount of edema present.
10. *Is the dietary requirement for the hypertensive patient essentially the same as in chronic heart disease?*
    Essentially, yes. However, we should get into the habit of distinguishing among "heart diseases." *Chronic* may mean many things to many people. It may include everything from a certain recurrent arrhythmia, the size of the heart with or without vascular changes, and in this case, we are referring to hypertension as a symptom often accompanying cardiovascular and renal disease. The diet will still remain low caloric for the same reason; sodium restriction and adjustments in protein and fluid content will require close watching if there is kidney involvement.
11. *What is a "sodium-restricted" diet?*
    A sodium-restricted diet is a normal adequate diet modified in sodium content, from a very low amount of 200 milligrams to 2,000 milligrams or more.
    The average diet normally used by us all, according to whether we add our own salt to taste at the table, usually provides about 3,000 to 7,000 milligrams of sodium daily. Most persons are surprised to discover this. Thus, for therapeutic purposes, sodium may be cut in the diet 200 to 2,000 milligrams or more. Diets in which sodium is limited formerly were called "low-salt" diets when salt was omitted only in preparation of the food, and "salt-free" when it was allowed neither in the cooking nor at the table. Such diets are now named in terms of the level of salt restriction, the most usual being the 500-milligram sodium, or strict; the 1,000-milligram, or moderate; and the 2,400–4,500-milligram sodium diet, or mild restriction. All these diets may be obtained from the Heart Association.
12. *Is salt different from sodium? Where are they found?*
    Sodium is an essential mineral nutrient required in small but significant amounts. Salt or sodium chloride (NaCl) is nearly half sodium. An average healthy person receives more sodium through food and water than he requires, and the excess is excreted by the kidneys to maintain the homeostasis or balance of salt and fluids. However, in certain disorders water is retained in the body and some sodium along with it. A reduction of the sodium in the diet under these conditions helps the body to reduce its salt content to approximately the amount it needs daily.

13. *Are there certain foods which contain more sodium than others?*
    The following list, adapted from diet booklets published by the American
    Heart Association, shows the sources of sodium in the diet:

## Natural Sources

Small amounts: fruits
Large amounts: meats; fish; poultry; milk and milk products; eggs; canned, smoked,
    salted, or seasoned meats
Small to large amounts: vegetables
High amounts: average drinking waters, "softened" waters
Low amounts: distilled waters
Read labels for sodium in cereals (some have no added sodium)

## Sodium Compounds Added to Foods in Processing and Preparation

Salt (sodium chloride)
Baking soda (sodium bicarbonate)
Brine (table salt and water)
Monosodium glutamate
Disodium phosphate
Sodium hydroxide
Sodium proprionate
Sodium alginate
Sodium benzoate
Sodium sulfite

Note:
1 level tsp. salt = 2,300 mg Na
1 level tsp. baking soda = 1,000 mg Na
1 level tsp. baking powder = 370 mg Na

14. *Then, one only need pay close attention to food products?*
    No, indeed. Many medicines and dentifrices contain salt also:

    "Alkalizers"            Pain relievers
    Antibiotics             Sedatives
    Cough medicines         Toothpastes and powders
    Laxatives               Mouthwashes

    It is a good habit to read all labels carefully.

15. *Briefly, then, what are the purposes and indications for sodium-restricted
    diets?*
    Briefly, we can sum up the purposes of the sodium-restricted diet as follows:
    a. To assist the body in eliminating sodium and fluids (to prevent edema)
       in disorders where there is abnormal retention
    b. To control sodium intake
    c. To relieve severely elevated blood pressure
    Sodium-restricted diet may be indicated in many instances; among the
    most frequent are:
    a. Hypertension
    b. Congestive heart failure
    c. Renal disorders with edema
    d. Edema from any cause
    e. Toxemias of pregnancy

    f. ACTH and cortisone therapy
    g. Cirrhosis of the liver
    h. Ménière's disease
16. *Can anyone prepare these special salt-modified or sodium diets?*
    Yes. As previously indicated, many booklets are available from local heart
    associations or the American Heart Association free of charge. Among the
    most useful to the person charged with the preparation of these meals are:

    "Your 500-Milligram Sodium Diet"
    "Your 1,000-Milligram Sodium Diet"
    "Your Mild Sodium-Restricted Diet"
    "Food for Your Heart"
    "Planning Low Sodium Meals"

# 10 ANTICOAGULATION

The use of anticoagulants in the treatment of patients with myocardial infarction or, more specifically, coronary artery disease remains an area of some controversy. Studies designed to evaluate the effectiveness of anticoagulants in the treatment of angina pectoris (by reducing the incidence of subsequent infarction), in acute myocardial infarction (by reducing death rate and thromboembolic complications), and in long-term prophylaxis after an acute myocardial infarction (by reducing reinfarction and mortality rates) have shown conflicting results.[1] Many of these studies have been criticized for their failure to select similar patients for control and treatment populations and to make follow-up treatment programs identical in all respects except for the selected variable. Controversy has also arisen over the adequacy of present laboratory procedures in evaluating the level of hypocoagulation, the optimum therapeutic level for maintenance of effective anticoagulation, the incidence and nature of hemorrhagic complications, and the danger that heparin administered early in an acute myocardial infarction might increase the chances for internal hemorrhage of the myocardium.

## Indications for Use of Anticoagulants

The administration of anticoagulants to the majority of patients with peripheral arterial emboli, deep venous thrombosis and sometimes superficial thrombophlebitis, and pulmonary emboli rarely produces any controversy. Definite criteria for the selection of patients with coronary heart disease do not exist, but the three groups listed are usually chosen for anticoagulant

1. Robert C. Packman. *Manual of Medical Therapeutics,* 18th ed. (Boston, Little, Brown and Co., 1964), p. 89.

therapy, providing there is careful follow-up and there are no contraindications to the use of anticoagulants.

1. Acute myocardial infarction.

   Antocoagulants are usually given to "poor risk" patients, for instance, those with previous infarctions, severe pain, shock, marked cardiac enlargement, heart failure, arrhythmias, and other complicating diseases such as diabetes or obesity.

2. Long-term therapy after acute myocardial infarction.

   It is believed that anticoagulant use does produce favorable results in reducing reinfarction and mortality rates, particularly in younger patients. For many patients, anticoagulant use may be continued from one to five years or longer.

3. Angina pectoris.

   Cases are reported where anticoagulants are given to a number of patients (the lower the age, the higher the percentage) with angina of less than one year's duration, especially if a recent[2] change (increased frequency and intensity) in the pain pattern has occurred.

## *Contraindications to Anticoagulant Therapy*

In general, anticoagulants are not administered to patients who have a predisposition to bleeding, severe high blood pressure (diastolic pressure higher than 115 mm Hg), suspected intracranial bleeding, dissecting aneurysms, active ulceration or any known bleeding from the gastrointestinal tract or genitourinary tract, bleeding from the respiratory system with the exception of hemoptysis due to pulmonary embolism or mitral stenosis, or threatened abortion.

In other cases, the physician must consider the risks against the urgency involved. Such cases would include subacute bacterial endocarditis, severe hepatic or renal disease, the presence of thoracic or abdominal aneurysms, surgery in general, pericarditis complicating myocardial infarction, and patients with moderate hypertension, vasculitis, or diabetes.

In general, anticoagulants are not employed under the following circumstances:

- a hemorrhagic diathesis (predisposition)
- severe hypertension
- cerebrovascular hemorrhage
- active ulceration or overt bleeding from the gastrointestinal, respiratory, genitourinary, or pulmonary tracts (exception of pulmonary embolism)

2. *Ibid.*, p. 88.

- surgery of the central nervous system
- inadequate laboratory facilities
- inadequate cooperation of the patient with the therapeutic regimen

In pregnancy the coumarin derivatives are generally contraindicated due to their ability to pass the placenta barrier.

Other contraindications, depending upon the urgency of the therapy, must be balanced against the risk of hemorrhage. These include moderate hypertension, diabetes, vasculitis, subacute bacterial endocarditis, renal and liver disease, surgery in general, but particularly of the biliary tract in the presence of hepatic failure, and surgery of the lung and prostate. Pericarditis complicating myocardial infarction deserves special consideration in view of the possibility of hemopericardium consequent to the use of the coumarin drugs. Extensive bleeding into the thyroid has also been observed in thyrotoxic patients who have received therapeutic I[131] while on anticoagulant therapy.

In addition, there is a group of disorders in which adequate preparation before anticoagulants are given may reduce the hazards of therapy. These include congestive heart failure, malnutrition, vitamin C and K deficiencies, ulcerative colitis, sprue, steatorrhea, and pancreatitis.

## Heparin

Heparin is a polysaccharide whose structure is only partly known; its sulfate groups are bound to smaller amino groups to sulfaminic linkages; its high content of ester sulfates gives heparin the highest negative electrical charge of any substance that can be safely injected into man; and its structure is such that it is the strongest organic acid occurring within the body.[3]

In the blood serum its action is said to be linked to its negative charge. Thus the anticoagulant action of heparin, attributed to its highly negative charge, depends upon its inhibition of certain interactions involved in thromboplastin production, in thrombin formation, and in thrombin disposition. In appropriate dosages, heparin also prevents platelet agglutination and, in addition, is said to potentiate the fibrinolytic system. Even in large doses heparin has no effect on blood pressure (except in rare cases), peripheral or coronary circulation, respiration, body temperature, renal and hepatic function, blood chemistry, or red and white cells.

The anticoagulant action is proportional to the dose, varies from patient to patient, and becomes evident within minutes following intravenous administration. The overall result is retarded coagulation *manifested by the*

3. Elsie Krug. *Pharmocology in Nursing,* 9th ed. (St. Louis, The C. V. Mosby Co., 1963), pp. 471–7.

*elevated clotting time* of the freshly drawn blood. *This is the cardinal guide to dosage.* A common way to titrate the therapeutic effect of heparin is to administer the amount necessary to double the base-line clotting time just before the succeeding dose. The bleeding time which reflects more the response of the microvascular tree to trauma is unaffected.

The anticoagulant effect of heparin is short-lived; for example, 6,000 units may prolong the clotting time for only two to four hours following intravenous administration. Peak prolongation occurs within minutes after injection, after which the clotting time gradually returns to normal.

However, when heparin is given by intramuscular or subcutaneous routes, the clotting time is more prolonged although the duration is occasionally erratic. This prolonged effect is a disadvantage in shifting from heparin to a coumarin compound for two reasons: sustained elevated blood levels of heparin interfere with the prothrombin time determination, and in patients on both heparin and coumarin drugs, the P & P time (prothrombin-proconvertin time) may be used to judge coumarin dose since it is not changed by heparin.

As far as any toxicity is concerned, heparin is essentially nontoxic. Alopecia (loss of hair) occurs rarely. In certain individuals the drug may cause untoward reactions ranging from mild urticaria to sudden, severe hypotension, respiratory distress, and chest pain. Most rarely, transient thrombocytopenia has been observed shortly after its administration. Heparin does not interfere significantly with the extravascular deposition of fibrin and so does not retard the healing of surgical wounds. Long-term use has been associated with osteoporosis.

### ABSORPTION, FATE, AND ADMINISTRATION (Heparin) *

Within 15 minutes after the intravenous injection of heparin, 30 percent is found in the liver, where it is inactivated by heparinase. Within 30 minutes, 2 percent, and within 24 hours, 40 percent appears in the urine largely as a breakdown product, "uroheparin." Elimination occurs both by way of the glomeruli and tubules, and if there is renal injury the amount eliminated is drastically reduced. The importance of both liver and kidney function in the disposal of heparin is such that physicians are cautious in its use when disease of these organs is present. Heparin, in contrast to coumarin drugs, does not pass the placental barrier and does not appear in milk.

The potency of heparin-sodium preparations varies from 120 to 150 USP units per milligram. Drug dosage, therefore, is preferably expressed in

* Ben Alexander, and Stanford, Wessler. *A Guide to Anticoagulant Therapy,* prepared for The Committee on Professional Education of the American Heart Association, 44 East 23 Street, New York, N. Y.

units rather than in milligrams. The usual therapeutic dose is 7,500 units every six hours.

Administered in the form of a soluble salt, heparin is best given intravenously, preferably intermittently but also continuously by infusion. The subcutaneous and intramuscular routes are also used sometimes. Heparin has little, if any, effect by mouth, sublingually, or applied dermally. Heparin cannot be added to the IV solution bottle and must be injected directly into the intravenous tubing. The high negative charge results in significant amounts being "trapped" inside the bottle.

### Abbreviated Clotting Sequence and Factors Involved

Phase I      Production of Thromboplastic Activity
Phase IA    Intrinsic (Blood) Thromboplastin: (Factors XII, XI, IV, V, VIII, IX, X, and Platelets)
Phase IB    Extrinsic Thromboplastin: (Factors III, IV, VII, and X)
Phase II     Production of Thrombin: (Intrinsic or Extrinsic Thromboplastin, and Factors II, IV)
Phase III    Production of Fibrin: (Factor I and Thrombin)
Phase IV    Dissolution of Fibrin: (Fibrin, Profibrinolysin plus Activator)

Heparin inhibits "intrinsic" thromboplastin formation, and also the action of thrombin. Coumarin-type compounds depress Factors II, VII, IX, and X.

Reproduced by permission of American Heart Association.

### ANTIDOTES FOR HEPARIN REVERSAL

The anticoagulant action can be promptly reversed, milligram for milligram, by an equivalent amount of protamine sulfate. This markedly basic protein has a strong affinity for heparin, thus combining with it to give a relatively insoluble product. Protamine is therefore extremely useful as an antidote and should be kept on hand whenever heparin therapy is being administered.

Protamine is available in 1 percent solution in 5 ml vials. It is slowly administered intravenously after dilution in physiologic saline, in an amount equivalent to the last dose of heparin but never in excess of 50 mg. Its antiheparin effect lasts about two hours. Some heparin activity may reappear if the anticoagulant was administered in large doses shortly before it was deemed necessary to reverse its action.

Recently, a new agent has been used effectively—hexadimethrine bromide (Polybrene). This antidote should be diluted to a final concentration of 1.0 mg per ml, and should be given over a period of 10 to 15 minutes at a dose of 1.0 mg per units of heparin.[4]

4. *Ibid.*

Blood or plasma transfusions, although of value in replacing blood lost from hemorrhage, are not specific antidotes against heparin as they are against the coumarin drugs.

## Coumarin Derivatives and Related Compounds

Since the discovery by Link and Campbell of bishydroxycoumarin, significant advances have been made in the basic and therapeutic aspects of this and related substances, termed "indirect anticoagulants." More than 100 chemically related compounds have been studied, but only a small number are generally accepted as reasonably safe agents [5] (Table 1).

### Properties of Some Coumarin-Type Compounds

| Class | Generic Name | Usual Initial Dose (mg) | Usual Maintenance Dose | Usual Onset of Peak Activity (Days) | Trade Name |
|---|---|---|---|---|---|
| **COUMARIN** | | | | | |
| | Bishydroxycoumarin | 300–600 | 25–100 | 1.5–3 | Dicumarol |
| | Ethyl Biscoumacetate | 1500–2400 | 600–900 | 1–2 | Tromexan |
| | Cyclocumarol | 100–200 | 15–40 | 1–2 | Cumopyran |
| | Acenocoumarol | 10–20 | 3–5 | 1–2 | Sintrom |
| | Phenprocoumon | 20–40 | | 3–5 | Liquamar Marcumar |
| | Warfarin | 40–60 | 5–10 | 1–2 | Athrombin-K Coumadin Panwarfin |
| **INDANDIONE** | | | | | |
| | Phenindione | 200–400 | 50–100 | 1–2 | Anthrombin Bindan Danilone Dindevan Dineval Hedulin Indema Indon PID Pindione |
| | Diphenadione | 20–50 | 2–3 | 1–2 | Dipaxin |
| | Anisindione | 500–700 | 50–150 | 1–2 | Miradon |

These agents depress the identical specific plasma clotting constituents concerned with the formation of thrombin from prothrombin. In contrast to

5. *Ibid.*

heparin, they have no direct action on coagulation. After a variable latent period they lead to a reduction in plasma factors II (prothrombin), VII (proconvertin), IX (PTC), and X (Stuart). Clotting is slowed by thus retarding and limiting the rate and amount of thrombin formation. Although the anticoagulant effect was initially attributed to diminution of plasma prothrombin per se, it now appears that depression of the other factors is at least equally important.

Coumarin-type compounds also decrease platelet adhesiveness, depress the activity of several platelet enzymes, and alter the fibrinolytic system. Other biological actions include an increase in capillary permeability, coronary blood flow, in vitro erythrocyte of $I^{131}$ triiodothyronine, and urinary uric acid excretion.[6]

Presumably all these agents act on the liver where they are fixed, metabolized, and degraded at variable rates, followed by excretion through the renal and biliary tracts.

Although the precise mechanism by which the "prothrombinopenic" effect is induced is obscure, it is likely that synthesis of the clotting factors is inhibited. The effect is in equilibrium with the patient's store of vitamin $K_1$, nutrient obtained from intestinal bacterial synthesis as well as by ingestion of foods containing vitamin $K_1$, such as mature grains, spinach, cauliflower, cabbage, and tomatoes. The coumarin drugs resemble the vitamin in chemical structure. They are thought to compete with the vitamin for the apoenzyme functioning in the synthesis of the pertinent clotting factors.

### ABSORPTION, FATE, AND ADMINISTRATION OF COUMARIN

The various factors which influence the individual reaction to a given dose are an important consideration. For example, bishydroxycoumarin is relatively insoluble, more slowly absorbed, bound longer in the plasma, remains for more prolonged periods in the liver, and is degraded there more slowly than some of the other related compounds. Accordingly, its prothrombinopenic effect is slow in appearance, more retarded in reaching peak activity, more cumulative, and more slowly dissipated. The net result is that bishydroxycoumarin when judiciously administered lends itself to maintaining a sustained effect.

Warfarin is at the other extreme. It is very soluble and is the only agent that can be given intravenously, intramuscularly, and rectally, as well as by mouth. This may be particularly advantageous, for example, when for any reason oral intake is temporarily precluded during the course of therapy.

6. *Ibid.*

The solubility characteristics which affect absorption and transfer to the liver also bear on the question of whether a particular drug should be administered in single or multiple daily doses. Some believe that the more soluble agents such as ethyl biscoumacetate, warfarin, and indandione derivatives should be given in divided doses for optimal sustained effect.

The variables inherent in a given individual are to a great extent responsible for the difficulties in maintaining the prothrombic activity at the desired level during therapy. Their importance cannot be overemphasized. These varying influences may be physiologic or may arise as a consequence of disease. Clearly the net effect of a given drug dose will depend somewhat on the initial stores of the pertinent clotting factors in both circulation and extravascular depots, on their rates of mobilization, and on their rates of synthesis and turnover. The latter are measured in terms of hours in contrast to other plasma proteins, such as albumin with a half-life of approximately three weeks. Accordingly, the momentary effect of an agent that only partially blocks synthesis of a rapidly consumed factor is subject to wide variations. On this basis alone fluctuations may be anticipated from day to day in a given individual.

Although the initial depressing effect of a single priming dose is fairly uniform for each compound, wide variations occur in the total duration of the effect among different individuals and in a given subject from time to time. Debilitated individuals are very sensitive to these drugs.

Variation in a given individual also occurs during the course of maintenance therapy. This has been attributed to fluctuations in gastrointestinal, hepatic, renal, and metabolic functions secondary to physiologic or pathologic disturbances. The physician tries to be alert to possible changes in the state of these organs, particularly during long-term therapy. Other pathologic states also influence the reaction to these drugs; for example, individuals with fever or scurvy are said to manifest increased sensitivity to the coumarin-type agents.

Also, there is considerable experimental evidence indicating that the thrombinopenic effects of the coumarin agents, as measured by the prothrombin time and hemorrhagic tendency, are enhanced by stressful stimuli and adrenocortical hormones.

Mention has been made of the antagonistic relationship between vitamin $K_1$ and the prothrombinopenic drugs. The patient's nutritional state with regard to this fat-soluble vitamin will therefore influence considerably the degree of prothrombinopenia induced. Body stores of the vitamin, initially or periodically supplemented from intake, can influence the ebb and flow of the pertinent factors dependent on this nutrient for synthesis. Here, again, the nature of the diet, hepatic function, gastrointestinal motility, and fat absorption will exert their effects, as well as intestinal bacterial flora which may be greatly influenced by antibiotics.

Although some anticoagulant effect of the prothrombinopenic agents is demonstrable within 24 hours after administration, peak activity may not be obtained until some time after that, depending upon the properties of the drug employed, the priming dose, and the metabolic processes just described.

An occasional patient is inexplicably resistant or sensitive to coumarin-type drugs. There are others who, after being steadily and satisfactorily maintained on a given dose for a long period of time, will develop hemorrhagic problems coincident with a marked drop in prothrombic activity, especially during acute infections.

Taking all that has been discussed this far, you can now realize that the physician treats each patient on an individual basis, especially in view of the many variables involved. It is for this reason, when acute disturbances arise, physicians wisely seek consultative advice from another physician schooled in these many variables.

As with heparin, toxic reactions to the coumarin-type drugs are rare, aside from bleeding. Nausea, vomiting, diarrhea, and leukopenia are sometimes observed. More serious, though unusual, reactions are hepatic and renal damage, fever, rash, jaundice, leukemoid reactions, and thrombocytopenia. The skin eruption, generally appearing prior to the other manifestations, may permit early recognition of toxicity. The physician can then shift to another drug. Untoward hematologic reactions are more frequent with the indandiones than with the coumarins. Bishydroxycoumarin is least toxic of all coumarin-type drugs.

One additional point regarding the indandiones is worth noting. The urine may be colored orange-red following the first day of therapy. This is attributed to the metabolic breakdown product of the drug. It can be avoided by a large intake of water, or by diluting and acidifying the urine to pH 4.2.

Albuminuria is not uncommon during the first few days of therapy. This soon disappears despite continued use of the drug.

Although not of toxic effect, coumarin-type compounds pass the placenta barrier and also appear in milk. For these reasons, they are considered to be contraindicated in pregnancy or in the puerperium. In general, the small amount of drug that may be ingested by the normal lactating baby is not likely to compromise hemostasis, but it can have dire consequences in premature infants.

### ANTIDOTES FOR COUMARIN-TYPE COMPOUND REVERSAL

Vitamin $K_1$ is effective in reversing excessive anticoagulant action. It may be administered intravenously, subcutaneously, intramuscularly, or by mouth in this order of preference for attaining most rapid anti-coumarin ef--

fect. Some correction is demonstrable within a few hours; full correction is usually acquired in 24 hours. Water-soluble derivatives are distinctively less effective in this regard than is the natural vitamin. However, large doses of vitamin $K_1$ may make the patient subsequently resistant to the coumarin drugs for several weeks.

Although vitamin $K_1$ correction of drug-induced prothrombinopenia is fairly prompt, immediate reversal of the clotting defect can be attained by transfusion with blood, plasma, or plasma fractions rich in the pertinent clotting factors. Because the involved factors are relatively stable, ordinary ACD banked blood, bank plasma, or lypolized plasma is fully potent and the clotting factors will exert their effects almost immediately. Usually three units of blood or plasma is enough, in conjunction with vitamin $K_1$, to set in motion the regeneration of the respective clotting factors. In patients with limited cardiac reserve, such volumes may be hazardous unless blood loss has been significant.[7]

## Laboratory Tests and Discussion

The most satisfactory laboratory test as a practical guide to the dosage of coumarin-type drugs until recently was the *Quick whole plasma prothrombin time.* The *Thrombotest,* recently devised by Owren, theoretically provides a more comprehensive assay of the pharmacologic effects of these drugs because it is said to assay factor IX in addition to the other factors, depressed by these agents (factors II, VII, and X). Owren and others claim that this test will alert the physician to possible hemorrhage earlier. It has further advantages in that it can be performed on capillary blood at the bedside, and stable standardized reagents are readily available. However, many physicians believe more experience is needed before it can be stated definitely whether it is superior to the Quick prothrombin determination as a guide either to the antithrombotic action or the hemorrhagic complications of coumarin-type drugs.

The results of the prothrombin determination should be reported by the laboratory *in seconds and percent of prothrombin activity,* even though this increases the amount of data to be recorded.

Reporting in seconds provides an indication of the potency of thromboplastin and at the same time indicates whether the desired level or elevation in prothrombin time has been achieved. It should be elevated 1½ to 2 times the value of the control plasma. Another advantage is that the results obtained in one laboratory can be compared with those obtained on the same patient in another laboratory, provided the control value of the other labora-

7. *Ibid.*

tory is known and the thromboplastin employed in the test is derived from the same species.

Reporting in percentage, on the other hand, permits a simple assessment of the day-to-day and week-to-week trend of the effect of the drug.

The question of *how often prothrombin times should be performed* has special significance with regard to long-term therapy. After the daily prothrombin time determinations establish the individual dose requirements (usually about a week), the tests are usually spaced to every other day, subsequently to twice a week, and eventually to every two weeks.

On long-term therapy, less frequent determinations are performed, but only after the physician has become sufficiently familiar with the patient's needs and stability, and after he is assured of the patient's capacity and willingness to cooperate. If the results indicate stability, determinations can be safely performed every two weeks. There is some difference of opinion as to the advisability of longer intervals. Intervals longer than three weeks incur substantial risk of inadequate control. Determinations spaced at more than four weeks are usually reserved for extremely few individuals under special circumstances.

Persons who are planning long vacations, or those who travel a great deal, should be referred by their physician to a reliable physician elsewhere; some kind of identification card stating the individual is on anticoagulants should be carried in the wallet or handbag in case of accident.

People often ask what other tests besides the prothrombin time should be done periodically on a patient who is on long-term coumarin therapy. It is suggested that the hemoglobin, as well as examination of the urinary sediment and stool for occult blood, should be determined periodically. Although the prothrombin determination is the cardinal laboratory guide to coumarin therapy, it is known that bleeding may occur in some individuals in spite of maintenance of the prothrombic activity at levels considered compatible with normal hemostasis. The reason for this is obscure; it is probably attributable to factors outside of blood clotting that play important roles in the overall hemostatic mechanism, or to the fact that some other clotting factor is affected which is not measured by the prothrombin assay.

As far as is known, neither heparin nor coumarin derivatives affect other important laboratory tests such as measurements of the formed elements of the blood, sedimentation rate, electrocardiogram, or agglutination tests. Heparin does, however, bind complement and thus may interfere with certain serologic tests. Also, heparin is said to increase the resistance of red cells to hypotonic salt solutions.

Since heparin is effective when administered both subcutaneously and intravenously, another question frequently asked by nurses working in coronary care units is whether it would be more advantageous to use the subcutaneous route rather than the intravenous route. However, in contrast to intravenous administration, the subcutaneous route occasionally results in a more erratic time elevation. Also local pain, ecchymosis, and, rarely, neuritis may occur at the injection site. These side effects may be compounded if other medications are also being administered by this route. Moreover, reversing the anticoagulant effect with protamine or hexadimethrine bromide, should this be necessary, is more difficult after subcutaneous than after intravenous administration. Finally, shifting from heparin to coumarin-type agents is less difficult when the route of heparin administration is intravenous. For these reasons the intravenous route is considered preferable, although it is recognized that satisfactory elevations of the clotting time may be obtained by subcutaneous or intramuscular administration.

Many observers have the impression that a significant incidence of recurrent thrombosis follows the abrupt discontinuance of anticoagulant therapy. It has been found that discontinuing heparin may result in an abnormally shortened clotting time. Also, after cessation of coumarin therapy certain clotting factors may attain abnormal high levels. These elevations are said to be even more pronounced if the termination of therapy is hastened by the administration of vitamin $K_1$. This has been interpreted as a "rebound" effect.

Whether this phenomenon is the cause of recurrent thrombosis is unknown. Nevertheless, these impressions and observations provide sufficient basis for the recommendation that both heparin and coumarins be discontinued gradually rather than abruptly and that the use of vitamin $K_1$ in stopping therapy be avoided whenever possible.

## Summary

There is much more that is significant in anticoagulant therapy. However, this chapter includes the pertinent information necessary for the nurse to understand the physician's objectives for his patient regarding anticoagulant therapy. Further studies and research findings are included in the bibliography for those who may wish to examine this therapy more closely.

## Review and Advance

1. *What is the difference between a thrombus and embolus?*
   An abnormal clot that develops in a blood vessel is called a thrombus. Once a clot has been formed, continued flow of blood past the clot is likely to break it away from its place of attachment, and then it is free to flow in the blood stream. Such a free-flowing clot is known as an embolus. Emboli do not generally stop flowing until they come to some narrow point in the

circulatory system where they lodge. An embolus originating in the large arteries or the left side of the heart might very well lodge in the smaller arteries or arterioles; an embolus originating in the venous system or in the right side of the heart will flow into the vessels of the lungs to cause pulmonary embolus.

2. *What are the causes of thromboembolic conditions?*

The causes of thromboembolic conditions in human beings may be due to several factors: mainly, any roughened surface of a vessel is likely to initiate the clotting process (arteriosclerosis, infection, or injury), and blood often clots when it flows very slowly through the blood vessels, for small quantities of thrombin and other coagulants are always being formed. It is important to recognize that immobility slows the blood flow, which is one reason for the importance attached to the practice of moving bed patients frequently. Presumably, sluggish blood flow allows thromboplastin to accumulate and, in turn, to reach a concentration adequate for clotting.

Once started, a clot begins to grow. Platelets enmeshed in the fibrin threads disintegrate, releasing more thromboplastin which, in turn, causes more clotting, which enmeshes more platelets, and so the circle continues. Clot-retarding substances have proved valuable for retarding this process.

3. *What pharmacological agents retard clotting?*

Commercial preparations of heparin are used as anticoagulants. This is helpful in preventing clot formation both inside and outside the body. This agent must be given parenterally. The anticoagulant Dicumarol and its derivatives have become well known because of their clinical value in lessening thrombus and embolus formation. It is thought to decrease prothrombin synthesis, perhaps by blocking vitamin K formation. Outside the body, citrate is used chiefly to treat blood to be used for transfusions. It combines with the calcium ions.

4. *How can a clot dissolve without breaking loose and flowing into the circulation?*

Fibrinolysis is the physiologic mechanism that dissolves clots. An enzyme, fibrinolysin, is known to be present in the blood and to be able to hydrolyze and thereby dissolve fibrin. Many other factors, however, presumably take part in clot dissolution, for example, substances that activate profibrinolysin formation, the inactive form of fibrinolysin. Streptokinase, an enzyme from certain streptococci, can act this way and so cause clot dissolution and even hemorrhage.

5. *Are anticoagulants dangerous drugs?*

Anticoagulant drugs require very careful regulation as to amount and continuity of dosage, and the nurse is given a responsibility in this. If too much is given, the patient may have a hemorrhage in a vital area such as the brain. If too little is given, he may have no beneficial effects from the drug and, in addition, may have additional thrombi formation.

6. *Exactly what is heparin?*

Heparin is obtained from the lungs and livers of animals. Its advantage is that its effects are almost immediate. The disadvantage is that it can only be given parenterally, since it is destroyed by the gastric juices. Also, its action is short-lived—three to four hours. Heparin dosage is expressed in units or milligrams and is calculated individually for each patient. When the patient is receiving this drug by infusion, the nurse must watch very carefully the rate of flow. If the rate cannot be regulated satisfactorily or if the solution stops dripping, measures should be taken immediately to restore it. In most coronary care units, nurses have been trained to start intravenous solutions and to adjust flow, including the irrigation of the intravenous cannula.

7. *Where does Dicumarol come from?*

Dicumarol was first isolated from spoiled sweet clover after it was observed that cattle eating this food experienced abortion and hemorrhage. It acts by suppressing the formation of prothrombin. The usual maintenance dose is 50 to 150 mg per day administered by mouth. Frequent determinations of the prothrombin level must be obtained and most physicians believe the prothrombin level should be maintained between 10 and 30 percent of normal. Dicumarol is widely used in the treatment of thrombophlebitis. It takes 12 to 24 hours to take effect, and, thus, it is not uncommon to see a patient on both heparin and Dicumarol at the same time before heparin is discontinued. Other synthetic drugs are now on the drug market which are believed to act more quickly.

8. *How is the dosage controlled once the patient has been discharged from the hospital?*

Although the benefits from anticoagulants enable patients to live useful lives, if the patient must remain on the drug indefinitely it can necessarily create a problem for him. Blood for the prothrombin time must be drawn from the vein, and this may have to be at least two or three times a week at first; later, depending upon the success achieved in stabilizing the prothrombin level, it may be spaced further apart. This is an unpleasant experience for the patient, and many nursing personnel are hesitant to emphasize the importance of his keeping apointments on time lest they cause more apprehension and fear in the patient. But, as a part of patient teaching, he must be taught not only the importance of keeping laboratory appointments but to recognize the symptoms of hemorrhage and to report them immediately to his physician. He should carry an identification card stating that he takes anticoagulant drugs so that, in case of accident, those who give him medical care will know this. The identification card should also have the name and phone number of his physician. Most coronary care units now issue these cards to patients even before they leave the unit for the medical complex.

# 11 X-RAY IN THE EVALUATION
## OF HEART DISEASE

The chest x-ray (roentgenogram), along with the patient's history, physical examination, and electrocardiogram, is very necessary in the evaluation of the patient who has known or suspected cardiovascular disease. It is well to keep in mind that x-rays may afford not only information about pathologic anatomy, but physiology as well.

### Background Information

In order to understand the potential of the x-ray for diagnosis, let us look at the physics of the formation of the final film. The completed picture is the result of the quantity of radiation that passes through the body and strikes the emulsion of the x-ray film. Radiation absorbed within the body plays no direct part in the formation of the picture; it is, however, important in the formation of "clear" areas on the film. Such clearer areas indicate minimal exposure of the emulsion. The useful picture results from the contrast presented by different degrees of radiation transmitted through the chest to impinge on the x-ray film.

There are four "screens," or densities, in the thorax through which the x-ray passes before reaching the film. The least dense is gas. Air in the tracheobronchial-alveolar system (or carbon dioxide, in right atrial cardiography) creates nearly black areas on the film because it "stops" only a minute quantity of radiation. Fat is the next most dense (radiolucent) substance. Therefore, the epicardial fat may cast on the film a shadow that can be separated from the surrounding tissues and structures; this phenomenon frequently is useful in the diagnosis of a pericardial effusion. Water is much more dense than fat. All soft tissues, heart, blood vessels, liver, spleen, pancreas, etc., basically are of equal density per weight. The pericardium, myocardium, endocardium, and the blood within the heart are also of equal density and, consequently, cast a uniform shadow. The densest material in the body is mineral. Normally, the only mineral present in quantities large enough to be appreciated is the calcium in the bones. The costal cartilages, unless they are calcified, cast no shadows on the conventional x-ray. Similarly, heart valves cannot be visualized unless they are calcified also.

The heart is seen only as it impinges on the lesser (gas) density of the lungs; therefore, only the borders of the heart can be identified on an x-ray. Certain patterns of change are diagnostic of anatomic or physiologic abnormality within the heart; e.g., left atrial enlargement may be appreciated as a double density. However, more frequently, left atrial enlargement is recognized only because the left atrium impinges on structures of different densities, such as the mainstem of the left bronchus and the esophagus filled with barium. Compared with this relatively unfavorable situation, the pulmonary vascular system can be seen in exquisite detail because of the excellent contrast afforded by the gas in the lungs surrounding the blood vessels which possess a considerably greater density. Almost all of the cross-sectional diameter of a small bronchus is made up of air; only the wall of the bronchus has a density comparable to water. On the other hand, a similar-sized blood vessel may be displayed, because both its wall and contents equal the density of water. The lines seen peripherally in the lung fields represent blood vessels, not "broncho-vascular markings," if the latter term means bronchi as well as vascular structures. Peripheral bronchi cannot be seen on the roentgenograms except in certain disease states.

## Routine Sets

Adherence to a set technique of radiography has advantages, both in terms of comparisons of structural dimensions and of one patient to another. Most commonly, all films for adults and children are made at a six-foot distance, with the subject erect and in inspiration. The technique for infants varies, but there are many devices used for securing the child in this same position. Four films are made for the initial examination; a PA and left lateral film suffice for follow-up studies. Barium sulfate, made into a creamy material, is used to fill the esophagus in all except the left anterior oblique (LAO) film, where the barium would obscure the important relationship between the left atrial wall and the left main-stem bronchus.

Because the heart is a three-dimensional structure with the individual chambers in part superimposed on each other, all four views are essential for

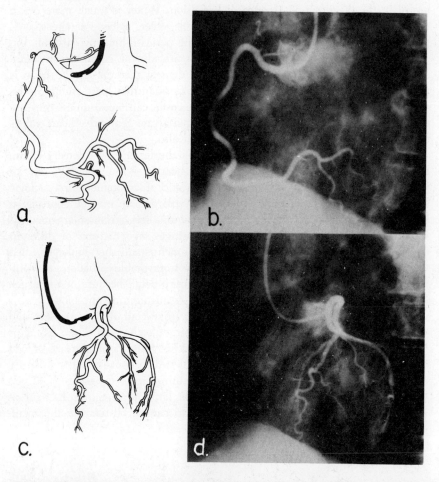

*FIG. 1* Schematic drawings and photographic prints of coronary arteriograms showing normal anatomy of coronary arteries—LAO view. a and b, right coronary artery. c and d, left coronary artery.

Dominance of the coronary artery circulation is determined by the arterial supply of the posterior left ventricle.

Dominate Right—Posterior intraventricular branch from right coronary artery.

Dominate Left—Posterior intraventricular branch from circumflex artery.

Equal—Balanced circulation.

(Courtesy of Cora and Webb Mading Department of Surgery, Baylor College of Medicine.)

a complete evaluation of cardiac enlargement. Findings for left atrial enlargement are the most reliable, and least so for the right atrial enlargement. Pure hypertrophy is difficult to tell on an x-ray; the electrocardiogram is much more reliable. On the other hand, chamber dilatation is defined clearly by radiographic techniques.

## Fluoroscopy

Despite the advent of image intensifications, the use of fluoroscopy as a part of the routine investigation of patients exhibiting heart disease has fallen into relative disrepute. Two reasons account for this reluctance to employ fluoroscopy: first, even image intensification requires a much greater radiation dose to the patient than an x-ray; second, the cardiovascular structures are seen in greater detail on the x-ray film.

There are, however, certain specific anatomic and functional abnormalities that can be best defined by the limited use of image intensification fluoroscopy. Calcifications, particularly of the valves, the coronary arteries, and the pericardium, appear with greater clarity by image intensification fluoroscopy than by static films. Pulsations, particularly of the pulmonary arteries, the aorta, and, in selected cases, of the cardiac chambers, can be appreciated only by fluoroscopy. In left-to-right shunts, increased pulsations are seen in the major branches of both left and right pulmonary arteries. On the other hand, significant pulmonary valvular stenosis results in a characteristic change consisting of increased pulsations of the left pulmonary artery with normal or diminished pulsations of the right pulmonary artery. In aortic stenosis, increased pulsations of only the ascending aorta are apparent, whereas in aortic insufficiency, increased pulsations of the entire thoracic aorta often are observed. In subaortic stenosis, the pulsations of the thoracic aorta are normal.

When indicated, the fluoroscopic study is restricted to less than two minutes of fluoroscopic time, always utilizing image intensification. Occasionally, it may be useful to record certain fluoroscopic findings on cine-strips for future study or demonstration.

## Selective Coronary Arteriography

Prior to the development of selective coronary arteriography, the diagnosis of coronary artery disease was based on clinical history and electrocardiographic findings. Experience with direct opacification of coronary vessels has demonstrated the potential error in diagnosing coronary heart disease without angiography in many cases. A poor correlation is frequently encountered between the angiogram and resting electrocardiogram in patients with angina pectoris.

Occasionally patients treated for coronary artery disease have been found by selective coronary arteriography to have normal coronary arteries.

Selective coronary arteriography permits precise delineation of the severity and distribution of atherosclerotic coronary artery occlusive disease. This technique is a reliable method of evaluating the coronary arteries as well as

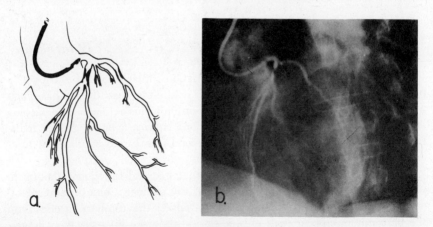

FIG. 2  a, schematic drawing of anterior descending coronary artery. b, photographic x-ray of same on left anterior oblique view (LAO).

(Courtesy Cora and Webb Mading Department of Surgery,
Baylor College of Medicine.)

the status of collateral circulation. A simultaneous ventriculogram allows evaluation of the left ventricular myocardium, particularly regarding the thickness of muscle and identification of areas of poor contractibility, fibrosis, or aneurysm formation. This arteriographic technique provides the basis by which candidates are selected for myocardial revascularization.

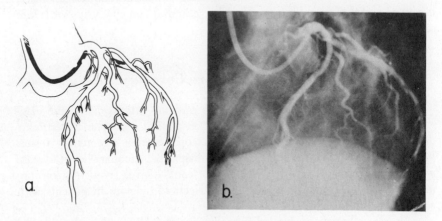

FIG. 3  a, schematic drawing of circumflex coronary artery.
b, photographic x-ray of same in left anterior oblique view (LAO).

(Courtesy of Cora and Webb Mading Department of Surgery,
Baylor College of Medicine.)

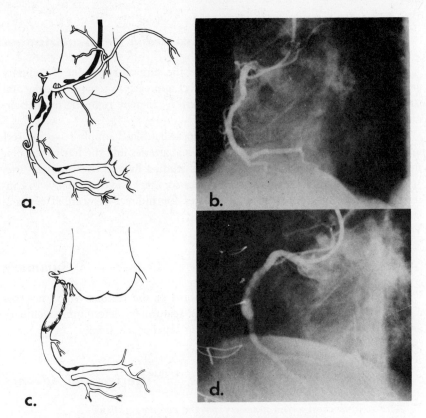

*FIG. 4*  a. Localized disease—right coronary artery in schematic.
  b. Photographic view of same with catheter in right coronary ostia.
  c. Postoperative arteriogram 2 years following surgical repair.
  d. Photographic x-ray of same.

(Courtesy of Cora and Webb Mading Department of Surgery,
Baylor College of Medicine.)

Patients presenting with typical or atypical angina pectoris, suspected of having coronary artery disease with or without associated valvular disease, are considered candidates for arteriography.

Selective catheterization of each coronary artery is performed with a Sones catheter inserted through the brachial artery. Hypaque (50 to 75 percent) is injected into each coronary ostium and the arteriograms recorded on spot films and 35 mm movie film at 35 frames per second. The electrocardiogram and arterial pressure are continually monitored.[1]

1. Richard G. Lester. Radiological Concepts in the Evaluation of Heart Disease (1). *Modern Concepts of Cardiovascular Disease,* published by American Heart Association (August, 1968), No. 8.

## Myocardial Revascularization

There are two operative approaches in the surgical treatment of coronary artery atherosclerosis. One method is a direct approach to remove a segmental stenosis or occlusion in a major coronary artery, thereby restoring normal circulation to the distal arterial bed.

The second method of improving myocardial blood supply is an indirect approach based upon implantation of systemic arteries into the left ventricular myocardium. Only five percent of patients studied by selective coronary arteriography are potential candidates for direct coronary endarterectomy. In contrast, the majority are potential candidates for indirect myocardial revascularization procedures.[2]

## Summary

In this chapter, we have presented some of the reasons why x-rays are a valuable part of the overall diagnostic feature in determining coronary artery disease. Two surgical remedies were touched on briefly.

## Review and Advance

1. *Are routine chest x-rays necessary for the coronary patient?*
   Routine chest x-rays are valuable to show the position and measurements of the heart. Inspiratory and expiratory films show how well ventilation is being performed and any displacement of the heart.
2. *What is the purpose of an intravenous angiography?*
   This is done to study and evaluate the structure and function of the cardiac chambers and the major blood vessels. It also can assist in establishing the diagnosis of a right-to-left shunt, a pericardial effusion, a dissecting aneurysm, or an arteriovenous fistula.
3. *What contrast mediums are usually used?*
   Various contrast mediums may be used, but the most common is 50 to 75 percent Hypaque.
4. *Can cardiac catheterization trigger an arrhythmia?*
   Catheterizations are usually performed with electrocardiogram monitoring. If there are many ventricular premature contractions, the catheter is pulled back temporarily. Injection of the contrast medium may cause ventricular fibrillation when injected near the aortic root. The blood pressure is watched carefully since the catheter can stimulate vagovagal reflexes and produce a drop in blood pressure.

2. Study by Herb Smith, Director, Baylor University College of Medicine, Texas Medical Center, Houston, Texas, reported in their brochure "Medical Communications."

5. *What studies may be done through catheterization?*

Aside from determining oxygen saturation studies, intracardiac ECGs can be taken and various pressure measurements may be obtained, such as the pulmonary wedge pressure (6–8 mm), pulmonary artery pressure (15 mm), right ventricular pressure (25/0 mm of mercury), right atrial pressure (plus or minus 4 mm), left atrial pressure (6–8 mm), left ventricular pressure (has a high systolic pressure; diastolic pressure (called end-diastolic) may go up to 8 mm of mercury, and cardiac output.

6. *What is the Fick principle?*

This is a procedure for determining the cardiac output. Using a dye dilution technique, a known amount of dye is injected into the circulation at any given point (vein, cardiac chamber, or artery). The concentration curve of the dye at a given spot distal to the injection site is recorded with a photomultiplier from changes in the optical densities in the blood. The area under the concentration curve can then be calculated to obtain the volume flow between the two points, that is, the site of injection and site of recording. This is usually the cardiac output. The shape or slope of the curve can give additional information on the presence and type of shunts and on valvular insufficiency.

The Fick principle is based on oxygen consumption and the arteriovenous oxygen difference. By knowing the amount of oxygen consumed and the number of milliliters of oxygen added to each unit of blood over a period of time, one can determine the cardiac output for that period. The arteriovenous difference is obtained by analyzing the blood sample from a systemic artery and from a vessel in a prepulmonary location, usually the pulmonary artery, on the venous side. Cardiac output is expressed as the cardiac index, or the liters of flow per minute per square meter of body surface. It is determined by the following formula:

$$\text{Cardiac output in liters} = \frac{O_2 \text{ consumption in cc per minute}}{\text{Arteriovenous difference in cc per liter}} \quad *$$

---

* Philip Cooper. *Ward Techniques and Procedures.* Appleton-Century-Crofts, New York, 1967, pp. 88–93.

# 12 ASSOCIATED PROBLEMS IN CORONARY HEART DISEASE

Many other problems may arise as the result of the heart failing in its function of pumping the blood into the great vessels to carry nourishment to all the cells of the body. Many symptoms arise due to secondary retention of salt and water. We have already touched on some of these, but there are several conditions which require a bit more attention. The nurse must have some knowledge and understanding of these conditions since they very often affect her planning or the nursing care of her patients.

## Congestive Heart Failure

With virtual control of bacterial infection, cardiovascular disorders have become the major cause of death among the general public. Among vascular disease, arteriosclerosis and hypertension are the most prevalent, and cause the largest number of deaths (Fig. 1). Both of these conditions may be involved in the etiology of congestive heart failure. Thus, congestive heart failure is not a disease in itself; it describes a group of symptoms that may be the result of any number of underlying processes. However, whether one subscribes to the classic view that congestive heart failure is the result of inability of the heart, as a mechanical pump, to maintain normal hemodynamic relationships, or to the view that congestive heart failure develops as a result of decreased renal flow, this process leads to decreased glomerular filtration, which results in retention of salt and water, which increases blood volume, which causes a congestive state. In this, the heart generally shows a certain degree of hypertrophy and dilatation as reflected by a thickening of the mus-

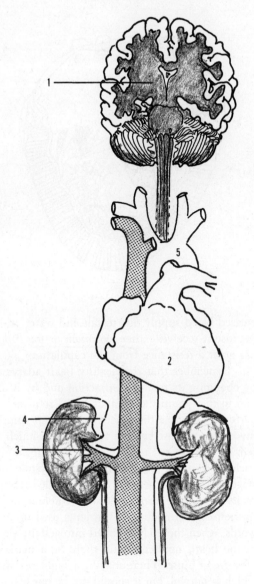

*FIG. 1* Ten percent of the specific causes of hypertension involve the brain and nervous system, the kidneys, or adrenal glands (as shown in perspective drawing). In the other ninety percent the condition is called essential hypertension, meaning the cause is unknown. The heart and large arteries are "target, or catchment" areas commonly damaged by hypertension.

cle fibers and by an increase in the volume of the heart chamber (Fig. 2). Seemingly, this should "clear up" the situation, but let us take a closer look at the physiology involved.

In congestive heart failure the heart is unable to receive its *normal* flow of blood from the venous system and to pump out the required amount through the arterial circulation. The preceding paragraph described an in-

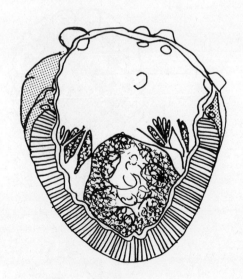

*FIG. 2* Cross-section of the heart in state of hypertrophy, or enlargement, due to excessive work loads imposed over a long period of time. Common causes of hypertrophy leading to cardiac failure include many etiological factors, among them rheumatic fever, bacterial endocarditis, pericarditis, myocarditis, and hypertension; those caused by anatomic change, such as valvular scarring and congenital anomalies of the heart; and those caused by physiological change, such as heart failure and arrhythmias.

Congestive heart failure is also known as cardiac decompensation, cardiac insufficiency, heart failure, and cardiac incompetency.

creased blood supply due to salt and water retention; thus, the heart may fail because it receives either too *much* or too *little* blood, or must pump against too great a resistance from the capillaries.

Remember that the healthy heart adapts to the demands made upon it by changing its rate of contraction and by adapting the force of the contraction to the quantity of venous blood returned to it. Therefore, to adequately perform its job as the mechanical pump running the circulatory system, the myocardium must be able to "eject" as much blood into the circulatory system as is delivered to it without holding any of that blood within the ventricles as residual blood at the end of systole, or at the end of the contraction stage. Secondly, when the body is called upon to adapt to increased activity by its owner, the heart must also be able to meet the needs of the body tissues in their call for additional nutrients used up or expended in activity. In other words, when the body is called into activity there should be no residual blood in the heart, neither should there be a marked or unexpected rise in blood pressure or pulse. There may be a slight rise in the pulse and respiration rate, which is normal, but it should not be out of proportion to the degree of activity. In a very short time, both can be expected to return to normal.

Medical researchers indicate the causes of failure in the pumping mechanism fall under three main headings: 1) failure to fill, 2) overloading, and 3) deterioration in functional capacity.[1]

1. Irene L. Beland. *Clinical Nursing: Pathophysiological and Psychological Approaches.* The Macmillan Company, New York, 1967, p. 111.

Failure of the heart to fill depends upon whether there is sufficient circulating blood volume to return to the heart for filling. In order for the heart to move the blood into the great arteries, it must receive it from the venous system, and it can only eject the amount returned to it. The blood volume may fall due to hemorrhage, shock, or excessive loss of fluid into the tissues. On the other hand, the blood volume may be within normal physiologic limits, but the blood vessels themselves may be in a dilated state causing the capacity of blood within the vessels to be greatly increased, thereby cutting down on the amount delivered to the heart.

Other causes which prevent adequate filling of the heart include obstruction to blood flow, such as mitral stenosis, or constrictive pericarditis which limits the amount of blood than can enter. Another vital factor is a reduction in the length of the interval during which the heart fills. Blood enters the heart only during the period known as diastole. If ventricular rates are high, the length of the diastole will be shortened in relation to systole. As a result, the period for filling will be considerably shorter than the period for ejection of blood. The main example of this is atrial fibrillation, when the volume of blood entering the heart during diastole is so minimal that, in spite of the ventricular contractions, there is little ejection power.

In complete reversal of failure due to inadequate filling of the heart (usually referred to as inadequate ventricular filling), the heart may fail because too much blood is being delivered to it or the resistance it must overcome in moving the blood into the arteries is too great. These are referred to as *high-output failure,* when a large volume of blood is delivered and ejected as in thyroid toxicosis, fever, and anemia, and *high-resistance failure,* when the site of resistance is located between the left ventricle and the peripheral arterioles. Examples of this latter include arteriolar stenosis associated with hypertension, aortic stenosis or coarctation of the aorta. The ventricle must exert more force to overcome the resistance of the narrowed channels.

With deterioration in the functional capacity, the myocardium is unable to perform adequately. This may be due to a number of myocardial diseases such as degenerative diseases, inflammatory diseases, metabolic diseases of the myocardium, and disturbances in the rhythm of the heart. Not to be overlooked is that with advancing age, even with no demonstrable disease condition, the myocardium can no longer handle a large volume of blood. This lessens the capacity of the heart to cope with any additional burden. Eventually, when the heart fails, it is unable to supply the tissues and vital organs with sufficient blood to carry on their activities. The outcome depends upon the completeness of failure and the rate at which failure develops.

The symptoms of congestive heart failure result from the congestion of fluid throughout the body. Edema, which is an excessive amount of fluid in the extracellular tissues and cavities of the body, may occur in the legs, the liver, the abdominal cavity, the lungs, the pleural cavity, or other spaces of

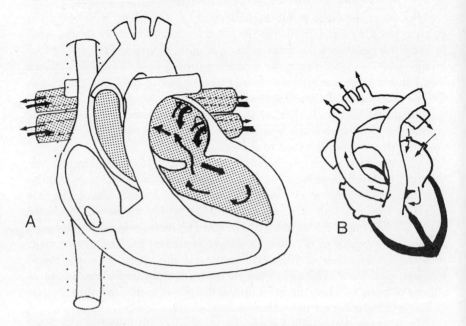

FIG. 3 A. In left-sided heart failure, the ineffective ejection of blood from the left ventricle causes back pressure in the left atrium, enlargement of the pulmonary veins, and increased pressure in the lung vessels. B. Normal circulation flow in the left side of the heart.

the body. With the backed-up blood comes the slowing down or cessation of blood flow, at times known as venous stasis; thus, the venous pressure increases. Because of this, fluid remains in the venous system intead of circulating to the kidneys where excessive sodium is excreted. When the patient consumes more salt than can be excreted, the excess is stored in the body. Thus, the more salt retained, the more water retained in the body. (Refer to chapter on electrolytes.)

Congestive heart failure is often referred to as *right-sided* or *left-sided* failure, although both are usually present to some degree. In left-sided failure (Fig. 3), the fluid accumulates in the pulmonary system for the most part; in right-sided failure, fluid accumulates in the systemic circulation (Fig. 4).

Symptoms of right-sided failure are distended neck veins, gastrointestinal disturbances, ascites, hydrothorax, hydropericardium, subcutaneous edema, hepatomegaly (enlarged liver), renal disturbances, and disturbances of the nervous system, such as confusion and hallucinations. Although left-sided failure is associated with the systemic circulation, it produces symptoms primarily of pulmonary congestion because of the back-up or pooling of blood in this area. Unusual tiredness, dyspnea upon exertion or at rest, cough,

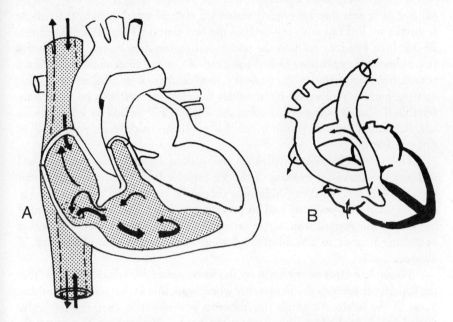

*FIG. 4* A. In right heart failure, the right ventricle has difficulty in delivering venous blood to the lungs. Blood backs up into the atrium and superior and inferior vena cavae, causing dilatation, with backing up of blood, increased pressure in veins in the upper and lower parts of the body and in the liver. B. Normal circulation of the right side of the heart.

hemoptysis, orthopnea, paroxysmal nocturnal dyspnea, cyanosis, hoarseness, and confusion are all symptoms of left-sided heart failure.

According to medical authorities, the goals for treatment of congestive heart failure are

- to bring back into balance the demand for blood with the supply of blood
- to remove and prevent accumulation of excess fluid and excess blood volume when the output of the heart cannot meet the requirements of the body (even the normal requirements)

These goals are accomplished by reducing the body's oxygen requirement, by eliminating the edema, and by increasing the cardiac output.[2]

Rest is one of the primary goals in nursing care for the patient with congestive heart failure. The requirements for oxygen are decreased with both physical and mental rest. However, the patient cannot tolerate adequate ventilation lying down since this position increases intrapulmonary blood

2. *Ibid.*, pp. 582–587.

volume in vessels that are already distended with blood; therefore, the patient is usually on bed rest with the head of the bed elevated from 60 to 90 degrees. In this high Fowler's position the abdominal organs drop down and allow for full pulmonary expansion. When the head of the bed is elevated, pillows are placed lengthwise under the patient's head and back as well as under his arms to prevent pulling on his shoulder muscles. He will also be more comfortable if a small pillow is placed at the small of his back. The knees should not be raised because pressure on the popliteal space may predispose to thrombi formation.

Use of the footboard will keep the patient from sliding down in bed and may also serve for exercise of the leg muscles later when the patient can press his feet against them. Side rails should be on the bed to assist the patient in changing positions and to prevent accidents. Position can be varied by having the patient lean across an overbed table padded with pillows, or by having him sit in a comfortable lounge chair by the side of the bed, if allowed.

Elastic bandages or stockings on the lower extremities channel blood from the superficial veins to the deep veins where muscular action aids in returning blood to the heart. Although this prevents venous stasis, they should be removed and reapplied at least every eight hours. At this time the nurse observes the color, temperature, and presence of numbness or tingling as an indication that the bandages have been applied too tightly. She also looks for beginning signs of thrombophlebitis, such as tenderness, redness, swelling, or warmth. When the feet are wrapped, the heels should also be wrapped.

Nursing care can be spaced to provide maximum rest. A complete bath every day is not necessary for a patient in severe congestive heart failure, but a partial bath is necessary for comfort and circulation stimulation.

A complete change of bed linen is not necessary as long as the bed is kept dry and free of wrinkles to prevent skin irritation. If the head of the bed cannot be lowered, the linen is changed from top to bottom rather than from side to side.

Sedatives and tranquilizers may be ordered by the physician to reduce apprehension and promote rest. Because many of these drugs are detoxified in the liver, the nurse watches for signs of overdose since hepatic congestion may cause them to accumulate in the body.

Oxygen is given to increase blood oxygenation when the usual concentration has been impaired by congestion and sluggish circulation through the lungs. This may be administered by cannula, nasal catheter, oxygen mask, or by tent. However, the physician may order intermittent positive pressure breathing if pulmonary congestion is severe. This helps to prevent further transudation of serum from the pulmonary capillaries by exerting pressure on the pulmonary epithelium during expiration. The doctor must determine the concentration of oxygen, the desired pressure, and the frequency of use.

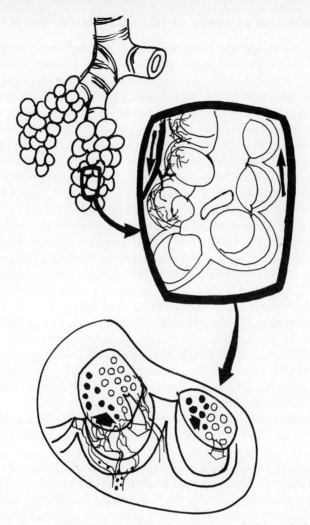

FIG. 5 A greatly magnified diagram shows the tiniest bronchioles and alveolar ducts which terminate in blind globular air sacs called alveoli. The bronchioles and alveolar ducts contain smooth muscle. The many millions of alveoli are microscopic air cells. Top: the pulmonary artery brings venous blood with carbon dioxide load to alveoli; pulmonary vein carries oxygenated blood back to the heart. Center: microscopic section shows blood vessels in thin walls of air-containing alveoli. Bottom: in the air cell, the oxygen molecules diffuse into blood, and carbon dioxide molecules diffuse out of blood.

The patient receiving this treatment needs attention to the skin from the mask which may cause irritation. On some positive pressure respirators, mouthpieces are used; frequent oral hygiene is necessary since oxygen has a drying effect on the mucous membrane of the mouth and upper respiratory tract (Fig. 5).

The nurse should use every opportunity to listen to the patient to find out what concerns him and makes it difficult to rest. During the evening and night hours she should visit him frequently just to let him know she is nearby, and if he is not sleeping, give him a chance to mention anything disturbing his rest. It may help to be in daily contact with a social worker to whom he can talk about his family, his job, and his plans for the future. Although the social worker cannot make extensive plans with him at this time, she may be able to take care of any immediate problems, thus helping to relieve his mind. Visits from the chaplain, or spiritual adviser, are comforting to some patients. However, these people should not make small talk which may only serve to make him think "people are holding something back."

During the early stages of congestive heart failure the diet should be liquid or soft and the foods served should be easily digested. He should be fed during the acute stage, and mealtime should be made as pleasant as possible. The work of the heart is increased during digestion, since blood is needed by the digestive tract to carry out its functions. Several small meals a day will be better tolerated and less tiring than three large meals. When the patient is allowed to feed himself, his appetite may improve as his morale improves with the feeling that he is progressing toward recovery.

As with the patient suffering from myocardial infarction, it is advisable for the patient to avoid straining in attempting to move his bowels. This is sometimes the most difficult adjustment many patients have to make. Therefore, some physicians allow the patient to slide off the bed onto a commode to have a bowel movement. The feces may be kept soft with a mild cathartic. If a small enema is ordered, the rectal tube should not be inserted any further than three or four inches. Many physicians disagree on giving cardiac patients even small enemas, or taking rectal temperatures, because of the involuntary contractions this involves. This is considered a strain on the patient. Try to allow the patient some privacy, if possible step outside the curtain or room for awhile, but reassure him that you will be within call should he need you.

After the acute phase, the patient may have a diet with foods low in bulk, caloric value, and fat, as well as sodium. The diet will decrease abdominal distention, help the patient lose weight, and prevent edema. Foods and drugs containing salt are reduced or eliminated according to the physician's evaluation of the patient's condition. Salt substitutes must be used cautiously since many of them contain potassium or ammonium chloride and should not be used in severe renal insufficiency or in hyperkalemia.

One of the most important methods in eliminating edema is the administration of diuretics. These drugs rid the body of the excess fluid that has been stored in the tissues by promoting the excretion of sodium, which carries water along with it. Since they produce polyuria, diuretics are administered early in the morning so that the patient's sleep will not be disturbed.

To summarize, the therapy of the patient in heart failure depends upon the degree and suddenness with which the heart fails. The objective of treatment is to restore the capacity of the heart to adapt or respond efficiently to the demands placed upon it, that is, to restore the pumping mechanism of the heart so that it can pump out as much blood as it receives. This requires two sub-objectives: (1) to increase the force or strength of the contraction of the myocardium, and (2) to reduce the demands upon the myocardium until the efficiency of the pumping mechanism can be restored. Later, the reserve power of the pumping mechanism will have to be evaluated and plans made with the patient and his family regarding any modifications of his living and working habits.

Digitalis contains an active principle in the form of a glucoside that has a number of important effects on the heart. Although this drug and other cardiac drugs are discussed in another chapter, a few points will be emphasized here. In congestive heart failure, digitalis increases the strength of ventricular contraction with the result that the volume of residual blood is reduced at the end of systole. In short, it increases the efficiency of the pumping mechanism of the heart. It has a second action that is modified by the level of potassium in the body. In the presence of normal amounts of potassium, it lessens the responsiveness of the conduction system of the heart. Digitalis increases the irritability of the heart muscle whether the level of potassium is normal or low, but the effect is more marked in the presence of low potassium levels. The mechanism seems to be related to the effect on intracardiac calcium concentration. Potassium levels can also be effectively lowered by intravenous administration of glucose in water. Increased myocardial irritability may be manifested by premature contractions and an increase in the pulse rate. This is called pulsus bigeminus, since an extra contraction is interspaced between the normal contraction. All changes in the pulse are important and should be reported to the physician, but this is particularly important for the patient taking digitalis. To prevent the possibility of digitalis-induced arrhythmias, potassium is frequently administered to patients who are under regular and prolonged therapy with diuretics, as they predispose to potassium depletion.

## Thromboembolic Disease

The body has natural defense mechanisms which respectively prevent, limit, or dissolve intravascular thrombi. These mechanisms include inhibitors, which have the function of suppressing the principal coagulation reactions, thus preventing the formation of clots; and fibrinolytic substances, which dissolve fibrin clots. To these natural homeostatic mechanisms, which serve to maintain the blood in the free-flowing state, has been added therapy with anticoagulant agents such as heparin and the coumarin derivatives, and, more recently, fibrinolytic agents such as streptokinase and fibrinolysin.

Intravascular clot formation is the result of disturbance of these mechanisms. The site of a pathologic clot formation depends on the existence of a local injury or deformation.

Essentially, clotting is a mechanism whereby the soluble blood protein fiibrinogen is changed into the insoluble protein fibrin. The nature of this mechanism is one of the most complex fields in physiology. However, if the nurse realizes that there are three major stages through which the process must pass, she may better understand why rest is the major goal of nursing care planning. These stages are[3]

- Thromboplastin formation
- Thrombin formation
- Fibrin formation

The first of these stages consists in a number of ill-understood chemical reactions that result in the formation of active thromboplastin (prothrombinase) from two sources, the tissues near the clotting area and platelets. The triggering mechanism is not entirely understood but apparently any roughened area, known as a wettable surface, is thought to begin the process. When platelets contact the wettened surface, they tend to distintegrate, releasing granules of a substance known as *platelet factor 3*. Platelet factor 3 then reacts with several blood proteins and calcium ions to form active thromboplastin. All this takes place in about three to six minutes.

In the second stage of clot formation, prothrombin comes into play. Prothrombin is one of the many complex globulin proteins in the blood. It combines with the thromboplastin formed in stage one and several other blood proteins and calcium ions to form thrombin. Vitamin K catalyzes prothrombin synthesis by the liver cells.

In the third stage, another blood protein synthesized by liver cells and involved in blood clotting is fibrinogen. Its molecules are long, fiberlike, and large. The enzyme thrombin formed in stage two catalyzes the formation of the gel fibrin from the fibrinogen. Fibrin appears as an interwoven network of fine threads. Red cells get caught in this network, producing the red color of clotted blood. The pale yellowish liquid left after a clot forms is blood serum.

The formation of intravascular clots, then, is thought to be prompted by one or more of the following factors:

- Prolonged bed rest or external pressure resulting in venous stasis

3. Catherine Parker Anthony. *Textbook of Anatomy and Physiology,* 6th ed. The C. V. Mosby Company, St. Louis, 1963, pp. 298–305.

- Local injury of the endothelium by ligature, operative manipulations, contusions, chemicals, bacteria, or the introduction of air
- An imbalance between the factors promoting flow and those favoring clotting

In view of this last factor, then, there must be something in the body that is opposed to clot formation, since it seems blood clotting goes on continuously. Several factors do operate to oppose clot formation and enlargement of intact vessels. First, the normal endothelial lining of the blood vessels is a smooth nonwettable surface. Therefore, platelets do not readily stick to it and disintegrate to release thromboplastin. Secondly, blood contains some substances, known as antithrombins, that tend to discourage clotting, that inactivate thrombin and make it unable to catalyze stage three, fibrin formation. Heparin is one substance that acts as an antithrombin. (Heparin is discussed in the chapter on anticoagulants.) Its normal concentration in blood, however, is too low to have much effect in keeping blood flowing. Where it comes from is not definitely known, but *mast* cells are known to contain considerable amounts of heparin. They themselves cannot synthesize, thus must act as storehouses. It was first prepared from liver (from which it gets its name), but various other organs also contain heparin.

The most life-threatening complication of phlebothrombosis or thromboembolic disease is pulmonary embolism, which occurs when a thrombus is dislodged or fragmented shortly after it is formed and before it has become firmly fixed in the vessel where it originates.

As yet, there is no satisfactory diagnostic aid to determine in advance which patients will develop thromboembolic disorders as the result of surgery or prolonged bed rest. However, clinical experience reports that the following types of patients will benefit from anticoagulant therapy: 1) those showing a history of such disorders, 2) those who have suffered an acute arterial occlusion, and 3) those who have atrial fibrillation.

The effectiveness of anticoagulants in arterial occlusions has already been discussed, although the prognosis of treatment depends greatly on the prompt initiation of treatment. The most beneficial medical approach to this condition at the present time seems to be the administration of heparin for immediate anticoagulant effect, then a long-acting anticoagulant to prevent thrombus re-formation. Studies on the effectiveness of postoperative anticoagulant therapy in the prevention of pulmonary embolism have firmly established its benefits in such patients. The use of anticoagulants in myocardial infarction is still controversial.

Blood clots in arteries differ structurally from those in veins. Arterial clots are usually crescent-shaped, relatively acellular, and have little tendency toward dissolution. On the other hand, venous clots usually entrap cellular elements, particularly platelets, and inhibit a strong tendency toward dissolution (retrograde progression). Since arterial occlusion is a much more serious matter than venous thrombosis, the quick restoration of circulation by an efficient agent is extremely important. The agent responsible for the normal, physiologic lysis of clots in the blood stream is the enzyme fibrinolysin. However, as previously noted, many factors take part in clot dissolution, for example, substances that activate profibrinolysin, the inactive form of fibrinolysin. Streptokinase, an enzyme from certain streptococci, can act this way and so cause clot dissolution and even hemorrhage.

## Cardiogenic Shock

Cardiogenic shock occurs in about 10 percent of patients with an acute myocardial infarction; the mortality rate is about 80 percent. Hypotension is not the lone criterion upon which to base the presence of shock; the brief drop in blood pressure that may occur following an acute myocardial infarction, if unaccompanied by clinical signs of shock or decrease in urine flow, generally does not require treatment with vasopressor drugs. Since we are concerned with the myocardial infarction patient, it is good to review the physiologic mechanisms which precede cardiogenic shock.[4]

Remember that adequate circulation of blood is in accordance with three major mechanisms: 1) a sufficient volume of blood, 2) a healthy cardiac muscle-pump mechanism, and 3) vascular tone. The failure of the second of these, the cardiac-pump mechanism, leads to *cardiogenic shock*.

Heart failure represents the ineffectiveness of the heart muscle to pump blood to all parts of the body. Thus, left myocardial failure is one of the most common causes of cardiogenic shock. Left-sided heart failure has been discussed earlier in this chapter but, in review, the following series of events occurs after a left myocardial infarction:

- Obstruction of the left coronary artery
- Left myocardial insufficiency
- Decreased strength of contraction of left myocardium
- Decreased systolic emptying of left ventricle
- Increased residual blood in left ventricle
- Dilatation of left ventricle
- Damming up of blood in left atrium
- Increased left atrial pressure and dilatation
- Damming up of blood in the pulmonary veins
- Pulmonary engorgement

4. Katherine J. Bordicks. *Patterns of Shock: Implications for Nursing Care.* The Macmillan Company, New York, 1968, pp. 115–135.

- Pulmonary edema
- Perfusion of pulmonary alveoli with plasma fluid
- Decreased diffusion of oxygen and carbon dioxide across the alveolar membranes
- Respiratory insufficiency
- Severe dyspnea

How does this affect the right side of the heart? Although left-sided heart failure is characterized by an immediate failure of the left atrium and ventricle to empty completely, it is important to remember that the right side of the heart will continue to function normally in the early part or stage of the attack. Later, when the right ventricle (right myocardium) becomes weakened because of the poor oxygenation from the right coronary artery, the following sequence of events results in the accumulation of blood in the right heart chambers with a damming up of blood into the great vessels, the superior and inferior vena cavae:

- Left myocardial failure
- Decreased cardiac output
- Increased pressure in left atrium and ventricle
- Decreased inflow of blood into left atrium from pulmonary veins
- Increased accumulation of blood and pressure in the pulmonary circuit
- Damming up of blood in the right side of the heart
- Incomplete emptying of blood into pulmonary artery from right ventricle
- Increased pressure in right ventricle
- Increased pressure in right atrium
- Decreased inflow of blood from systemic veins into right atrium
- Elevation of venous pressure in systemic cricuit

It is important that the above events indicate that heart failure involves peripheral failure also; when massive dilatation of the peripheral vessels occurs, the blood inflow into the right atrium is low. In all other kinds of heart failure, the cardiac output decline is relative to the inflow load of venous blood. This re-emphasizes that, while absolute decline in cardiac output is not present in all cases, decline in cardiac output relative to venous inflow load does occur in all instances.

General measures of treatment include giving oxygen nasally, relieving pain promptly, and treating any cardiac arrhythmias promptly. The nurse who cares for cardiac patients knows that treatment must be prompt, but is faced with the question of which problem has first priority. The ability to make quick, accurate decisions increases with her professional growth and experience.

First, the nurse knows that such signs as cyanosis, semiconsciousness, and confusion mean that blood in insufficient quantities or with too little oxygen is reaching the brain. Therefore, she places the patient in the supine position; but, considering that the patient's shock is due to a heart failure, a low Fowler's position is indicated. The brain will receive better oxygenation since the blood can move more freely to the brain. Also in considering the low Fowler's position, she remembers the diaphragm will be somewhat lower, which provides for greater expansion of the lungs, making more alveolar surface available for the diffusion of oxygen and carbon dioxide. The slight degree of gravity favors pulmonary venous emptying into the left atrium which tends to relieve the congestion in the pulmonary circuit. There is less resistance to the return of venous blood from the brain by way of the superior vena cava to the right atrium. Result: anoxia of the brain tissues is prevented.

Anoxia prevention will not be effective if only poorly oxygenated blood reaches the brain; thus, it is imperative that increased oxygenation of the pulmonary blood stream be assured. Immediate treatment with administration of both oxygen and digitalis (as ordered) will strengthen myocardial contractions and greatly (and dramatically) improve both the respiratory status and the circulation of oxygenated blood to the brain.

The low Fowler's position has another beneficial effect: the return of venous blood from the lower part of the body to the right atrium will be decreased. It is for this reason that the physician sometimes assists the body compensatory mechanisms by ordering the use of tourniquets on three extremities (Fig. 6). It not only decreases the right atrial inflow load, but relieves pressure in the pulmonary circuit. To further assist in increasing the force with which the oxygen enters the alveolar-capillary system in the lungs, some physicians prefer that intermittent positive pressure respirators be used for these patients. Fluid that has perfused from the blood stream into the alveoli will be pushed back into the blood stream. In spite of the decreased cardiac output, what blood it does put into the circuit will be much more heavily laden with oxygen.

Since the respiratory insufficiency is one of the major problems of the patient, and since severe anginal pain cuts down on respiratory excursions of blood, it is logical to relieve the chest pain as soon as possible. Opiates (morphine and codeine) are believed to interrupt the reflex arcs set up by the rising venous pressure; they are usually ordered and should be given immediately. Nitroglycerin under the tongue helps relieve the pain. This drug dilates the coronary arteries, thereby allowing increased circulation in the myocardium, and tends to limit the size of the infarct. It also favors the development of a collateral circulation in the myocardium. The patient is usually permitted to have a supply of nitroglycerine tablets at his bedside, to be taken as needed.

To review, the nurse takes steps to provide for increased circulation of blood to the brain, increase oxygenation of the pulmonary blood stream, and

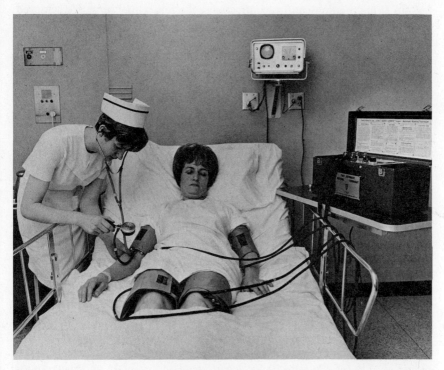

FIG. 6 Automatic rotating tourniquet operates without further attention on the part of the nurse or physician. Tourniquets are rotated so that each extremity is free, in sequence, for twenty minutes. Restrictions of venous return by application of tourniquets presumably lowers pulmonary blood flow and volume, reduces gradient for capillary alveolar transudation and probably intracardiac volume, thereby improving cardiac or myocardial efficiency.

(Courtesy of JOBST Institute, Inc., Toledo, Ohio.)

relieve the patient's pain. All of these are extremely important; however, if no measures are taken to increase the strength of myocardial contractions and increase the output of the heart, all of these measures would be useless.

Medically, the physician orders digitalis or one of its derivatives to establish a rhythm, rate, and output compatible with life. Digitalis is discussed elsewhere, but briefly: Digitalis decreases the heart rate and strengthens myocardial contractions, which results in increased cardiac output. For immediate results, the physician may administer the drug intravenously. If left ventricular fibrillation is also present, he may give quinidine or isopranolol to establish a more rhythmic beat. The nurse should always be on the alert for signs and symptoms of digitalis toxicity. These include depression, nausea and vomiting, or disturbances in the heart rhythm. They should be reported at once.

In strengthening cardiac contractions, the following events are achieved:

- Cardiac output is increased.
- Left ventricular-atrial-pulmonary-venous high-pressure dam will be relieved, and the blood in the left circuit resumes a more normal flow through the systemic arterial circuit.
- Pressure within the pulmonary capillary blood stream will decrease considerably, with a subsequent discouragement of perfusion of plasma fluid into the pulmonary alveoli.
- Myocardium receives a greater quantity of oxygenated blood.
- All tissues of the body receive greater amounts of blood.

As the patient becomes digitalized, the signs and symptoms of myocardial failure decrease. Cyanosis and pallor disappear; the skin becomes warmer and dry; cyanosis is relieved; mental faculties clear; pulse becomes stronger and more regular, and the blood pressure rises.

In order to achieve the return to balance, the physician gives attention to the peripheral circulation also. Increased cardiac output does not necessarily mean that an adequate supply of blood is being delivered to all parts of the body. If peripheral constriction has been replaced by dilatation, the amount of blood delivered to the body tissues would not be adequate to maintain proper cell functioning. For this reason, vasoconstrictor drugs may be ordered in intravenous solutions. Such drugs are given well diluted and at a very slow rate. Examples of these drugs are levarterenol (Levophed) and metaraminol (Aramine). Whenever the patient is on such a drug, the nurse must be very careful to check and record the patient's blood pressure reading every two to five minutes, since there is danger of increasing the blood pressure too much. In short, the nurse must be alert to changes and must act accordingly. Many of the drugs of vasoconstriction, if allowed to seep into the tissues, cause severe sloughing since the blood vessels will be greatly constricted allowing no blood into the site. A complete absence of blood from any area will result in necrosis. For this reason, the intravenous site must be watched closely to make sure the needle does not slip out of the vein or there is no leaking.

With peripheral vasoconstriction and increased cardiac output, improved circulation of blood to all parts of the body is usually achieved.

### Cardiac Arrhythmias

Cardiac arrhythmias exclusive of premature ventricular contractions occur in 20 to 40 percent of patients with acute myocardial infarctions; the mortality in this group is 7 to 15 percent higher. The treatment does not differ from that in the patient without acute infarction. The arrhythmias are discussed in a separate part of this text.

## Post Myocardial Infarction Syndrome

Although this syndrome may not appear frequently, it is characterized by pericarditis, pleuritis, pneumonitis, severe precordial pain which worsens with inspiration, an elevation of the white blood count, all running a lengthy course and varying in intensity. Therapy is symptomatic. It should not be confused with the anterior chest wall syndrome, which is sometimes an accompaniment of postcoronary syndrome.

## Rupture of the Ventricle

Rupture of the ventricle results from the weakening of the necrotic area of the myocardium. No treatment is available for rupture since when this catastrophe occurs, blood immediately fills the surrounding pericardium. This condition is called cardiac tamponade. Death follows within a few minutes.

## Summary

In this chapter we have discussed only a few of the disorders that may be associated with acute myocardial infarction. Other problems involving papillary muscles are assuming more importance now and will continue to do so in the future with the advent of surgical intervention in acute myocardial infarction. However, a discussion of this problem is beyond the scope of this book.

In discussing the treatments of the diseases associated with infarction, it serves to reinforce the concept that the basic elements of treatment of the cardiac patient are essentially the same. The emphasis remains on keeping the patient at rest both physically and mentally, and avoiding some aspects of "routinizing" nursing care. The patient must remain the focal point, and all nursing care activities are adapted to meeting his needs.

## Review and Advance

1. *What are the aims of treatment for congestive heart failure?*
   The principles of treatment are to bring back into balance the demand for blood and the supply of blood and to remove and to prevent the reaccumulation of excess fluid and excess volume when the output of the heart cannot be made to meet near normal requirements of the body. This is accomplished by reducing the requirements of the body for oxygen, by increasing the cardiac output, and by eliminating the edema.

2. *What are the early symptoms of congestive heart failure?*
The early symptoms are shortness of breath, usually apparent on exertion such as climbing stairs or walking rapidly; a slight cough, more of a hacking type; a tendency to become easily fatigued; slight abdominal discomfort; and swelling of the feet. The edema of the feet and ankles subsides at night when the person is in a supine position.

3. *What are the symptoms of advanced congestive heart failure?*
As congestive heart disease becomes more advanced, the dyspnea may be of a panting type and may be so severe that the person must remain in an upright position (orthopnea). The cough becomes productive with foamy, blood-tinged sputum. The edema may extend to the face, neck, sacrum, and extremities, and is of the pitting type. There may be cyanosis, enlargement and tenderness of the liver, and decreased urinary output. Abnormalities of the pulse may be found, and the patient may or may not complain of pain in the chest and abdomen. When left-sided failure occurs, acute pulmonary edema may occur. Dyspnea is increased, cyanosis occurs, and a productive cough is present. This is always a serious emergency and immediate treatment is necessary. Right-sided heart failure, briefly, involves visibly distended neck veins, gastrointestinal disturbances, ascites, hydrothorax, hydropericardium, subcutaneous edema, enlarged liver with some tenderness, renal disturbances, and some disturbances of the nervous system manifested by mental confusion and hallucinations.

4. *What is the "backward" theory of congestive heart failure?*
Remember that congestion of the tissues or capillaries is due to a failure of the ventricle to eject as much blood into the circulation as is delivered to it. Output may or may not be reduced below normal limits. At first, the myocardium will be stimulated to contract more forcefully. This is the normal homeostatic mechanism by which the body attempts to take care of its own problem. Accordingly, this is expected when the residual blood within the heart causes the myocardial fibers to stretch. According to Starling's law of the heart, within physiologic limits, the longer the muscle fiber is at the end of diastole (or the beginning of systole), the more forceful the contraction of the heart. The force of the contraction is a function of the length of the fiber at the end of diastole. In other words, the more it is stretched, the more forcibly it contracts, within the limits of its extendibility. But, eventually, when the residual blood in the heart becomes so great that the heart is over-dilated, the heart can no longer keep this pace; it is no longer effective as a pump. As blood accumulates in the heart, the intraatrial pressure rises and offers resistance to the inflowing blood. This increase in venous pressure is reflected by elevation of the pressure in the great vessels—the inferior and superior vena cavae—and in the small veins as well. As the pressure in the veins rises (venous hydrostatic pressure), the tissues drained by these veins become congested with blood and fluid.

5. *How are the kidney disorders involved in congestive heart failure?*
This question involves the theory of forward failure to explain the series of events leading to the retention of fluids. According to Guyton (Arthur Guyton. *Textbook of Medical Physiology*, 3rd ed., W. B. Saunders Company, 1968, p. 330), the premise on which the theory of forward failure is based is that, as the heart fails, its output falls, and causes a relative ischemia of the tissues. This low cardiac output has a profound effect on renal function. The kidney responds to diminished blood flow by a reduction in glomerular

filtration. Renal blood flow is further decreased by the activation of sympathetic reflexes which cause a marked constriction of afferent renal arterioles. Although it has been suggested that one of the factors in edema formation in congestive heart failure is an increase in the secretion of aldosterone, chronically elevated levels of aldosterone do not lead to edema, even though the total circulating blood volume may be increased. Blood volume may possibly be further increased by the release of the antidiuretic hormone by an ischemic posterior hypophysis (pituitary gland).

According to the forward theory of failure then, the increase in the blood volume and the congestion of tissues primarily result from the inability of the heart to eject as much blood into the circulation as is needed by the tissues to maintain their function. There are still many speculative theories.

6. *What makes the sputum blood-tinged in congestive heart failure?*
Cough with clear or blood-tinged sputum may accompany pulmonary edema. The cough is a mechanism for maintaining a clear airway. Although blood-tinged sputum is not uncommon in left heart failure, larger amounts may appear. Hemoptysis may result from an increase in the pulmonary pressure, which leads to the rupture of a pulmonary vessel, and any quantity of blood in the sputum is likely to frighten the patient. Blood coming from the lung is bright pink or red and frothy in appearance. Frothing is due to the air passing through it. The patient should be encouraged to lie still in whatever position is comfortable. The physician usually orders morphine because it helps allay apprehension. Whenever possible, the nurse should remain with the patient to enhance his feeling of safety and to further determine the extent of bleeding.

7. *What are some of the diagnostic aids the physician might use to assist in his diagnosis of congestive heart failure?*
Diagnostic procedures specific to the heart include electrocardiogram, x-ray of the heart, and the circulation time. As in all medical diagnosis, the history and physical examination are important.

# II  Electrocardiogram and Electrical Tracings

# 13 THE ELECTROCARDIOGRAM

For many years physicians have been using electrical potential on the surface of the body to make increasingly complete and reliable diagnoses of the heart. Now, nurses find that they are called upon to know and recognize variations that have long been known to the physicians. Physicians can read electrocardiograms with confidence because thousands of these records have been correlated with other findings in the clinic and in autopsies.

## Electrical Conductivity

At the laboratory of the School of Medicine, University of Washington, there has been developed a multi-tip extracellular electrode with which the electrical events within the muscle of the heart are observed. The studies trace the pathway of the wave of electrical excitation that controls and coordinates the rhythmic contractions of heart muscle. What contribution such direct study of cardiac potentials can make to diagnostic electrocardiography is not yet clear. But it considerably enhances the picture of the physiologic events that give rise to the electrocardiogram.

During the recording of a conventional electrocardiogram (which will be referred to as "ECG") the body acts as a volume conductor, as though it were a container of salt solution. Such a conductor extends the potential field around a current source in a manner analogous to the extension of a magnetic field around a magnet. Just as a piece of iron that is not in direct contact with the magnet is attracted and repelled by the proximity of a magnetic pole, so distant recording electrodes, affixed to the skin with a conducting paste, respond to the potential field set up by the action of the heart.

A typical ECG shows a characteristic potential change in time. The various waves are known respectively as the P *wave,* the *QRS complex,* and the T *wave,* after the designations given them near the turn of the century by Willem Einthoven, the Dutch physician who devised a galvanometer sensitive enough to permit routine recording of the electrocardiogram.

## *The Conductivity Pathway*

The onset of the P wave closely follows the firing of the pacemaker, a knot of highly specialized muscle cells that set the rhythm of the heart. The P wave is produced by the movement of a wave of electrical activity through the atria (auricles), the two thin-walled chambers at the top of the heart. A single mass of muscle forms the outer walls of these chambers, and the inner space is partitioned by a sheet of muscle called the interatrial septum.

Electrical activity always precedes mechanical contraction, and almost immediately after the wave of electrical activity moves through a portion of atrial muscle, the muscle contracts. During contraction, the blood contained in the atria flows into the ventricles, the lower chambers of the heart. From the right atrium oxygen-poor venous blood flows into the right ventricle; simultaneously from the left atrium, oxygen-rich blood from the lungs moves into the left ventricle. The atria are separated from the ventricles by a ring of electrically inert connective tissue that contains the atrioventricular valves.

After the P wave there intervenes a pause of 80 milliseconds. During this interval the atrioventricular node and the attached conducting bundles, which

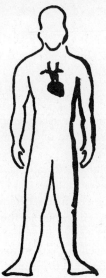

FIG. 1 The relative size of the heart and position within the chest.

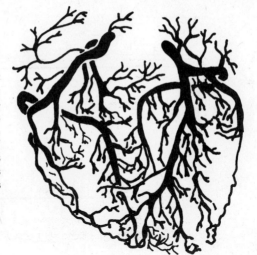

*FIG. 2* The myocardium, or heart muscle, receives its own blood supply through the coronary arteries and the blood is returned by the coronary veins. "The coronary arterial tree" branches from the major vessels into finer and finer subdivisions that bring blood to local groups of muscle fibers.

furnish the only electrical connection between the upper and lower chambers of the heart, carry the wave of excitation to the ventricles. The ECG now records the QRS complex. This is produced by the electrical activity of the massive muscles of the ventricular walls and of the interventricular septum. This electrical activity leads to contraction of the two ventricles; the right ventricle discharges venous blood into the pulmonary artery and the left ventricle discharges arterial blood into the aorta for distribution to the systemic arteries. Then follows the T wave, which marks the recovery of the ventricles for the next cycle.

The potential changes recorded by the electrocardiogram represent the summation of the electrical activity of thousands of individual cells of cardial muscle. As in all muscle cells (See Chap. III), the contraction of these cells is initiated by potential changes that occur across the cell membrane. Between the interior of the resting cell and its external environment there is a difference in electrical potential that is set up by a difference in the concentration of ions in the interior of the cell and in the fluids that bathe the cells. Inside the cell the concentration of sodium is low and that of potassium high with respect to the concentrations of those ions outside. A chemical "pump" somehow maintains the concentration gradients and a consequent potential of 80 millivolts across the membrane of the resting cell; the inside of the cell is negative with respect to the outside.[1] When a cell goes into the active, or depolarized, state, there is a rush of ions across the membrane and the inside now becomes about 30 millivolts positive with respect to the outside. How this "depolarization" of the membrane triggers mechanical contraction remains unexplained (Fig. 3–16).

1. Heinz Holter. How Things Get Into Cells. *Scientific American*, September, 1961.

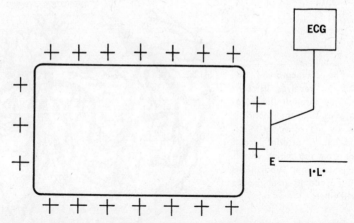

*FIG. 3* In a resting state all the positive ions are presumably on the outside of the cell membrane. There is no difference in electrical potential and no electric current is flowing. Electrode E is facing the right side of the resting muscle, and connected to a galvanometer (the electrocardiograph machine), will record no current; the isoelectric line remains undisturbed. E = electrode; ECG = electrocardiograph machine; Isoelectric line = straight line on ECG tracing.

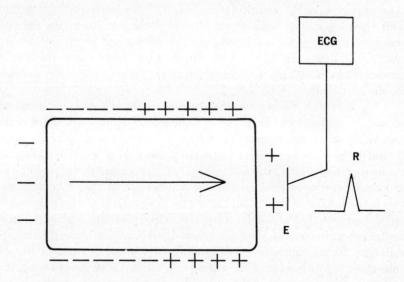

*FIG. 4* A muscle may be stimulated electrically, chemically, or mechanically. Such stimulation will produce a change of membrane permeability permitting the reorientation of the ions. Such a muscle is in the state of *depolarization*. In other words, between the interior of the resting cell and its external environment there is a difference in electrical potential that is set up by a difference in the concentration of ions in the interior of the cell and in the fluids that bathe the cells. Inside the cell the concentration of sodium is low and that of potassium high with respect to the concentration of those ions outside. When a cell does into the active, or depolarized, state, there is a rush of ions across the membrane and the inside now becomes about 30 millivolts positive with respect to the outside. How this "depolarization" of the membrane triggers mechanical contraction remains unexplained. But, once initiated, or "sparked," the process of de-

polarization will spread rapidly through the entire length of the muscle without additional stimuli.

Activation may begin at any point and wherever this "depolarization" begins, the nonpermeability of the membrane is disturbed, and the *negative* ions now appear on the outside of the cell membrane. There is now current flowing because negative and positive ions are present on the outside of the membrane. The positive ion is facing the direction of the current, and the negative ion is following it. As soon as the entire muscle strip (only one of many) is depolarized—that is, as soon as it becomes electrically negative—electrical activity again stops for a short period of time.

The electrical potential has disappeared because all of the ions on the outside of the muscle membrane are now electrically negative. This state of contraction cannot long persist, and the muscle will start to relax, or "repolarize."

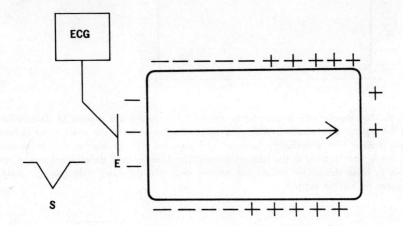

FIG. 5   The same muscle strip is stimulated again from the left, and now electrode E is facing the negative side of the current and therefore will write a negative deflection, the S wave.

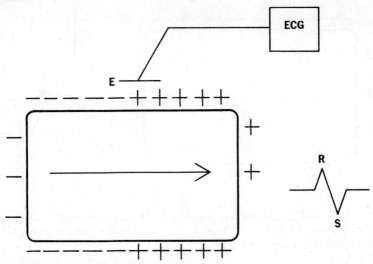

FIG. 6   Again the muscle is activated from the left. Electrode E facing the center of the muscle strip will first write a positive and then a negative deflection, an RS complex.

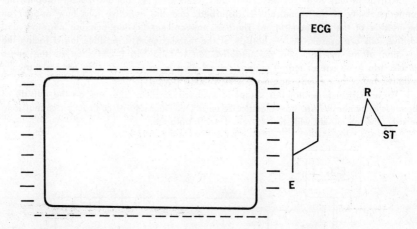

*FIG. 7* The muscle strip is completely depolarized. During the process of depolarization the R wave was recorded. With completion of depolarization the entire outer surface of the muscle strip presumably becomes negative; the flow of electric current ceases, and the R wave returns to the isoelectric line (ST). A completely depolarized muscle, as shown in these demonstrations of one muscle strip, like the completely resting muscle, produces no electric current.

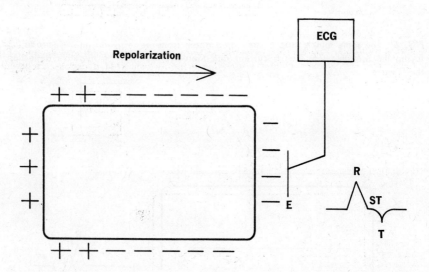

*FIG. 8* While skeletal normally will repolarize in the same direction in which it was depolarized (producing an inverted T wave), the heart muscle repolarizes in the opposite direction (producing an upright T wave).

This strip of *skeletal* muscle has been completely depolarized from left to right. During this process E was facing the positive end of the electric current, and the ECG recorded a positive deflection R. With completion of depolarization, the flow of electric current ceased and the R wave returned to the isoelectric line ST.

Presumably the outer surface of the muscle strip remained negative throughout, while the muscle was in a state of contraction. No electric current was flowing, and the isoelectric ST segment was written.

Then, the muscle strip starts to return to the resting state (repolarization) in the same direction in which it was activated: from left to right. The left end of the muscle will be the first to become positive at a time when the right end is still activated and electrically negative. An electric current is flowing again. The electrode E facing the right side of the muscle strip is exposed to the negative potential of this current and therefore will write a negative deflection T. The T wave then represents a normal *skeletal* muscle tissue returning to the resting state (repolarization).

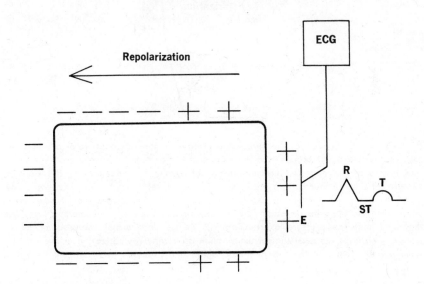

*FIG. 9* Can repolarization, or direction of electrical current flow be disrupted or disturbed? As in the previous example, the muscle strip was depolarized from left to right. The R wave is the result of this electrical current. The ST segment, isoelectric as in the previous example, is written while the entire muscle is in a state of contraction (electrically negative).

If we apply pressure to the left end of this strip, this will prevent repolarization from starting in this area. Then the muscle will start to relax on the opposite side, or from right to left. The right end of the muscle strip will be the first to become positive. During this process of repolarization, the electrode E is exposed to the positive end of the current and will write a positive deflection, the T wave, upright.

We learn from this experiment that repolarization, unlike depolarization, is disturbed easily. Slapping one end of the muscle strip, pinching it, or applying ice water will prevent repolarization from beginning in this area.

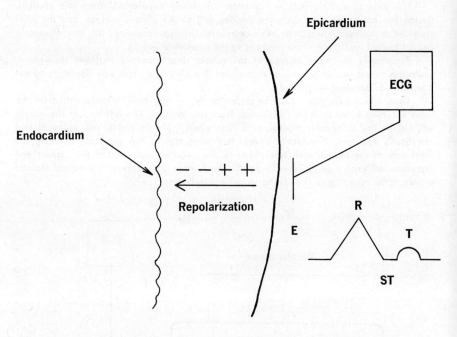

*FIG. 10* Depolarization of the myocardium begins in the subendocardial or inner surface of the heart and proceeds to the subepicardial or outer surface area. Repolarization travels in the opposite direction: from epicardium to endocardium. The previous experiment showed that certain pressures disturbed skeletal muscle repolarization. Why, then, or rather, what accounts for the disturbance causing myocardial muscle to repolarize in the opposite direction of depolarization? Physicists and experimentors have theorized that the pressure exerted against the subendocardial myocardium during systole is perhaps the most logical explanation as to why repolarization of the myocardium *normally* starts in the subepicardial region and proceeds from there to the endocardium.

From these experiments we learn the following: If repolarization travels in the same direction as depolarization as shown in the skeletal muscle strip, the T wave will move in the opposite direction from the R wave. If repolarization travels in the opposite direction from depolarization as in myocardium, the T wave will move in the same direction as the R wave.

When any cell in the heart depolarizes, current flow into it from adjacent cells. The current flow lowers the resting potential of adjacent cells, and these cells thereupon depolarize explosively. Thus, like a flame sweeping through gunpowder, a wave of excitation sweeps through the entire mass of muscle. Excitable cells, unlike grains of gunpowder, spontaneously return to the polarized resting condition and are ready to become active again. Nerve cells spend less than .001 second in the depolarized state after firing. Heart cells are comparatively slow to recover. They remain in the depolarized state

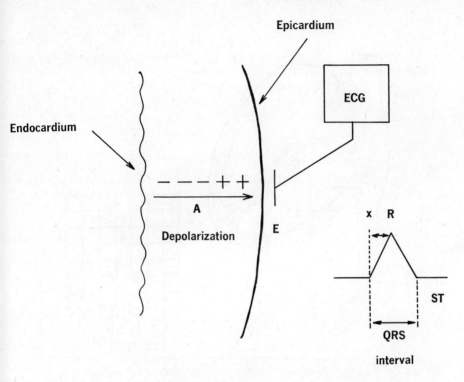

*FIG. 11* Intrinsicoid deflection represents the time it took for the depolarization to travel from endocardium to epicardium in this particular position. Electrode E is facing the positive end of the current and will record a positive deflection—the R wave. As soon as the forces of the depolarization wave arrive under E, the electric current will cease to flow and the ECG stylus will return to the isoelectric line ST segment. This is the intrinsicoid deflection, and X represents the time it took this force to travel from endocardium to epicardium. The QRS interval is the time it took for the entire myocardium to be activated.

for a quarter of a second to half a second before returning to the polarized, resting and relaxed stage.

From the point of view of the recording electrode of an electrocardiograph, each segment of heart muscle acts as if it were a large single cell. A resting cell—and resting tissue—induces no potential at the electrode. Generally speaking, the influence that an aggregation of charges exerts on an electrode is a function of the distance to the electrode. The positive and negative charges in resting tissue cancel each other.

The movement of a wave of activity through heart tissue causes potential changes at the electrodes. As the wave of activity starts, an electrode near its origin registers a negative potential representing the combined influence of

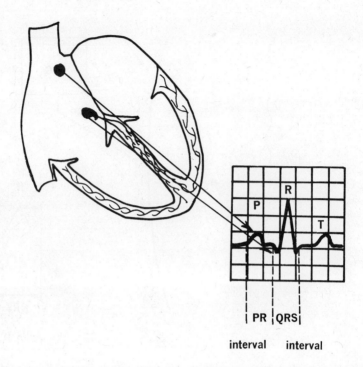

*FIG. 12* Cardiac conduction system. The cardiac impulse arises at the SA node, which is the natural pacemaker of the heart. From there it spreads through the atrial musculature, producing the P wave in the ECG, representing depolarization of the atria (time = no more than 0.10 second). This is followed by an isoelectric line which represents the slowing down of the impulse through the AV node. The PR interval is the time it takes to travel through the AV node. It is measured from the beginning of the P to the beginning of the QRS complex (time = 0.12 to 0.20 second in adults). After breaking through the AV node the impulse travels rapidly through the bundle of His, the right and left bundle, the Purkinje's fibers and through the ventricular myocardium from endocardium to epicardium. This ventricular activation is represented in the ECG by the QRS complex (time = 0.1 second or less). This is followed by the ST segment. This segment represents complete depolarization of the entire heart and, because no electric forces are usually apparent during this period, the ST segment is isoelectric. With the beginning of repolarization, or the return to the resting state, from epicardium to endocardium, the T wave is written as a positive deflection. After complete repolarization, electric forces are again absent, and an isoelectric line is seen after the T wave. This is diastole.

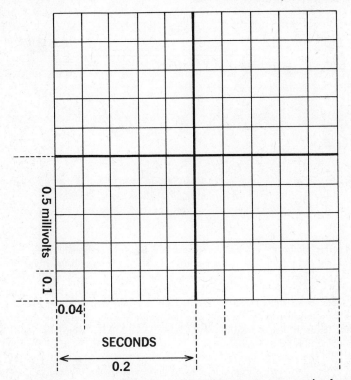

*FIG. 13* It is important to correlate the speed of the tracing across the face of the cardioscope with normal paper speed in an ECG in order to estimate rates thereby. For instance, the ECG machine drives the paper at 2.5 cm per second. The grids, or squares, are used for timing events. The larger squares measure 0.5 cm and the smaller squares 0.01 cm, or 1 mm. Therefore each large square represents 0.2 seconds of time at normal paper speed and the small squares represent 0.04 seconds. Five large squares move under the writing stylus each second; thus, 300 squares go by in one minute, a fact most useful in quickly determining heart rate or heart beats per minute. Simply count the number of large squares between identical points on adjacent complexes and divide the number of these 0.5 cm squares into 300. The heart rate is the result. For example, if there is one complete cycle from P to P in one large square, the heart rate will be 300.

| Number | Heart Rate | Number | Heart Rate |
|--------|-----------|--------|-----------|
| 1.5 | 200 | 6 | 50 |
| 2 | 150 | 7 | 43 |
| 2.5 | 120 | | |
| 3 | 100 | | |
| 3.5 | 86 | | |
| 4 | 75 | | |
| 4.5 | 67 | | |
| 5 | 60 | | |

Another way less confusing to many nurses is: to count the R waves in a 6 inch ECG strip and multiply by 10. The result is the number of beats per minute.

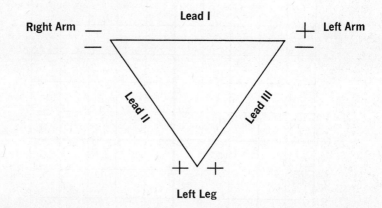

**FIG. 14** This Einthoven triangle is represented by three extremities: the left arm, the right arm and the left leg. Lead I is made up by the left arm and the right arm. The left arm is the positive pole and the right arm is the negative pole. Lead II is made up by the right arm and the left leg, and the right arm is the negative pole, the left leg the positive pole. Lead III is made up by the left leg and the left arm, and the left leg represents the positive pole, the left arm the negative pole. These are the so-called bipolar limb leads. It is most helpful for the nurse to be familiar with these leads and their potentials (positive and negative poles). It is useful also to think of the potential as derived from the roots of the respective limbs, that is, from the right and left shoulder and the groin. The heart is approximately in the center of the triangle so formed, and is commonly referred to as the Einthoven triangle, named after the great cardiologist.

the negative charges accumulating outside the depolarized muscle cells closest to it and the negative charges inside the cells in the still-resting tissue beyond. Conversely, an electrode near the termination of activity registers a positive potential set up by positive charges outside the cells of the resting tissue closer to it and the positive charges inside the more distant cells that have been fired by the approaching wave. An electrode affixed to the skin or planted directly in the heart thus "sees" the movement of a wave of activity as a sequence of potential changes. It records receding activity as a negative potential and approaching activity as a positive potential. The system is arranged so that a wave moving toward a recording electrode is registered as a positive deflection while a wave moving away from an electrode is recorded as a negative deflection. From the shape of the potential recorded at any given point on the body, therefore, one may determine the direction in which the wave of activity traveled through the heart with respect to that point.

The ECG, like any other amplifier, has two input electrodes. Its output is a record of the difference in potential between them. For many records it is necessary to nullify one of the two inputs, to make it effectively indifferent to potential change. This is accomplished by a network that connects electrodes

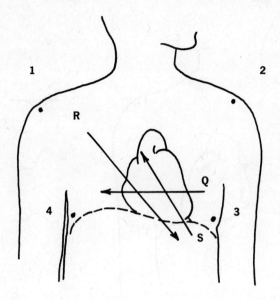

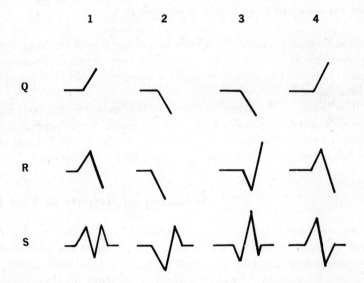

*FIG. 15* Movement of depolarizing wave through the ventricles (arrows) produces a variety of curves of potential change when recorded through electrodes located at four different spots around the heart. The changes of potential are so complex that the movement of the Q, R, and S waves cannot be analyzed by this standard technique.

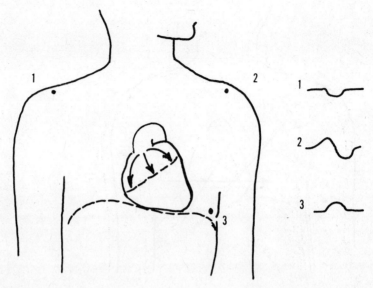

*FIG. 16* Atria are depolarized by waves that move downward and to the left (shown by arrows). P waves produced by this activity (far right) are negative when recorded at left shoulder 1, positive and negative from electrode at 2, and positive when recorded at 3. These differences come about because the activity wave is moving away from 1, toward and away from 2 and toward the electrode at 3.

placed at three extremities of the body to a single side of the input amplifier. The potentials at these three sites are therby averaged to approximate a zero potential to which the positive or negative change recorded by the active input can be compared.

The shapes of the waves recorded on the surface of the body from the thin-walled atria were sufficiently clear to enable English physiologist Sir Thomas Lewis to plot the pathway of atrial activity in 1914. Later work in other laboratories has not significantly modified his conclusions.[2]

### Summary of Activity at This Point

An electrocardiogram, commonly referred to as "ECG" or "EKG," represents electrical activity of the heart. Through electronic instrumentation, the approximately one millivolt electrical signal (1/1,000 volt) available from the patient is amplified to produce tracings permanently on electrocardiograph paper, or temporarily on the cardioscope, the "heart monitor." The ECG does not picture or trace out mechanical contractions taking place, but presents

2. Allen M. Scher. The Electrocardiogram. *Scientific American*, November, 1961.

the sequence of electrical events preceding actual mechanical contractions. The sequence follows a definite pattern in the normal ECG:

$$P \ Q \ R \ S \ T$$

The classic tracing consists of three major waves designated as:

| | Designation | Characteristic |
|---|---|---|
| 1st Wave | P | low amplitude |
| 2nd Wave | QRS | high amplitude, sharp and short duration |
| 3rd Wave | T | broad and prolonged |

## *Precordial Leads*

The standard leads that we have been discussing up to this point have two disadvantages: (1) each is derived from two points distant from the heart and (2) the three electrodes are all in the frontal plane of the body. Additional information is obtained by placing electrodes closer to the heart and moving across and around the thorax to obtain tracings of the heart from different angles. There are six precordial leads or electrode positions, and sometimes more if the physician desires tracings from the right side of the thorax and a posterior tracing from the back (Fig. 17). In addition, it may be useful to unravel difficult arrhythmias, to obtain a tracing from behind the left atrium by means of an esophageal electrode, or from the cavity of the right atrium by means of a transvenous wire electrode.

Since the standard leads are equally distant from the heart, they both contribute equally to the tracing. However, when one electrode is placed in one of the precordial positions and the other remains attached to the limb, it is natural that the electrode closer to the heart should contribute more than the lead attached to the limb. For this reason, the limb electrode of such a lead is called the "indifferent electrode," and the chest lead is referred to as the "exploring electrode,"[3] since it is moved in an exploring fashion from point to point across the chest. If the indifferent electrode is attached to the left leg the connection is called the CF; if to the right arm, CR; if to the left arm, CL.

According to the point on the chest where the precordial electrode is placed, a subscribed number is added to the CF, CR, or CL label. For example, a lead labeled $CF_5$ indicates that the exploring electrode is placed at point 5 in the anterior axillary line while the indifferent electrode is attached to the left leg.

---

3. Henry J. L. Marriott. *Practical Electrocardiography*, 4th ed. (Baltimore, The Williams & Wilkins Co., 1968), pp. 44–45.

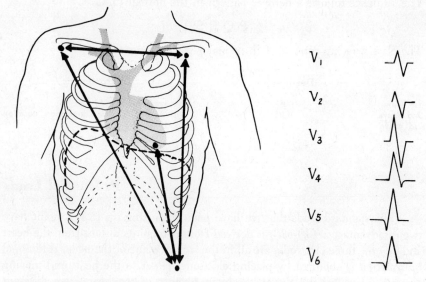

*FIG. 17* Position of the precordial (V leads) leads:

$V_1$—in the fourth interspace at the right border of the sternum
$V_2$—in the fourth interspace at the left border of the sternum
$V_3$—midway on a straight line between $V_2$ and $V_4$
$V_4$—in the fifth interspace in the midclavicular line
$V_5$—in the anterior axillary line at the level of $V_4$
$V_6$—in the midaxillary line at the level of $V_4$ and $V_5$.

These are called "vector" or V leads. Their positioned electrode represents a positive pole. Any electric force traveling toward one of these positions will write a positive deflection; one traveling away from it will write a negative deflection. These are called the precordial leads and represent the horizontal plane of the heart.

## V Leads

In review, the standard limb leads are strictly bipolar and the two poles involved exert equal influences; CF, CR, CL leads are also bipolar since they record the difference in potential between two points. However, the precordial point is more influential than the distant limb lead. In the V leads, the distant limb lead influence is practically nonexistent since all three limb leads or electrodes have been connected to form a common central terminal. Hooked up in this manner, the central terminal potential is practically zero throughout the cardiac cycle; this leaves the exploring electrode as sole dictator of the pattern. Now, you can see why the precordial leads are called *unipolar* precordial leads. Once this is understood, it is a short transferral to the unipolar limb leads. The central terminal is used as the *indifferent* connection and the exploring electrode is placed on one limb; the result is expected to yield a tracing that records the potential at the root of the explored limb exclusively. These leads are labeled VR, VL, or VF according to the limb with which the exploring electrode is connected. Although the deflections in such a lead are small, the amplitude of complexes may be amplified by disconnecting the central terminal attachment to the explored limb. This increases the size of the deflections, making them more readable without altering their shape. This augmentation of potential is designated by a prefix "a," thus: aVR, aVL, aVF.

## *Directional Forces*

Up to this point in discussion of electrocardiographs, that essential information which makes the nurse aware of the importance of the electrocardiogram in diagnosis and following the course of disease has been presented. She has been in the habit of seeing others performing electrocardiographic records. On the other hand, she might be one of the many nurses whose responsibility now is to perform this function as a part of her regular duties. Later, discussion of the advantages of recognition of the normal patterns and certain other patterns will be presented. For the moment, let us look at *vectorcardiography*.

### VECTORCARDIOGRAPHY

The electrocardiogram records the electromotive forces generated by the heart from moment to moment, as projected onto various areas of the body. Since the electrocardiogram represents magnitude in voltage and polarity of positive and negative charges, it is strictly a scalar reading . . . a scale delineation of those forces. It does not show the direction of those forces. The vector is said to denote not only magnitude and polarity, but also direction (Figs. 18 and 19).

In the cardiac cycle, the impulse is initiated in the sinoatrial node in the wall of the right atrium. Depolarization, or action, follows throughout the atria; the depolarization wave front generates a voltage. These voltages are represented by the vectors, and the term used as a complement to the scalar precordial leads is vectorcardiogram.

### SPATIAL VECTORCARDIOGRAPHY

We now know that vector is a word for *force* and as applied to electrocardiography it means "electrical force." As all electrocardiography deals exclusively in electrical forces, all electrocardiography is necessarily vectoral.[4]

4. *Ibid.*, p. 53.

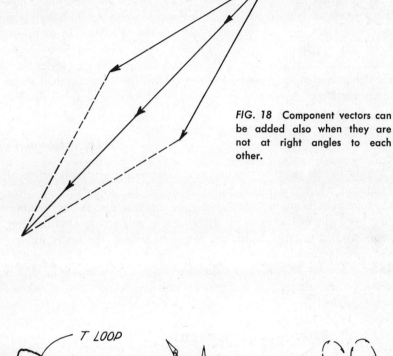

*FIG. 18* Component vectors can be added also when they are not at right angles to each other.

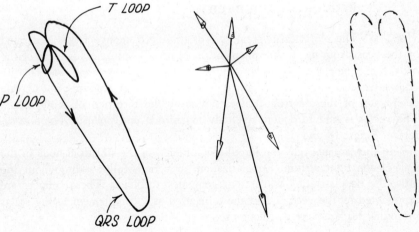

*FIG. 19* The normal spatial P, QRS, and T loops. Arrows show the direction of electrical beams resulting from ventricular activity. Formation of spatial vector loops are the result of connecting the tips of the vectors.

But, the term is reserved for that form of electrocardiography in which the heart's forces are represented by straight lines or arrows showing the direction of the forces and loops. Spatial vectorcardiography indicates that arrows or loops are "fired," or disposed, in three-dimensional space, not just two-dimensional symbols on paper like the complexes of the scalar tracings of the electrocardiogram.

### INSTANTANEOUS VECTOR

The vector, as any other force, has size and direction; these can be conveniently embodied in an arrow whose length is proportional to the size of the force (Fig. 20). An instantaneous vector represents the resultant of all the heart's electrical forces at a given moment. The mean vector is the average or resultant of all the instantaneous vectors. The loop substitutes for a set of innumerable arrows a single continuous line and is obtained by joining up the heads of the arrows. In the same manner, the instantaneous vector for

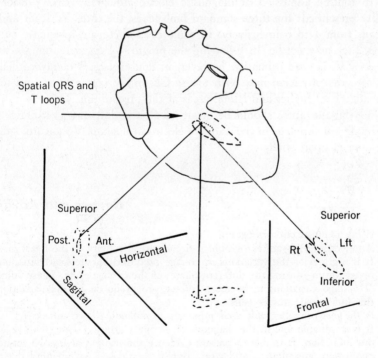

*FIG. 20* Projection of the spatial QRS and T loops on the frontal, the sagittal, and the horizontal planes of the body.

any given moment can be obtained from the loop by drawing an arrow from the center of the loop to a point at its periphery.[5]

However, it is only fair to say that there is much controversy about vectorcardiographs, but it is not within the scope of this book to give more than a brief concept of vectors so that the nurse who is interested may continue further study. There is no question that the understanding of the vector concept is of value in understanding electrocardiography. Vectorcardiologists are convinced that the vector concepts serve as a short-cut or simplification for the student in that hundreds of different electrocardiograph patterns may be resolved into fewer than a dozen basic vector patterns or spatial loops.[6] The reader is encouraged to investigate the footnote references for more thorough information on this subject.

## Summary

In routine admission or diagnostic electrocardiograms twelve leads are usually prescribed: the three standard limb leads, the three aV leads and six V leads from 1 to 6 inclusively. In some cases these are adequate, but, in others, they may not be. In following the progress of an arrhythmia a single lead 2 or $V_1$ is used primarily; however, in doubtful cases of myocardial infarctions, the physician may wish to use CF and V connections, and to explore additional higher and lateral areas of the precordium. There is no rigid routine, but the nurse should be aware of all the different possibilities that may modify or supplement the standard electrocardiogram. Vectorcardiography was touched upon briefly.

## Review and Advance

1. *What is an electrocardiogram?*
   An electrocardiogram is a graph of the electrical activity of the heart muscle. It is a graph of the variations in voltage produced by the heart muscle—the myocardium—during the different phases of the cardiac cycle. These voltages, or voltage variations to be more correct, are produced by depolarization of the individual muscle cells.
2. *Is the electrocardiograph used primarily to diagnose "heart attacks"?*
   It is a valuable tool in the diagnosis of coronary artery disease, with or without infarction. It is able to present evidence that cannot always be found by percussion, auscultation and x-ray. But, it should be kept in mind that it is

5. *Ibid.*, p. 54.
6. Herman N. Uhley. *Vector Electrocardiography.* (Philadelphia, J. B. Lippincott Co., 1962), p vii.

not necessarily infallible or positively diagnostic. In other words, it is an aid to diagnosis, but not a substitute for a careful history and physical, just as the monitor is not a substitute for nursing care.

3. *What is meant by electrical potential across a cell membrane?*
In the normal resting state, a difference in electrical potential exists across the cell membrane, the outside having positive charges, the interior having negative charges. The difference of potential of about 90 millivolts is maintained by the so-called sodium-potassium pump mechanism. The concentration of sodium on the outside of the cell membrane is 30 times higher than that on the inside.* On the other hand, potassium is about 30 times greater within the cell than in extracellular fluid.

If one end of a normal muscle cell is stimulated, the barrier of the cell membrane is broken at that point. Sodium flows in with its positive charges, and very transiently the polarity across the cell membrane is reversed, that is, the outside becomes negative to the inside by about 20 millivolts. Almost immediately, this polarity is neutralized so that the potential across the cell membrane is zero. Still, as compared with the still-resting portion of the cell, there is a potential difference of about 90 millivolts, the portion which is still polarized being positive, the depolarized are negative. This difference draws positively ionized sodium along the electrical gradient, so that a wave of depolarization passes from one end of the cell to the other and from one muscle to the next.

4. *What determines how this depolarization will be traced on the electrocardiograph?*
If an electrode is placed on the side facing the advancing wave of depolarization, a positive deflection will be produced, the magnitude of which will depend upon the thickness of the muscle involved. At the same time, an electrode placed on the side from which the wave of depolarization is receding will show a negative deflection. If electrodes are placed at right angles to the wave of depolarization, there will be either a diphasic deflection or no change at all.

5. *Does the depolarization wave sweep over the ventricles from the top down in one swoop?*
No, it must be understood that in the ventricles the wave of depolarization passes from the endocardium to epicardium. Since the magnitude of deflection depends upon the thickness of the muscle through which the wave of current must pass, the thicker left ventricle will overbalance the right ventricle. Therefore, during ventricular systole, a positive deflection (R wave) will appear in an electrode that faces the left side of the heart, while a negative deflection (S wave) will appear in an electrode facing the right side of the heart.

6. *Do physicians routinely order several electrocardiograms in succession?*
When the physician orders several tracings on the same person at certain specified times, these are referred to as serial tracings and enable him to follow the course of the disorder. However, it must be remembered that the first electrocardiogram after the "attack" might show no changes whatsoever. A single electrocardiogram often is not significant; repeated tracings may be necessary before evidence of disease may be detected.

* Charles K. Friedberg. *Diseases of the Heart,* 3rd ed. W. B. Saunders Company, Philadelphia, 1966, pp. 24–45.

# 14 INTERPRETING THE ELECTROCARDIOGRAM

In every electrocardiogram ten features should be examined systematically. They include the following:

1. Rhythm
2. Rate
3. P wave
4. P-R interval
5. QRS interval

6. QRS complex
7. ST segment
8. T wave
9. U wave
10. Q-T duration

Some of these salient features will be discussed in detail; others will be touched upon lightly since the nurse is not expected to minutely interpret all she observes. She must be expected to recognize any deviation or abnormality to preclude unexpected crises (see Chap. 13, Fig. 13), and to institute appropriate measures until the physician arrives. In order to be able to recognize drastic changes in ECG, rhythm strip, and oscilloscope pattern, she must be familiar with the normal. This chapter will aid her in this.

## *Conductivity Pathway in Brief*

An impulse begins in the SA node (pacemaker) and spreads through the atria and gives rise to

- *P wave* which represents atrial depolarization.
    The impulse causes a second and major depolarization only after
    1) time required for the impulse to cross the atria and the
    2) delay time in the AV node.

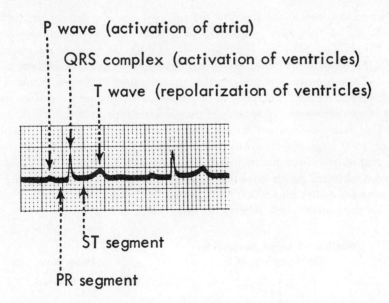

P wave (activation of atria)

QRS complex (activation of ventricles)

T wave (repolarization of ventricles)

ST segment

PR segment

*FIG. 1* Anatomy of the ECG.
(Reprinted with permission from Marriott, CCU Nursing Slides, 1967,
Tampa Tracings, Oldsmar, Fla.)

- P-R *interval*
    The AV node is a relay station at the junction of atrial and ventric-
    ular tissues and passes the impulse to special conducting fibers, then
    to ventricular muscle giving rise to
- *QRS complex* which represents ventricular depolarization.
    The ventricles have a recovery phase after depolarization followed by
- T *wave* which represents ventricular repolarization (Fig. 1).

## *Rhythm*

The nurse is expected to do much more than merely notice whether the
rhythm is regular or irregular. She must know that certain variations are considered normal; for instance, SA, AV, or idioventricular rhythms are all considered normal, not irregular rhythms.

## *Rate of Timing*

Although many methods are offered to establish heart rates, this can be
done fairly simply. When the patient is attached to a monitoring device, it is

important to correlate the speed of the tracing across the face of the cardio-scope with normal paper speed in an ECG. One can thereby estimate rates.

The ECG paper is marked off in vertical lines; the speed of the machine drives the paper at 2.5 cm (25 mm) per second, or so that the lines are 1/25 or 0.04 seconds apart. The grids on the paper are used for timing events. The larger squares measure 5 mm and the smaller squares are 1 mm; therefore, each large square represents 0.2 seconds of time at normal paper speed.

Five large squares per second move under the writing stylus. In one minute, 300 large squares go by, a fact most useful in quickly determining rate, that is, heart beats per minute. Simply count the number of large squares between identical points on adjacent complexes and divide the number of these 5 mm squares into 300. The heart rate is the result. In order to clarify this, an appropriate guide follows.

| Number of Large Squares for One Complete ECG | Heart Rate |
|:---:|:---:|
| 1 | 300 beats/min. |
| 1.5 | 200 |
| 2 | 150 |
| 2.5 | 120 |
| 3 | 100 |
| 3.5 | 86 |
| 4 | 75 |
| 4.5 | 67 |
| 5 | 60 |
| 5.5 | 55 |
| 6 | 50 |
| 7 | 43 |

After suitable experience in the examination of tracings, both on chart paper and on the cardioscope, it is surprising how well one can estimate rate with just a glance at the cardioscope simply by quickly noting the distance between the complexes. However, it is important that cardioscope observers be certain of the sweep rate setting of the cardioscope (the speed of the trace across the face of the cardioscope in cm/seconds).

## P Wave

As discussed earlier, the base line is referred to as the isoelectric line; that is, the straight line upon resting phase. Therefore, there are terms applied to the tracings which fall below or reach above the isoelectric line. When a complex is partly above, it is diphasic or biphasic. When it traces a line approximately the same distance above the line as below, it is isodiphasic or equiphasic.

The P wave—the first wave of the ECG—represents the spread of electrical impulse through the atria (activation or depolarization). It is normally upright in leads 1 and 2, but is frequently diphasic or inverted in lead 3. However, it is easier to think of the P waves as

> Normally upright in 1, 2 and aVF
> Normally inverted in aVR
> Variable in 3, aVL and chest leads

The abnormalities that should be looked for in P waves are:

- Inversion where it normally should be upright, or upright where it should be inverted.
- Increased amplitude which usually indicates right atrial hypertrophy, dilation, and is found especially in AV valve disease, hypertension, cor pulmonale, and congenital disease.
- Increased width which may indicate left atrial enlargement or diseased atrial muscle. The normal P wave does not exceed 0.11 seconds in duration.
- *Diphasicity* which is an important sign of left atrial enlargement when the second half of the P wave is greatly negative in lead 3 or $V-_1$.
- *Notching*—along with widening, the P wave appears taller in lead 1 when the left atrium is involved as in P-mitrale. Notching is noteworthy when the distance between peaks is over 0.04 sec.
- *Peaking*—right atrial strain usually produces pointed P waves taller in lead 3 than in lead 1 in P-pulmonale.
- Absence of P waves occurs in some AV nodal rhythms and in SA block.

*The P-R interval* is measured from the beginning of the P wave to the beginning of the QRS complex. It measures the time taken by the impulse to travel all the way from the SA node to the ventricular muscle fibers; this is normally from 0.12 to 0.20 seconds. It is customary to examine several intervals and record that which appears the longest.

The P-R interval is abnormally short when the impulse originates in the AV node instead of the SA node, and also when the passage of the impulse to the ventricle is accelerated, as in Wolff-Parkinson-White syndrome. It shortens and lengthens for many reasons; although you will not be expected to memorize these, briefly they include:

| Prolonged | Shortened |
|---|---|
| In AV block | In AV nodal and low atrial rhythms |
| Coronary disease | In Wolff-Parkinson-White syndrome |
| Rheumatic fever, etc. | In glycogen storage disease |
| As a rare normal variation | As a normal variation |
| Some cases of hyperthyroidism | In some hypertensive patients |
| | In corticosteroid administration |

## QRS Complex

The QRS complex is the most important in the ECG (Fig. 2). It represents the spread of the impulse through the ventricular muscle (activation or depolarization of the ventricles).

This can show up in many different forms or shapes so you should be familiar with the terms applied to it:

- If the first deflection is downward, it is negative and is labeled the "Q wave."
- The first upright deflection is the "R wave," whether or not it is preceded by a Q.
- A negative deflection following an R wave is an "S wave."
- Any other deflections above the line are labeled R', R'', etc.; any other deflections below the line are labeled S', S'', etc.

The points at which the complex begins and ends are labeled Q and S, respectively, even when there are no actual Q or S waves. When the complex consists exclusively of a Q wave it is described as a QS complex. To simplify which is predominant, the use of small and large letters are used to signify the relative size of the component waves; for example, qRs means "a small Q, a tall R, and a small S wave (Fig. 3). In interpreting the QRS complexes, several things should be scrutinized:

- The duration (0.05 to 0.105 sec.)
- The amplitude (approx. 5 mm although some precordials up to 30 mm)
- The presence of Q waves
- Their electrical axis in the frontal plane (limb leads)
- The relative prominence of the component waves in the precordial leads, $V_1$ to $V_6$, noting the transitional zone (point where negative deflections rule or cancel out positive deflections)
- The timing of the intrinsicoid deflections (downstroke in precordial leads)
- The general configuration of the complex, including the presence and location of any slurred component

*The ST segment* is that part of the tracing immediately following the QRS complex. The point at which it separates from the QRS is called the "J" (junction) point.

The two features to be observed with the ST segment are its level relative to the base line and its shape. Normally it is level, as is the T-P segment, or only slightly above or below the base line. It is never elevated more than

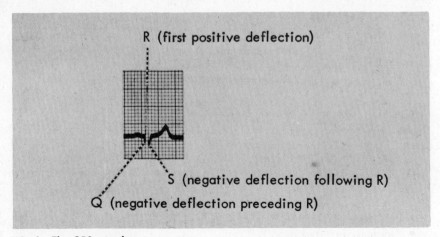

R (first positive deflection)

S (negative deflection following R)

Q (negative deflection preceding R)

*FIG. 2*  The QRS complex.

(Reprinted with permission from Marriott, CCU Nursing Slides, 1967, Tampa Tracings, Oldsmar, Fla.)

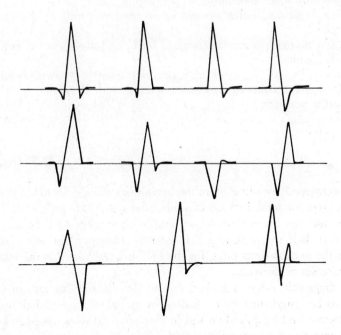

*FIG. 3*  Variations in QRS complex. The QRS complex can take many different forms: A q wave is negative and precedes the R; the S wave is negative and follows the R. Small letters signify small deflections; large letters signify large deflections. There may be no Q or S wave observable, and there may be no R wave. If two R waves are present in one complex, the second one is called R prime, or R'. The same world go for the S prime, or S'.

1 mm above the base line in the standard leads, and perhaps 2 mm in the chest leads. On the other hand, it is never depressed more than half a millimeter. It should curve gently into the near limb of the T wave. Any sharp angle or flattening may indicate myocardinal ischemia.

## T Wave

The T wave represents the recovery period of the ventricles, or repolarization. Three features should be noted: its direction, its shape, and its height. In the normal adult, the T wave is as follows:

- Normally upright in 1, 2 and $V_3$ to $V_6$
- Normally inverted in aVR
- Variable in 3, aVL, aVF, $V_1$ and $V_2$
- Shape is slightly rounded and slightly asymmetrical
  (Notching sometimes found in pericarditis)
  (Sharply pointed either upright or inverted may indicate myocardial infarction)
- Height normally 5 mm in standard leads, and not above 10 mm in precordial leads
  (Unusually tall T waves may be indicative of myocardial infarction, potassium intoxication, myocardial ischemia without infarction, or cerebrovascular accident.)

## Q-T Duration

This interval, measured from the beginning of the QRS to the end of the T wave, gives the total duration of ventricular systole. It varies with the heart rate, sex, and age. Some cardiologists simply say that the Q-T interval should be less than half the preceding R-R interval. However, this may hold good only for the normal sinus rates, for the Q-T interval varies as the rate of the heart increases or decreases.

Its diagnostic value is limited due to the difficulty in measuring. It is known to be lengthened in congestive heart failure, myocardial infarction, hypocalcemia, and by quinidine and procainamide. It is shortened by digitalis, calcium excess, and potassium intoxication.

*The U wave* is a small wave sometimes seen following the T wave. Its normal polarity is the same as the T wave; if the T wave is upright, it is upright; if the T wave is inverted, the U wave is inverted. It is most easily seen in lead $V_3$, is made more noticeable in potassium deficiency, and is seen inverted in myocardial ischemia. There are other conditions which alter it, but this is sufficient to make you aware of its presence. Its significance is uncertain.

## Summary

In the preceding chapter we have discussed the electrocardiogram, vectorcardiogram, and now, the interpretations of the actual tracing itself. The nurse may make an electrocardiographic diagnosis when competent to do so; she is expected to distinguish certain abnormalities from the normal. This chapter has attempted to give her that information which will make her duties more meaningful and understandable.

## Review and Advance

1. *What are the various waves on the electrocardiographic tracing called?*
   The various waves on the electrocardiographic tracing are arbitrarily designated by the successive letters of the alphabet P, Q, R, S, T, and U.
2. *Do the lines on the tracing paper mean anything specific?*
   The paper upon which the electrocardiogram is recorded is ruled in lines 1 millimeter apart, both horizontally and vertically. Each fifth line in both directions is heavier than the rest.
3. *What do the vertical lines indicate?*
   Vertically, the lines indicate change in voltage. When properly standardized, each one-millimeter space represents 0.1 millivolt. Each 5 mm space between heavy lines represents 0.5 mv.
4. *What do the horizontal spaces indicate?*
   The horizontal spaces designate the passage of time. A one-millimeter space represents 0.04 second. The distance between heavy lines (5 mm) equals 0.2 second.
5. *What does the P wave indicate?*
   The first wave, the P wave, in the tracing is produced by atrial depolarization. This wave, usually measured in lead 2, does not normally exceed 3 mm in height or 0.11 second in duration (less than 3 mm spaces measuring the inside of the wave). Except in aVR, the P wave is upright.
6. *What are some examples when change might be expected in the P wave?*
   The P wave might be tall and peaked in right atrial hypertrophy, average height in left atrial hypertrophy, but notched and wide. In atrial fibrillation, it shows as fine irregularities along the isoelectric line; in atrial flutter, a sawtoothed pattern replaces the single P wave. Others will be discussed later.
7. *What is the P-R interval?*
   The P-R interval (or it may be P-Q interval) represents the delay in transmission of the impulse from atria to ventricles in the bundle of His, but chiefly in the atrioventricular node.

8. *Is the P-R interval isoelectric?*
Normally, the P-R interval, the time between atrial depolarization and ventricular depolarization, is nearly isoelectric, because the voltage of repolarization of the atrium is too weak to register.

9. *Does this mean it is always isoelectric?*
No. In chronic cor pulmonale (right ventricular hypertrophy and congestive heart failure), repolarization of the atrium produces a definite negative deflection in leads 2 and 3.

10. *What is the significance of the QRS complex?*
It is usually considered the most important in the electrocardiogram. The relative heights of these three waves vary with the lead examined, the position of the heart, and the degree of abnormality present. It represents the spread of the depolarization impulse through the ventricular muscle.

11. *What is the duration of the QRS complex?*
The duration of the QRS complex, measured from the beginning of the Q to the end of the complex, usually ranges from 0.06 and 0.08 second, and does not exceed 0.10 second normally. Occasionally, it may be 0.11 or even 0.12 second in an individual with an apparently normal heart. It is usually shorter in children, ranging from 0.04 to 0.08 second under the age of five, and 0.05 to 0.09 second between the ages of five to fourteen.

12. *What is the S-T segment?*
The S-T segment and T wave reflect the repolarization of the ventricles.

13. *The cardiac conduction system consists of myocardial fibers that are specialized for rapid transmission of impulses. What structure in this system conducts impulses more slowly than the rest?*
This structure is the atrioventricular node, from where normal impulses pass directly into the bundle of His. The delay of impulses at the AV node allows the ventricles to fill before ventricular contraction. Since impulses normally pass through the AV node immediately before depolarization of the ventricles, this is portrayed on the electrocardiogram immediately before the QRS complex, in the P-R interval.

14. *What is the normal pathway of cardiac conduction?*
The parts of the cardiac conduction system are the sinoatrial node (SA node), the atrioventricular node (AV node), bundle of His, right and left bundle branches, and Purkinje system.
The depolarization wave originates from the SA node and travels through the atrial myocardium. It reaches the AV node next, from which it is transmitted to the bundle of His, to the right and left bundle branches, to the Purkinje system. The fibers of the Purkinje system terminate in the ventricular myocardium.

15. *Is there any way of calculating heart rate other than by counting the large squares?*
There are probably several other methods. One is to count the R's in a six-inch rhythm strip and multiply by 10; for example, if there were 6 R waves in a 6-inch strip of electrocardiogram tracing, multiplied by 10 this would give a rate of 60. Other nurses prefer to count the number of R-R intervals in 3 seconds (15 spaces of 0.2 second each: one heavy line every 5 small), then multiply that number by 20 to give the rate per minute. For example, if there were 3.5 R-R intervals in 15 time spaces of 0.2 second each, 3.5 multiplied by 20 would equal 70 beats per minute.

16. *Haw can the heart change position in the chest?*
    This can be a perfectly normal phenomenon. Actually, the heart can rotate around an anteroposterior axis, a transverse axis, and an anatomic axis which runs from the base to the apex. The heart can rotate from front to back, side to side, and around the anatomic axis, all simultaneously. It is enough to recognize that all of these variations are normal.

# 15 MYOCARDIAL INFARCTION AND ECG TRACINGS

Many nurses have been privileged to observe clinical experiments on a dog's heart in the "dog lab." It is from actual observation of experiments of this kind that one really begins to understand the phenomenon of the injuries to the heart and the resultant electrical pattern which may be evoked.

When a branch of the dog's coronary artery is tied off and an electrode is placed over the myocardium in the area of the now occluded vessel, the resultant tracing almost immediately becomes changed; the *T wave becomes inverted* (Fig. 1). When the tie is removed and the blood allowed to resume its course, the T waves revert to normal. The implication is that a change in the T wave is a direct result of simple ischemia, therefore, inverted T waves form the basis of the pattern of ischemia in the clinical tracing.

If the tie is allowed to remain, in addition to the inverted T wave, another change occurs within a very few minutes; as evidence of injury, the ST segment becomes elevated to the point that it obliterates the inverted T wave. If the tie is removed, the pattern gradually reverts to normal; elevated ST segment recedes, the inverted T wave becomes upright, the pattern returns to normal. Therefore, it appears that at this point, ischemia is still reversible even though it has crossed over into the zone of injury; thus this stage is known as the *pattern of injury*.

If the tie is left in place beyond the pattern of injury, a further drastic change occurs: the entire QRS becomes inverted to produce a QS complex, while the ST segment comes back to the base line and the T wave may or may not revert to its upright position. If this pattern is allowed to continue—that is, the tie is kept in place—irreversible structural changes will have occurred and it will not be able to return to normal; thus, with irreversible structural changes, a QS pattern will continue after the tie is removed. This is known as the *pattern of necrosis*. The deep QS complex is proof that necrosis, or death of the myocardium, has occurred. The absence of any R wave indi-

218

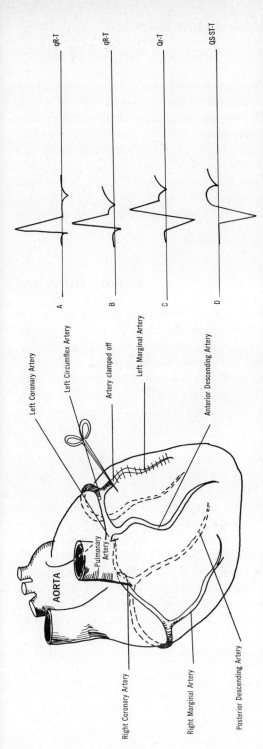

FIG. 1 Progressive myocardium pattern. A branch of the coronary artery is clamped off in a dog: The T waves become inverted in leads facing this area of ischemia. A. If the clamped artery is freed and circulation allowed to resume, the condition can be relieved and the T wave will revert to its original, upright position. We know from this experiment that ischemia changes the direction of repolarization which is normally from epicardium to endocardium.

B. If the clamp is left in place instead of being released, the T wave remains inverted, and, in addition, the ST segment soon becomes elevated. This represents the current of injury. The process is still reversible, and removal of the clamp will allow the return of the ECG tracing back to normal.

C. If the clamp is left in place after ischemia and injury effect have become apparent, this part of the myocardium having been deprived of its blood supply, and death of that part will ensue. It is unable to produce an electric potential, and so the R wave, which represents activation, will disappear either in part, or completely and be replaced by Q waves.

D. If the death of that part of the myocardium involves the entire thickness from endocardium to epicardium, there will be no R waves at all. Thus is referred to as a transmural infarction.

219

cates that the myocardium has been injured by a transmural infarct, from epicardium to endocardium.

As previously mentioned, electrical current flows through a channeled pattern; if something happens to the tissue so that it cannot continue to pass along the electrical impulse, the impulse must either be thwarted or must find another pathway. An electrode placed over the "dead" myocardium receives no electrical forces from the underlying muscle, and this results in a negative deflection, or Q wave. The infarct is then a window into the chamber, revealing forces directed away from the dead area; and this may be indicated by an increase in the size of the positive deflection, or R wave, in leads taken from the opposite surface of the heart. This concept is helpful in explaining some of the less classical patterns of infarctions.

## *Clinical Infarction*

For many years, the two main types of infarctions were called anterior and posterior. However, it is now recognized that the term posterior is somewhat anatomically incorrect since this side actually rests on the diaphragm; thus, the term has been discarded in favor of "diaphragmatic," or "inferior." However, it is very clear to anyone examining a heart that there are no clear-cut lines between any of the four walls, or sides, so they are called merely anterior, lateral, inferior, and true posterior (to distinguish from former posterior).

The three changes observed in the experimental dog form the basis of the clinical pattern of myocardial infarction, i.e., T wave inversion, ST elevation, and the appearance of Q waves. Surrounding any small area of necrotic myocardium, there is a less damaged area which produces the pattern of injury; and outside this is an even less-affected area which produces the pattern of ischemia. Since the electrode cannot be placed directly over the infarcted area as could be done in the experimental animal, the nearest it can get is over the area on the chest wall; thus, the ECG tracing picks up through this electrode a composite picture combining the patterns of ischemia, injury, and necrosis all in one QRST sequence. In short, the relatively distant electrode is influenced by all three areas or circles instead of only one. Here, then, lies the difficulty of seeing a true pattern as we have seen in our experimental dog.

The first step in recognizing an infarction on the ECG tracing, then, is to know what to look for:

- the fresh appearance of Q waves
- ST segment elevations
- T wave inversions

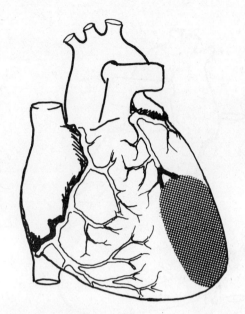

*FIG. 2* Antero-lateral infarct. Occlusion of anterior inter-ventricular branch of left coronary artery.

Remember that only Q waves are diagnostic of necrosis, or true infarction, with the other two features only providing suspicions. The Q, ST and T changes are all special characteristics:

- The Q wave is often wide as well as deep.
- Any Q wave measuring 0.03 sec. or more is highly suspicious.
- The deviated ST segments typically show an upward convexity.
- The T waves are pointed and are asymmetrical on both sides, resembling an arrowhead.

These changes are all noticeable in leads that face the area of damage. Opposite changes appear in leads facing the diametrically opposed surface of the heart, i.e., some increase in the height of R wave, no Q wave, depressed ST segments, and tall upright T waves.

In anterior infarction indicative changes occur in precordial leads and in leads 1 and aVL, while reciprocal changes develop in leads that face the inferior posterior surface, leads 2, 3 and aVF (Figs. 2, 3, and 4).

In lateral wall infarction, leads aVL and $V_5$ and $V_6$ are most likely to show indicative changes, and reciprocal changes may sometimes develop in leads farthest to the right, $V_1$, $V_{3R}$, etc.

None of the leads—the 12 basic—face the true posterior surface of the heart; infarctions of this wall must be inferred from reciprocal changes occurring in anterior leads, especially $V_1$ and $V_2$.

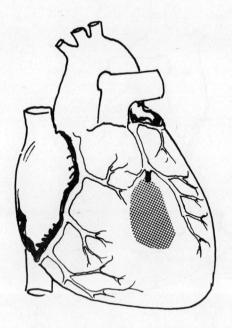

*FIG. 3* Anterior infarct. Occlusion of right division of anterior inter-ventricular branch of left coronary artery.

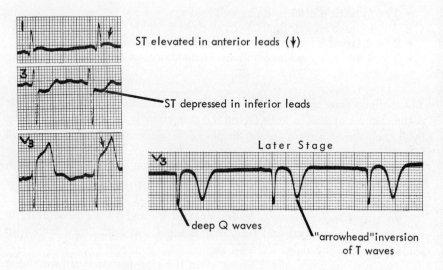

ST elevated in anterior leads (↓)

ST depressed in inferior leads

Later Stage

deep Q waves

"arrowhead" inversion of T waves

*FIG. 4* Acute anterior infarction.

The limb leads indicative of anterior and inferior infarction are summarized as follows:

*Anterior Infarction* (Figs. 5 and 6)

- Changes in lead $1 = Q_1T_1$ type of infarction
- Changes in aVL with reciprocal changes in 3 and aVF

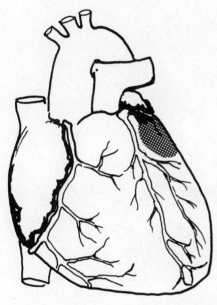

*FIG. 5* Small apical infarct. Occlusion of terminal portion of anterior inter-ventricular branch of left coronary artery.

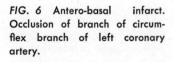

*FIG. 6* Antero-basal infarct. Occlusion of branch of circum-flex branch of left coronary artery.

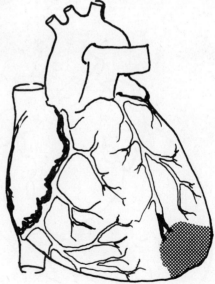

*Inferior Infarction* (Figs. 7, 8, 9, 10, and 11)

- Changes in lead 3 = $Q_3T_3$ type of infarction
- Changes in 2 and aVF with reciprocal changes in 1 and aVL

It must be remembered that changes of infarction may appear only in the precordial leads, while the limb leads remain normal or near normal.

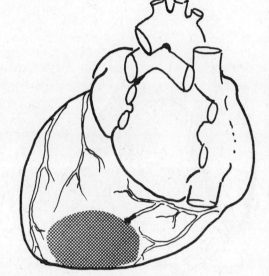

FIG. 7 Postero-inferior infarct. Occlusion of posterior inter-ventricular branch of right coronary artery.

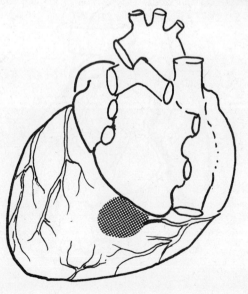

FIG. 8 Posterior infarct. Occlusion of right coronary artery, or its posterior inter-ventricular branch.

ST elevated in inferior leads

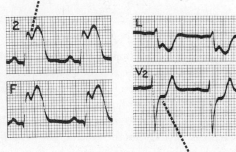

FIG. 9 Acute inferior infarction.
(Reprinted with permission
from Marriott, CCU Nursing
Slides, 1967, Tampa Trac-
ings, Oldsmar, Fla.)

ST depressed in anterior leads

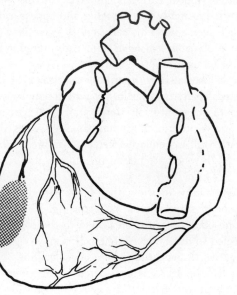

FIG. 10 Postero-lateral infarct.
Occlusion of circumflex branch
of left coronary artery.

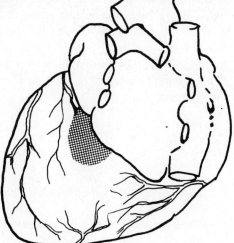

FIG. 11 Postero-basal infarct.
Occlusion of circumflex branch
of left coronary artery.

## *Other Considerations*

The brief description of the infarction patterns here is by no means complete, but that is not the function of this book. It is enough that you be aware of the typical pattern of myocardial infarction and probable changes that might occur on the cardioscope.

It is important to note that time relationships are important. Rarely, no changes develop in the tracing for several days, and sometimes, even in two or three weeks. Usually, they begin to make their appearance within the first few hours. ST segment changes appear early and progress. At this stage the T waves, later to become inverted, actually become taller and appear as an upward extension of the rising ST segments. This early tall T wave may be mistaken for the later tall T wave of reciprocal leads, and early anterior infarction may be thus wrongly labeled as inferior.

Sometimes this tall T wave is associated with striking depression of the ST segment, and then the reciprocal pattern of an inferior infarction is even more closely simulated. To add to the confusion similar tall T waves are occasionally seen in an early stage of inferior infarction; in such cases this may mean a stage of diaphragmatic wall ischemia before actual infarction has occurred. Similar but persistent tall T waves are not an uncommon finding in patients with angina.

These variables are mentioned only to show that great experience is necessary for anyone to attempt diagnosing from an ECG tracing. The nurse must merely note the changes she observes and bring these to the attention of the physician; she is not expected to diagnose. Although this may begin to sound like a broken record, it is worth repeating often since legalities can sometimes have dire consequences. The ECG is considered confirmatory of the physician's clinical impression. If the patient is suspected clinically of having suffered a myocardial infarction, he is usually treated accordingly even if his tracing is completely normal. The changes may appear later, or may never appear.

## *Summary*

In summary, it is merely noted that a sequence of changes within the myocardium develops a distinctive pattern. Although the pattern may vary, there is always some evolution of the pattern along similar lines, and before the physician diagnoses an acute infarction, this evolution is usually in evidence. The indicative features of acute myocardial infarction are:

| Changes | Anterior | Inferior |
|---|---|---|
| 1. Q, ST elevations, T inversion in leads | 1, aVL, anterior chest | 3, aVF, posterior chest |
| 2. Reciprocal changes in leads | 3, aVF, posterior chest | 1, aVL, anterior chest |
| 3. Progressive changes in pattern from day to day | | |

## Review and Advance

1. *What are bipolar leads?*
   When a lead is paired, that is, when a lead is secured by pairing one electrode on the body with another electrode on the body, this is called a bipolar lead. Customarily, these leads are taken with electrodes placed at the extremities or on the chest wall, but they may be placed elsewhere.
2. *What is the unipolar lead?*
   In contrast to the bipolar lead, a unipolar lead is one that represents the heart voltages present at one particular spot on the body with respect to a nonfluctuating reference point. This reference point is secured by connecting the limb electrodes together through three equal resistances of 5,000 ohms or more; [1] the junction is the reference point, or central terminal, which is usually embodied in the lead selector of the electrocardiograph, or in a special switching box.
   The electrodes placed on the body are then paired, in turn, with this reference point or central terminal, to secure the unipolar leads which represent the actual voltages present at these single points on the body.
3. *Is there any particular technique of assuring good chest leads?*
   The technique of taking acceptable chest leads depends upon three conditions: (1) the size of the electrode, (2) preparation of selected positions, and (3) methods of holding the electrode in place.
4. *What size should the electrode be?*
   The American Heart Association in specifying the physical size or area of a chest electrode, states that it may be 3 cm in diameter, or smaller.
5. *How should the skin be prepared for chest leads?*
   If an electrode paste is to be used, some slight friction will be required, as opposed to shaving the area. When several chest areas are to be used, care must be taken that the paste does not overlap between one location and another.
   Whatever device or method is used to hold the electrode in place, the contact should be firm and steady. It must not be so loose that it will rock

---

1. *Technician's Guide to Electrocardiography,* published by Hewlett-Packard Company, Waltham Division, Waltham, Mass., 4th ed., 1966.

with each breath the patient takes, yet not applied with such great pressure as to cause discomfort and muscle tremor.

6. *Is there a "best" method for holding the electrode on the chest?*
   There are a number of devices or means for holding chest leads or electrodes in place, such as vacuum cups, straps, sand bags, adhesive tape, or specially prepared paste and applicator supplied by the manufacturer of the monitoring device or electrocardiograph machine. Choice of these will depend on the frequency with which precordial leads are to be left in place.

   It is important in precordial leads, regardless of the type of electrode used, to insert the patient cable tips so there is no pull on the chest electrode.

7. *Is it always possible to diagnose myocardial infarction by electrocardiogram?*
   The diagnosis of myocardial infarction is sometimes impossible because of the location of the infarct. In the case of a small infarct not involving the epicardium or endocardium—that is, a small intramural infarct—it cannot be detected by either electrocardiography or vectorcardiography.

8. *Can angina pectoris be revealed by oscilloscope?*
   With an acute attack of angina pectoris, ischemia and injury of the heart occur, but *no* infarct. As a consequence, there are changes in the S-T segments and T waves which develop during the attack, but characteristically disappear when the pain has subsided. If the patient is attached to an oscilloscope, it is likely to show these transient changes.

9. *Then, an infarct has to be large to show up on the monitoring scope?*
   Remember that an infarct can be subendocardial, subepicardial, intramural (confined to the interior of the myocardium), or transmural (involving the full thickness of the myocardium), as well as full thickness infarct (from epicardium to endocardium).

   A shallow subendocardial infarct in the ventricular wall produces a depressed S-T segment with no particular alteration of the QRS complex in all leads facing the epicardium. If it has penetrated a little deeper, the R waves are lowered.

   A shallow infarct beneath the epicardial surface may only lower the R wave in the overlying electrode. If deeper, almost to the endocardium, the initial R wave may be replaced by a QS in the lead overlying the infarct.

   A transmural infarct, destroying the entire thickness of myocardium, will produce QS waves in the lead overlying the infarct. However, if the transmural infarct is small, it may produce no significant change at all in the QRS complex, but T wave changes may occur. The important thing to remember is that an infarct may be so small that it can only be detected by an electrode placed directly upon the heart; a precordial lead overlying it may show no change whatsoever.[2]

10. *What are the stages of myocardial infarction and the changes in electrocardiogram associated with the stages?*
    Zone of ischemia causes inversion of T wave due to altered repolarization. Zone of injury in myocardium causes elevation of S-T segment. The zone of infarction or area of death of muscle causes Q or QS waves due to absence of depolarization current from the dead tissue and opposing currents from other parts of the heart. During the recovery stage—the subacute and chronic stages—the S-T segment is often the first to return to normal, then the T wave, due to disappearance of zones of injury and ischemia.

2. J. Harold Walton, and Frank H. Netter. *The Electrocardiogram in Myocardial Infarction.* Ciba Pharmaceutical Company, Summit, New Jersey, 1968.

11. *What is meant by the "mirror" effect?*

    Remember that in the area of infarction, the heart muscle is dead and the cells cannot be either polarized or depolarized. Therefore, an electrode placed over the infarcted area will look through it as through a window and record deflections caused by the depolarization on the opposite side of the heart. There, the wave of depolarization will be receding from the endocardium to the epicardial surface, and the electrode over the infarcted area will show a Q wave. On the opposite side of the heart, unopposed by the infarct, an R wave will be written.

12. *Review briefly the predisposing factors of myocardial infarction.*

    Some of the causes increasing the risk of "heart attack" include age, heredity, obesity, high blood pressure, smoking, lack of exercise or too vigorous exercise when the body is unaccustomed to it, food, working habits, and emotional stress. These and other factors are presumed to have occurred over time to lead to changes in the coronary arteries that eventually are manifested as a myocardial infarction.

13. *What are the signs and symptoms of impending infarction?*

    The first sign many people notice is that they have a feeling of discomfort or mild pain in the chest which they attribute to dyspepsia or dietary indigestion. Soon, walking becomes a chore and the individual becomes quite fatigued upon walking short distances. He may experience chest pain as well as shortness of breath upon walking, or be awakened at night with chest pain. These are all serious warning signs and symptoms and should be more than enough to warrant immediate medical advice. When the nurse is consulted by an employee or neighbors and friends asking about such signs, she should encourage them to see their physician promptly.

14. *What are the positive symptoms of myocardial infarction?*

    The foremost and predominant symptom will be the sudden onset and intensity of pain. Pain intensifies shock and, for this reason, prompt relief of pain is important. Besides intense pain, the patient feels weak, is perspiring, and his color will look somewhat grey or cyanotic. Shortness of breath is usually present, and some nausea and vomiting. There may be a sudden drop in blood pressure; if the patient is a known hypertensive, this may be indicative of shock. It is important to remember that during the period following the onset of symptoms of myocardial infarction, the patient is in danger of ventricular fibrillation and shock. Neither the heart nor the peripheral circulation can be depended upon to respond favorably to increased demands of movement or stress. Even minor stimuli can worsen the patient's condition.

15. *What will be the course of treatment for a patient admitted with myocardial infarction?*

    You will remember that the body has certain defense mechanisms which are called into play immediately when the body balance or equilibrium is disturbed. These are regulatory mechanisms to enable the body to maintain function of the cells, tissues, organs, and systems within a central range described as normal.

    With the injury to the myocardium, as a result of obstruction in the coronary system, the sympathetic nervous system is activated. When sympathetic reflexes are effective, arteries and veins in the peripheral circulation constrict, and the blood pressure and circulation is maintained within reasonable limits. If the myocardial injury is large or the mechanisms for adapting the diameter of the blood vessels are defective, cardiac shock develops. When this happens, the effectiveness of the peripheral circulation must be increased or restored as soon as possible. Otherwise, tissue hypoxia, as well as myocardial muscle hypoxia, occurs, with progressive deterioration of cell function. Therefore, restoration of the circulation to the tissues has high priority; this is essential to the recovery of the heart and to prevention of injury to other tissues.

To decrease the demands upon the patient's heart, bed rest is ordered for at least 48 hours. The patient will do almost nothing for himself. Since he will be unaccustomed to this, the nurse must explain as briefly and as often as necessary that these are temporary measures of support until he is able. He is washed if necessary (a complete bath is not necessary if the patient is critical), turned, fed, and attached to the monitoring leads. All the while the nurse explains what she is doing and why in a quiet, firm, and confident manner. Usually a complete electrocardiograph is done by the physician, technician, or nurse, so that an initial record is obtained upon which later readings may be based or compared.

Since pulmonary edema often accompanies severe myocardial infarction, the patient is dyspneic. The head of the bed is elevated and his arms are supported to remove drag from his shoulders. A small pillow in the small of his back will add to his comfort. As soon as he is positioned and supported, pain medication should be given. If two nurses are working together, one gives priority to pain medication while the other sees to the patient's immediate needs and hooks up the oscilloscope.

If, after pain relief, the patient's blood pressure does not rise, a vasopressor may be prescribed. It may be given intravenously by slow drip. One is usually chosen which causes constriction of all vessels except the coronaries. Levophed (levarterenol) constricts all vessels and dilates the coronaries.[3]
It also increases the force of cardiac contraction and stroke volume, and cardiac irritability. It diminishes renal blood flow. Remember that this drug may cause tissue slough should the infusion infiltrate, so the physician will want to use a cannula rather than a straight needle. It must be watched carefully, not only for infiltration signs, but since this is a powerful vasopressor, it must be kept at a drip rate to regulate the blood pressure within the limits indicated by the physician. Other vasopressor agents are metarminal (Aramine), and the epinephrines. The drug prescribed depends upon the condition of the patient and the experience and preference of the physician. The nurse's responsibility is twofold: (1) to lessen the demands made on the patient to respond to his environment, and (2) to observe the effects of treatment. When the rate is too slow, clots may form in the cannula; if it is too fast, toxic reactions may be precipitated. In addition, the already overburdened heart may be overwhelmed and the capacity of the blood vessels to deliver blood restricted by overconstriction.

Besides giving attention to pain, positioning, and support to the heart and circulatory system, the next important supportive measure is the administration of oxygen. Congestion of the lungs decreases their efficiency in oxygenating the blood. The level of the oxygen concentration must be maintained at a therapeutic level; some physicians prefer to place patients in a

3. Irene L. Beland. *Clinical Nursing: Pathophysiological and Psychosocial Approaches.* The Macmillan Company, New York, 1967, pp. 628–648.

tent to ensure maintenance of concentration at the prescribed level. When the weather is hot and humid, the patient is more comfortable in an oxygen tent.

For the first 24 to 48 hours, nursing care and medical therapy are both planned to eliminate any stress to the patient in adapting to his new environment. Care is directed toward relieving shock and restoring adequacy of circulation to the tisssues. These objectives take precedence over all others for, unless they are accomplished, the patient will not recover. The length of time the patient remains on bed rest depends upon many factors. The more severe the injury or state of shock, the longer will be the time on bed rest. Other measures are regulated according to the condition of the patient. Fluids are usually restricted. (You remember that urinary output is a sensitive index to shock; it should be at least 30–40 ml per hour.) The diet will consist of fruit juices at first.

After approximately 24 to 48 hours, when the patient has recovered from initial shock, the plan of treatment will be reviewed and adapted. Rest still continues to be important, but may now be modified to include use of bedside commode. The patient should be instructed not to strain (Valsalva maneuver) or bear down during defecation. The physician usually orders a mild laxative or a stool softener. If the patient is allowed up in a chair, his position should be checked so that he is adequately supported. The chair should be of proper depth to avoid pressure at the popliteal spaces or on the calves of the legs. A footstool may help (although it has been a long time since footstools have been seen around the hospital with the new electric Hi-Lo beds).

16. *What are the true threats to the patient with myocardial infarction within the first 24 to 48 hours?*
The most frequent threats during the first 24 to 48 hours include ventricular fibrillation and arrest, pulmonary edema, extension of infarct, and shock. There is always the threat of other arrhythmias. In some patients, pulmonary edema or shock continues for several days or until the patient dies; in others, the patient may feel well within a few hours. Nursing care during this acute period should never be taken lightly. It is constantly directed toward preventing shock, preventing increase in prevailing shock or pulmonary edema, and supporting efforts for their relief.

# 16   DRUGS USED IN ARRHYTHMIAS

The cardiac arrhythmias present many challenging problems to the physician in diagnosing and treatment. Certain of them are life-threatening and require prompt and precise treatment. For this reason, he must rely upon the nurse to observe, recognize, and record disturbances in his absence, alert him at the earliest possible moment, and, at times, institute appropriate treatment. The mechanism of action, cardiotoxicity, and indications for use of the various antiarrhythmic drugs must be fully understood. The decision as to which drug to use and by what route will depend upon the type of arrhythmia as well as the severity of the clinical situation, ventricular rate, age of the patient, electrolyte values, previous administration of digitalis or other cardiac drugs, etc.

Since the emphasis is now on the importance of the nurse's role in assisting the physician as a member of the medical team in the coronary care unit, the available agents for the treatments will be discussed; sections dealing with specific arrhythmias follow.

## *Antiarrhythmic Drugs*

### DIGITALIS

The main pharmacologic effects of digitalis are due to its ability to increase the force of myocardial contractions; the manner in which digitalis influences cellular biochemical events to produce these effects is not established. Numerous studies, although yielding inconsistent results, show that digitalis influences the movement of sodium and potassium ions across heart-muscle membrane resulting in a loss of cell potassium; affects the contractile proteins; and, possibly, induces shifts in intracellular calcium concentration.

232

The specific relationship of these actions to increase in contractile force of the myocardium is not known. Let us look at the effects of digitalis administration, in low-output congestive heart failure, on certain organs and their function:

- On heart muscle—Increase in the force of systolic contraction resulting in more complete emptying and decrease in diastolic size of the heart; increase in the mechanical efficiency of the heart muscle, that is, less oxygen consumption per unit of work. Thus, you can see that the myocardial action of digitalis is its most important action.
- On heart rate—In sinus rhythm, the slowing of the ventricular rate is primarily a result of circulatory improvement from the beneficial effects on the myocardium. There is some slowing of the heart rate from a direct vagal action. Effects on the AV node increase the refractory period and slow the rate of conduction.
- On cardiac output—Increase in cardiac output is seen only in the failing heart and is secondary to improvement in cardiac contraction and emptying. In the normal heart digitalis usually does not change cardiac output.
- On venous pressure—The reduction in venous pressure is due to improved circulatory conditions and lessening of ventricular and diastolic pressure.
- On the kidney—There is some evidence that digitalis has a direct effect on the kidney, inhibiting renal reabsorption of salt and water directly, without changes in renal blood flow or glomerular filtration rate; these effects are of doubtful nature to clinical significance. Diuresis then results from increased renal plasma flow, secondary to improved cardiac output.

*Signs of digitalis effect* after administration can be noted in subsidence of dyspnea and orthopnea; disappearance of rales; slowing of ventricular rate, especially in atrial fibrillation; decrease in heart size; disappearance of "gallop" rhythm; and diuresis.

Certain ECG changes are considered classic in digitalis toxication prediction. These changes, however, are nonspecific and may be seen with myocardial disease: depression or scooping of the ST segment, followed by inversion of T wave, the Q-T interval is shortened, and the P-R interval prolonged. Their absence does not preclude recent digitalis administration.

There is always danger of *toxic manifestations* of digitalis, with gastrointestinal symptoms and cardiac irregularities among the commonest findings. Because purified glycosides may have minor local gastrointestinal irritating properties, intermittent cardiac irregularities may be the first evidences of digitalis excess; thus, toxicity may go unrecognized until serious arrhythmias develop. Some of the manifestations of digitalis toxicity are outlined here for quick reference:

- Cardiac alterations.
    In *irritability*, with tachycardias or premature systoles from any focus
    In *rhythmicity*, with occurrence of any arrhythmia, commonest of

which are ventricular premature contractions, paroxysmal atrial tachy-cardia with block, and atrial fibrillation
    In *conductivity,* with any degree of heart block
- Gastrointestinal.
    Anorexia, nausea, vomiting, diarrhea, and abdominal pain
- Visual (uncommon).
    Blurred vision, yellow vision, white halos around dark objects, di-plopia, blind spots
- Cerebral and neurologic (rare).
    Headache, fatigue, malaise, drowsiness, disorientation, confusion, delirium, dizziness, rarely convulsions, and neuralgias
- Other signs may be skin rash, vague symptoms of weakness and insomnia.

Digitalis usually is indicated for treatment of certain arrhythmias, and congestive heart failure of any etiology. It is of greatest value in low-output cardiac failure and systolic overload, but it is also given to patients with myocarditis and heart failure, or those with high-output congestive failure, even though beneficial effects in the latter may be negligible. Therapy in these situations is directed primarily at the underlying disease. Some physicians routinely administer digitalis before major surgery in patients with compensated heart disease; others feel it is not necessary since these patients obtain no significant hemodynamic effects, and the treatment of arrhythmias which might develop postoperatively becomes complicated.

Digitalis preparations are derivatives of the foxglove plants, *Digitalis purpurea* and *Digitalis lanata.* They may be whole leaf, purified glycosides, or mixtures of purified glycosides. The glycosides are said to offer certain advantages:

- They are given by weight, not biologic units.
- Absorption from the gastrointestinal tract is relatively complete and constant.
- Gastrointestinal symptoms after oral administration may be less.
- Injectionable forms are available.

Chemically, the digitalis nucleus is a phenanthrene ring. When an unsaturated lactone ring is added to the 17 position, the resulting compound is called an aglycone, which has weak cardiotonic actions. When a sugar is added in the form of a monosaccharide to the 3 position of aglycone, the resulting compound is the cardiac glycoside.[1] All nurses should be familiar with the more common forms of digitalis and their trade names (Table 1).

1. Jessie E. Squire. *Basic Pharmacology for Nursing,* 4th ed. The C. V. Mosby Co., St. Louis, 1969, pp. 9, 127.

## Table of Digitalis Preparations

| Prepa-ration | Trade Names | How Supplied: Oral Tablets Unless Specified | Parenteral | Comments |
|---|---|---|---|---|
| Digitalis, Powder U.S.P. | Digitalis | 0.05 and 1.0 gm; Tincture: 0.1 gm/ml | Available, but rarely used | If tincture is used, measurement should be made with calibrated droppers; increases in potency with standing. |
| Powd. Leaf | Digifortis | 0.1 gm (Capsule) | IM or IV 0.1 gm/ml | |
| Digitoxin | Purodigin | 0.05, 0.1, 0.15, 0.2 mg | IM or IV: 0.2 mg/ml in 40–50% alcohol | Main disadvantage is the long period of dissipation. |
| | Crystodigin Digitaline Nativelle | Same 0.1, 0.15, 0.2 mg | | |
| Digoxin | Lanoxin | 0.25 and 0.5 mg | IM or IV: 0.5 mg/2 ml in 40% propylene glycol and 10% alcohol | Rapid action and excretion makes this the favored drug for parenteral maintenance, especially if renal insufficiency present; IM inj.s painful. |
| Gitalin | Gitaligin | 0.5 mg | | |
| Lanatoside C (tabs) | Cedilanid | 0.5 mg | | |
| Deslanoside (parenteral) | Cedilanid-D | — | 0.2 mg/ml in 2 & 4ml amps.; for IM or IV use | A widely used preparation for rapid digitalization; it is not often used for maintenance. |
| Lanatoside mixture | Digilanid | 0.33 mg | | Erratic absorption. |
| Glycoside mixture | Digifolin | 0.1 gm | | Contains natural mixture of glycosides with the therapeutically inert material removed. |

Response to digitalis varies widely and is influenced by many factors. Because assay is difficult, blood levels are not available to assist in the adjustment of digitalis dosages. The physician must rely solely on the clinical status of the patient in the treatment of congestive heart failure, and any plan of therapy requires studied consideration on the dosage of the drug to produce the desired effect. In administration of digitalis to the patient, consider:

    1. Clinical status—very sick or not acutely ill: would use rapid-acting drug in former and parenteral route; slowly excreted oral drug in latter.

2. Route of excretion and rapidity of elimination: half-life of digoxin 44 hours, of leaf 14–21 days. In renal failure this is severely altered.
3. Electrolytes—diuretic administration: potassium and digitalis are antagonistic and low potassium makes patient more susceptible.

The amount of drug required to attain full digitalization depends upon the rate of digitalization; if rapid, the dose is large, the absorption time is reduced accordingly. Rapid digitalization is usually avoided when slower methods will bring the expected response; oral administration is considered safer than parenteral. As mentioned previously, a major problem for the physician is that of determining a digitalization dose for any given patient. Some physicians give the drug in moderate dosage until toxic symptoms develop, then omit it for several days before starting maintenance therapy; others administer somewhat less, and then "titrate" the patient to what is considered a maximum clinical response. Although this latter approach seems vague, it is considered the preferable approach; toxicity must be avoided, if possible, for the initial manifestations may be severe or result in a fatal cardiac arrhythmia.

*Digitalis toxicity* is estimated to occur in more than 5 percent of patients taking the drug. The most serious manifestations are cardiac arrhythmias; paroxysmal atrial tachycardia with block and nonparoxysmal nodal tachycardia are common. Others which may not be uncommon are multifocal ventricular premature contractions, ventricular tachycardia, and complete or incomplete atrioventricular dissociation. Prolonged tachycardia may bring on pulmonary edema and cerebral or coronary insufficiency.

A high degree of AV block may cause Adams-Stokes attacks. Unfortunately, digitalis intoxication is very difficult to anticipate. The ECG may give little indication of the digitalis effect, gastrointestinal symptoms may be minimal or absent, and transient cardiac irregularities may be the first evidence of digitalis excess. Because of this, digitalis is usually stopped at the first suspicion of toxicity. The serum potassium is measured to exclude hypokalemia. Methods of treatment used usually include the following:

- *Mild symptoms*—or occasional ectopic beats—usually require no treatment; withdrawal of the drug for several days is usually sufficient. If ectopic beats are very frequent, however, potassium chloride (5.0–8.0 g) may be given orally in divided doses each day for several days; Dilantin or procainamide may be given.
- *Cardiac toxicity* in most instances is treated with administration of potassium, but when high degrees of AV block are caused by digitalis intoxication, potassium salts are not given; in this case (except for paroxysmal atrial tachycardia with block) potassium may potentiate the effects of

digitalis on the conduction system, thereby further depressing AV conduction and ventricular responsiveness, and inducing more dangerous arrhythmias. (The treatment of PAT with block is discussed later in the chapter on arrhythmias.)

- *First-degree block,* common with digitalis administration, does not require specific therapy unless the P-R interval is markedly prolonged; the drug may be discontinued for several days. Complete AV block, when digitalis-induced, may be treated by infusions of disodium versenate or molar sodium lactate; isoproterenol is given cautiously for fear of developing further arrhythmias.
- *For life-endangering arrhythmias* the following may be used:

1. Potassium.

   40 mEq KCl in 500 ml 5 percent d/W over 1–2 hours; [2] monitor the ECG frequently. Intravenous use of potassium is preferred since more exact control of the drug may be maintained. However, 5 g KCl may be given orally in one dose, followed by 2 g every 3–4 hours as needed.

   *Remember:* The serum potassium level should be determined; if marked hypokalemia is present, larger amounts of potassium are given.
2. Procainamide (Pronestyl).

   Especially valuable for ventricular tachycardia; may be used in addition to potassium. Usually given intravenously, 100 mg every 1–2 hours until the arrhythmia converts, but total dose usually does not exceed 1.5–2.0 g; may be given intramuscularly, 0.5 g every 2–3 hours; orally, 1 g immediately and again 2 hours later, then 0.5 every 4–6 hours.
3. Lidocaine.

   This will be discussed later in this chapter.
4. Propranolol.

   This will be discussed later in this chapter.
5. DC countershock.

   May restore sinus rhythm in patients with digitalis-induced arrhythmias, but sudden death has been reported after attempts at cardioversion in these patients, and other methods of treatment are more often preferred.

   *Remember:* Do not give diuretics (which cause kaliuresis) or large infusions of carbohydrate (which causes intracellular shift of potassium with the deposition of glycogen) to a patient suspected of having digitalis intoxication before checking with the physician; the resultant lowering of the serum potassium concentration may aggravate the cardiac manifestations.

2. Henry J. L. Marriott. *Practical Electrocardiography,* 4th ed. The Williams and Wilkins Co., Baltimore, 1968, p. 255.

### QUINIDINE

This drug exerts beneficial antiarrhythmic effects by depressing myocardial excitability and thus ectopic impulse formation, slowing conduction speed (ECG shows widening of QRS complex), and prolonging the refractory period (ECG shows prolongation of Q-T interval).[3] Therapeutic levels also depress myocardial contractility, produce vagolytic effects, and cause varying degrees of peripheral adrenergic blockade with resultant peripheral vasodilation and hypotension.

Absorption from the gastrointestinal tract begins within 15 minutes after a single oral dose. Peak plasma concentrations occur in 2–4 hours; 40 percent disappears from the blood in 6 hours, 75 percent in 12 hours, and 90 percent in 24 hours. If repeated doses are given in a single day, the loss in blood level is slower. When quinidine is given every 2 hours, for instance, there are progressively smaller increases in blood levels after each successive dose through the fourth; no increases occur after the fifth or sixth dose because of balance between absorption and metabolic breakdown. When given every 4 hours, the maximum serum concentration occurs in 48–96 hours, then remains stable. Essentially all of the drug is excreted in the urine.

The most common side or toxic effects from quinidine are diarrhea, nausea, and vomiting. Other symptoms of salivation, ringing in the ears, dizziness, headache, visual disturbances, and confusion may occur. Administration of the drug is usually continued if the symptoms are mild. Idiosyncratic reactions such as fever, thrombocytopenic purpurea, and scaling dermatitis are uncommon. Respiratory paralysis and sudden death are rare but recognized complications of quinidine administration.

Hypotension most commonly follows parenteral administration but, rarely, vascular collapse may occur after administration of small doses orally. Myocardial toxicity may be manifested by VPCs, AV block, 50 percent or greater increase in QRS duration, ventricular tachycardia, or ventricular fibrillation. All of these are indications for stopping the drug. Unfortunately, these reactions may occur without any other preceding indications of toxicity or widening of the QRS complex on ECG. Quinidine may decrease the refractory period and conduction time of the AV node by its vagolytic effects; this action may cause undesirable increase in ventricular rate in atrial fibrillation or flutter, particularly if quinidine is administered alone.

The drug is usually administered orally; intravenous administration is usually reserved for exceptional life-endangering arrhythmias, such as ventricular tachycardia with circulatory collapse because of the high incidence of cardiovascular toxicity. With the advent of cardioversion equipment there

3. *Ibid.*, pp. 252–3.

are few, if any, circumstances in which quinidine is given parenterally. The drug is contraindicated in patients with known quinine sensitivity; it is given cautiously, if at all, in the presence of incomplete or complete AV block.

## PROCAINAMIDE (PRONESTYL)

We discussed this briefly under digitalis reaction, but there is more to be known about this sometimes "magic" preparation. As far as the cardiac actions of procainamide go, they are essentially the same as quinidine.

Absorption from the gastrointestinal tract is rapid; highest plasma concentration occurs *within 60 minutes* after administration of a single dose orally. Effects occur immediately after intravenous administration, and almost as rapidly (5–10 minutes) after intramuscular injection. Plasma level decline about 10 to 15 percent per hour. About 60 percent of the drug is excreted in the urine.

*Toxic effects* of procainamide are *severe hypotension,* which may occur after intravenous administration, much less common in intramuscular injection, and rare when administered orally. Other side effects include nausea, vomiting, anorexia, drug rash, ventricular fibrillation, or cardiac standstill. ECG changes include prolongation of the P-R, QRS, and Q-T intervals. Although the cardiotoxic effects of quinidine and procainamide are similar, the QRS widening due to quinidine may be accompanied by depression of the atrial pacemaker and AV dissocation, whereas procainamide more often includes premature beats and/or paroxysmal tachycardias. Severe cardiotoxic manifestations due to quinidine and procainamide may be treated by the administration of molar sodium lactate or EDTA.

Procainamide is most commonly used for the treatment of VPCs or other ventricular arrhythmias, especially those due to digitalis excess.

Procainamide may be given to patients who require quinidine but are sensitive to that drug. It is supplied in capsules of 250 mg and 500 mg for oral administration, and in 10 ml vials containing 100 mg/ml for parenteral use.

### LIDOCAINE

This drug has a mode of action similar to that of procainamide, but in contrast to procainamide, equivalent doses cause no fall in blood pressure or decrease in myocardial contractility. Its onset of action after intravenous administration is rapid (within 45 to 90 seconds) and duration of action brief (effects are spent within 20 minutes). The drug has been used most frequently for the treatment of ventricular arrhythmias developing during anesthesia, but more recently has been used for the treatment of unresponsive ventricular tachycardia (or, occasionally, supraventricular tachycardia) in unanesthetized patients. It may be administered in addition to procain-amide. The usual dosage is 1 mg/kg body weight intravenously by bolus and IV drip of 1–5 mg/minute, if necessary, until a maximum of 750 mg has been given. The drug is contraindicated in patients with Adams-Stokes attacks with AV dissociation and a slow nodal or idioventricular pacemaker. Side effects in unanesthetized patients include analgesia, drowsiness, discomfort in breathing or swallowing, blurred or double vision, numbness, and sweating. High doses may precipitate convulsions or respiratory arrest. Care must be taken in patients with impaired liver function since lidocaine is metabolized there and toxic levels occur rapidly.

## DIPHENYLHYDANTOIN (DILANTIN)

This drug may be very effective in treatment of certain cardiac arrhythmias, particularly those due to digitalis toxicity. Its onset of action is very rapid and toxic effects appear to be few. Clinical data are relatively limited, however, and the current literature should be studied closely. The precise mode of action is unknown, but probably related to effects of diphenyl-hydantoin on ion movement across cell membranes.

Indications for the use of diphenylhydantoin in the treatment of cardiac arrhythmias are *not well established* at present; reports indicate that a number of arrhythmias may be terminated or well controlled. Ventricular arrythmias, particularly multifocal VPCs and bigeminy, respond well, as do arrhythmias precipitated by digitalis excess. Ventricular tachycardia may be terminated; the incidence of ventricular arrhythmias associated with acute myocardial infarction or thoracic surgery may be reduced by prophylactic administration of diphenylhydantoin. Supraventricular tachycardias and APCs may also cease; atrial flutter and fibrillation are not converted to sinus rhythm, but the ventricular rate may slow significantly because of the effects of di-phenylhydantoin on increasing the degree of AV block. This drug may be administered orally in dosage of 100–200 mg three or four times daily for maintenance therapy. For acute arrhythmias 250 mg may be injected intravenously over a 5-minute period; response, if it is to occur, is usually noted within 5 minutes. Maintenance therapy is then started, but the IV dose may be repeated if the arrhythmia reoccurs.

The toxicity of long-term diphenylhydantoin therapy is reviewed in standard sources. Toxicity reactions usually occur after IV therapy and include tremors, ataxia, nystagmus, drowsiness, and confusion. Sinus bradycardia and defects in AV conduction (second degree heart block) may rarely occur; they are usually transient. Hypotension is infrequent. The drug is not usually given in the presence of marked bradycardia or high degrees of AV block.

### VASOPRESSORS

Rapid cardiac arrhythmias (especially atrial, nodal, and ventricular tachycardias) are often associated with varying degrees of hypotension. Restoration of the systemic blood pressure with vasopressor agents may terminate such arrhythmias in a significant percentage of patients, and administration of such drugs is often the first therapeutic measure employed by many physicians. The antiarrhythmic effects of pressor drugs are most likely to improve in some way the coronary perfusion, effects on the carotid sinus and arch, and, perhaps, a direct myocardial action. Blood pressure must be carefully monitored, for elevation to excessive levels may be complicated by the development of serious ventricular arrhythmias.

### PROPRANOLOL (INDERAL)

To understand the action of propranolol the nurse should remember that the norepinephrine drugs are still sometimes referred to as catecholamines. They mimic the sympathetic nervous system, thus also are referred to as sympathomimetics. Propranolol is a beta-adrenergic blocking agent that blocks catecholamine actions on the heart. Receptors in the myocardium are mainly of the beta category. These respond to the endogenous adrenergic stimulators, such as epinephrine and norepinephrine, and the exogenous stimulators, such as isoproterenol. Circulating catecholamines from the adrenal medulla also stimulate the beta-adrenergic receptors of the myocardium.

While sympathetic nervous stimulation is a significant component in supporting cardiac activity, it may also mediate the occurrence of several types of cardiac arrhythmias. Propranolol, by selectively blocking beta-adrenergic stimulation of the myocardium, will reduce increased cardiac activity, that is, the rate and force of contraction and irritability, and thereby act to abolish, control, or prevent certain arrhythmias. Another important response to beta-adrenergic blockage is the significant reduction in increased heart rate and cardiac output during exercise.[4]

Oral administration of propranolol is the preferred route of administration; intravenous administration is usually reserved for life-threatening acute arrhythmias when cardioversion techniques are not available. Orally, doses vary from 20 to 80 mg three or four times a day; intravenously, they are carefully regulated at 1 mg per 3 to 5 minutes up to a total dose of 5 mg.

The nurse must remember that propranolol is a myocardiac depressant and should not be used in the presence of bradycardia or AV block. It is contraindicated in congestive heart failure since sympathetic stimulation is a

4. Ayerst Laboratories. *Inderal, Brand of Propranolol HCl.* New York, Dec., 1967.

significant component in supporting circulatory function and propranolol would further depress the myocardium, precipitating acute heart failure. The manufacturer cautions that if propranolol is used in frank or incipient cardiac congestive failure, treatment be carried out cautiously and preferably under the protective cover of concurrent digitalization. Propranolol acts selectively without abolishing the inotropic action of digitalis on the heart muscle. In patients without a history of cardiac failure, continued depression of the myocardium over a period of time can, in some cases, lead to cardiac failure. Therefore, at the first sign or symptom of impending cardiac failure, the patient should be fully digitalized, and the response observed closely. If cardiac failure continues, propranolol is immediately withdrawn; however, if tachycardia is being controlled, the patient is usually maintained on combined dosage and closely observed until the threat of cardiac failure is over.

Propranolol also blocks the bronchodilator effects of the catecholamines; therefore, it should not be given in the presence ôf chronic lung disease or bronchospasm.

Brief mention might be made of *edrophonium* (Tensilon). This drug acts as an antagonist to curare-type drugs and is also a sympathomimetic drug. When respirations are acutely depressed, it is used to assist respirations. It should not be used in place of artificial respiration but as a supplement to it.[5]

## *Digitalis Intoxication or Toxicity*

Gastrointestinal symptoms:

- Anorexia, nausea, vomting, abdominal pain, diarrhea

Cardiovascular symptoms:

- Any arrhythmia or block, but especially
  1. Ventricular premature beats (multifocal, bigeminy)
  2. Atrial tachycardia with or without AV block
  3. AV tachycardia with or without AV dissociation
  4. AV block
  5. Ventricular tachycardia
  6. Atrial fibrillation
- Increasing heart failure

Neurological symptoms:

- Common—headache, drowsiness, dizziness, restlessness and irritability, confusion and fatigue

5. *Ibid.*

- Less common—neuralgic pains in teeth, face jaws, arms, legs, feet, epigastrium, and generalized in muscles; vertigo; hallucinations; confusion; delirium
- Rare—mood disturbances, convulsions, coma

Ocular symptoms:

- Common—blurring of vision, flashing of white light
- Rare—photophobia, oscillatory movements of eyeballs, reduced acuity, blindness, paresis of ocular muscles, diplopia

### *Treatment of Digitalis-Induced Ectopic Rhythms*

- Discontinue digitalis
- Potassium (avoid if AV block present unless low K)
- Chelation (EDTA, citrate)
- Diphenylhydantoin (Dilantin)
- Procainamide or quinidine (avoid if AV block present)
- Propranolol (avoid if AV block present, except APT with block)
- Lidocaine
- Magnesium sulfate
- Lactones
- Artificial pacing
- Cardioversion (as last resort)

### *Treatment of Digitalis-Induced Blocks*

- Discontinue digitalis
- Atropine
- Isoproterenol (Isuprel)
- Chelation (EDTA)
- Diphenylhydantoin (Dilantin)
- Intracardiac pacing

### *Summary*

In this chapter, a fairly comprehensive coverage of drugs most commonly found useful in cardiac cases has been presented. New drugs are being used in experimental units and the nurse is urged to keep a current "data" card file of her own, since many effects formerly referred to as side effects of drugs are now acceptable as the preferred action of the drug. No list of cardiac pharmacologic drugs is considered complete in our modern scientific age where new pharmaceuticals are being discovered every day.

*Review and Advance*

1. *Are certain arrhythmias associated or expected with certain types of heart conditions?*
   Although most arrhythmias can be due to a variety of physiologic, pharmacologic, and pathologic factors, certain types of heart disease are associated with certain arrhythmias frequently. For instance, some of the more common associations are: atrial fibrillation in advanced rheumatic heart disease, with mitral stenosis or mitral insufficiency, hyperthyroidism, chronic constrictive pericarditis, and in the aged patient with chronic ischemic heart disease. Ectopic beats of atrial origin are associated with advanced chronic cor pulmonale.
2. *Are certain drugs frequently associated with specific arrhythmias?*
   Among the most common arrhythmias caused by digitalis toxicity are: premature ventricular contractions occurring as bigeminal rhythm, ventricular tachycardia, various degrees of AV block, and ectopic supraventricular tachycardia with block.
   Quinidine toxicity occasionally is associated with intraventricular conduction disturbances and ventricular fibrillation. Hyperpotassemia also may produce intraventricular conduction disturbances, and hypopotassemia may produce supraventricular and ventricular ectopic beats. In addition, Adams-Stokes disease may be due to severe drug-induced bradycardia, ventricular standstill, paroxysmal ventricular tachycardia, ventricular fibrillation, and infrequently, supraventricular ectopic tachycardia or atrial flutter with a 1:1 block.
3. *Is the nurse really expected to know all these effects?*
   When a nurse elects to work in a coronary care unit, she already has been well prepared to function as a person able to make good judgments, depending upon her recognition of signs and symptoms expressed subjectively by the patient or objectively by her observations of patient and monitoring equipment. Nowhere else has she been placed as a true "teammate" of the physician since the advent of intensive care units. The last few years have seen a growing interest in other specialized units, such as cardiovascular, respiratory, and burn units; currently, emphasis is on stroke units. In the future there will be many more. The nurse should not be too critical of herself during her learning period, nor should she allow herself to be overwhelmed by the knowledge and skills she thinks she is expected to have. As she gains experience in the clinical setting, and works closely with physicians and her nursing supervisor-instructor, she may very well become very proficient in recognizing many signs that she felt beyond her capacity. As long as the nurse has the interest and enthusiasm to know all she can about her patient's disease and how she can best serve him, she will continue to learn and grow herself—even if it is by a process of osmosis. You cannot work in such a positive learning atmosphere without learning. However, if after a reasonable time, the nurse still feels overwhelmed, she should ask for a transfer.
4. *What direct action does digitalis have on the heart?*
   Digitalis is a cardiac stimulant; that is, it strengthens the heart and stimulates

it to beat more forcefully, yet more slowly. This improves circulation to all organs of the body, including the heart.

5. *What precautions must be taken in administration of digitalis?*
The pulse is always counted first, before each dose of digitalis or its derivatives is given. If the pulse is below 60 beats per minute, the nurse should check with the physician unless he has left express orders covering specified limits.

6. *What are some of the relatives or derivatives of digitalis most frequently used?*

| | |
|---|---|
| Digalen | Digifolin |
| Digitoxin | Tincture of digitalis |
| Digoxin | Cedilanid |

There are others, but these are the most common. (Refer to Tables.)

7. *What are some of the clinical symptoms of digitalis drug toxicity?*
   a. Nausea and loss of appetite; usually early symptoms.
   b. Diarrhea and vomiting: vomiting, a later symptom.
   c. Slow pulse, perhaps below 60 beats per minute, and irregular in its beat; a sudden pulse change.
   d. Headache, drowsiness, and sometimes blurred vision.

8. *What is the treatment for digitalis overdose?*
Treatment has been outlined in the Table of Digitalis Preparations. However, as ordered by the physician, the drug should be stopped immediately. Keep the patient quiet and at bed rest until improved. Increased elimination of the drug will be encouraged by the use of laxatives and enemas and the giving of more fluids by mouth. Drugs usually ordered according to the severity of overdose may include atropine, potassium salts, an anticonvulsant, a chelation, an adrenergic blocking agent (propranolol), and lidocaine. Cardioversion may be used as a last resort.

9. *Why is quinidine considered a cardiac depressant instead of a stimulant?*
Quinidine, also known as quinine derivative, acts on the muscles of the atria, or upper chambers of the heart, decreasing the irritability and the rate of conduction of impulses. In this way it slows the heart, or changes a rapid, irregular pulse to a slow, regular pulse. Quinidine aids in correcting both atrial and ventricular fibrillation and restoring the normal rhythm of the heart.

10. *What is a vasoconstrictor?*
A vasoconstrictor drug contracts the muscle fibers in the walls of the blood vessels and stimulates the vasocenter in the medulla. It is used to stop minor hemorrhage of small blood vessels, raise blood pressure, relieve nasal congestion, and sometimes increase the force of the heart action. Several vasoconstrictors are epinephrine (Adrenalin), levarterenol (Levophed), ephedrine, phenylephrine (Neo-Synephrine hydrochloride), and Pituitrin.

11. *Why is a vasoconstrictor different from a vasopressor?*
Remember we mentioned that drugs have different emphasis in treatment for different disorders? Vasopressors are drugs given definitely to raise the blood pressure; that is, they are given to prevent definite hypotensive states. For example, they are given to prevent shock postanesthesia or acute hemorrhage, reaction to drugs, coronary shock, surgical complications, and shock associated with brain damage caused by trauma or tumor.

One would assume that a drug may be classified as both vasoconstrictor and vasopressor and the assumption would be perfectly true. Such drugs include metaraminol bitartrate (Aramine) and levarterenol (Levophed).

12. *What is the difference between a vasodilator and a hypertensive drug?*
    Nothing. It is a matter of semantics again. If calling a hypertensive drug "antihypertensive" will keep it clear to the nurse, then she should label it so in her mind as well as her card file.
    The nitrites are good examples of vasodilators and hypertensives. They act on the smooth muscle of blood vessels and lower the blood pressure. They cause the fibers of the blood vessel to relax, increase the width of the vessel, and thus give vasodilator action. They relax muscle spasm in the coronary blood vessels of the heart and overcome pain of angina pectoris.

13. *What is an inotropic drug?*
    The term "inotropism" refers to the quality of influencing the contractility of muscle fibers, thus an inotropic drug influence on the heart would be one affecting the force or energy of muscular contractions. If the effect is negative, it will weaken the strength of muscular contraction; positively, it increases or strengthens the muscular contraction. Some examples of inotropic drugs are epinephrine, isoproterenol (Isuprel) ephedrine, levarterenol (Levophed), and metaraminol (Aramine). Vasoxyl is a poor inotropic.

14. *What is a chronotropic drug?*
    Again, the term "chronotropism" refers to interference with the regularity of a periodic movement such as the heart beat. Since it affects time and rate, any medication affecting the nerves whose stimulation or agents influence the rate of heart contraction can be called chronotropic. Positively, it increases the rate of contraction; negatively, it decreases the rate of contraction. The best example of a chronotropic drug is quinidine; others are procainamide (Pronestyl) and propranolol (Inderal).

15. *What are the indications for propranolol?*
    1. Cardiac arrhythmias
       a. Paroxysmal atrial tachycardia.
       b. Sinus tachycardia and extrasystoles (atrial and ventricular).
       c. Atrial flutter and fibrillation.
       d. Tachyarrhythmia of digitalis intoxication.
       e. Tachyarrhythmias associated with anesthesia.
       f. Ventricular tachycardias.
       g. Occasionally in severe tachyarrhythmias, the reduction of ventricular rate with use of propranolol may permit a more accurate electrocardiographic diagnosis of the arrhythmia.
    2. Hypertrophic subaortic stenosis
    3. Pheochromocytoma

16. *How are the dosages regulated?*
    For arrhythmias, dosages recommended are 10 to 30 mg three or four times a day, before meals and bed time; for hypertrophic subaortic stenosis, 20 to 40 mg three or four times daily, before meals and bed time. For pheochromocytoma, 60 mg is recommended daily in divided doses for three days prior to surgery, along with an alpha-adrenergic blocking agent. For management of an inoperable tumor, the recommended dosage is 30 mg daily in divided doses.

# 17 SA NODE AND ATRIAL ARRHYTHMIAS

You now know that the normal electrocardiograph tracing consists of a repetitive pattern of the P, Q, R, S, and T waves, which conform to an established standard of size and shape, and occur from 60 to 100 times each minute. If these conditions prevail, the heart is said to be in normal sinus rhythm. When rhythm is absent, or the variation from the normal rhythm differs, the disorder is called an *arrhythmia*.

## Types of Arrhythmias

There are two principle types of cardiac arrhythmias:

1. Abnormalities of cardiac impulse formation including those arising at abnormal sites (ectopic rhythms)
2. Disturbances of impulse conduction

In other words, this involves arrhythmias classified according to the site of initiation and by the type of mechanism responsible for the disorder.

At times, for therapeutic purposes, the arrhythmias are classified as either those requiring emergency treatment or those in which treatment may safely be more deliberate. Following this form, we can break them down into three categories:

1. Minor—those not of immediate concern; do not affect the circulation, but do reflect irritability of the heart (paroxysmal disturbances).
2. Major—those which reduce the efficiency of the heart or warn of im-

pending danger and require prompt treatment (premonitory rhythms, serving as a warning).

3. Death-producing—those which require immediate resuscitation necessary to prevent death.

### Interpreting a Rhythm Strip

We will leave the arrhythmias for a while and look at methods of interpreting what we see on the rhythm strip, to improve ability in recognition of "off-beat" patterns. It is not easy to know where to start but, fortunately, experience has given us some helpful guidelines. It is easier if you learn things in a sequence until it becomes second nature to you; then, you will be surprised that soon you will be able to "spot" abnormalities out of the corner of your eye, as well as estimate rate and rhythm. One word of caution, however; most electronic monitors have variable speed settings which will speed or slow the tracing "write-out." It is important to know what the particular speed is and if it has been changed from the normal.

The following order of study is suggested:

1. Run off a 6-inch ECG strip from the recorder.
2. Count the R waves in the 6-inch strip.

    Multiply this number by 10 to get the rate of heart beat in one minute. (The ECG paper is notched at the top into 3-inch strips; this becomes the easier and faster way.)

3. Note the regularity or rhythm of the R waves.

    If the R's occur at regular intervals, that is, with less variance than 0.12 second per beat, the ventricular rhythm is normal. This division of ventricular rhythm into regular or irregular will help in identifying the mechanism of the arrhythmia.

4. Examine the P waves.

    Does every P wave precede a QRS complex? If it does, the heart beat originates in the sinoatrial node and a normal sinus rhythm exists. (Caution: appearance of P wave will indicate if impulse originates elsewhere in atrium.) The normal duration is 0.11 second.

    Are the P waves shaped normally? Peaked? Notched? How? Or are the P waves all present? Absence of, or an abnormal configuration in respect to their positioning to the QRS complex indicates that the electrical stimulus started outside the sinoatrial node; an ectopic pacemaker is present.

5. Measure the PR interval.

    Normally this interval should be between 0.12 and 0.20 second. Anything longer or shorter indicates a defect in the conduction system

between the atria and the ventricles and represents a specific problem.
6. Measure the QRS complex.

Study it closely. Normally the width between the beginning of the Q wave and the end of the S wave should be no more than 0.1. If it is longer, an intraventricular defect of conduction is present.

Is the QRS complex preceded by a P wave on every beat? Is the P wave following the QRS complex?

If the ventricular complex is normal, you know that an arrhythmia is *supraventricular*; that is, either atrial or AV nodal.

If the ventricular complex is abnormal and widened, you know the arrhythmia is either *ventricular*, or *supraventricular with aberration* (abnormal conduction through ventricles).
7. Examine the T waves.

Notice direction, shape, and height. The shape is normally slightly rounded; when the waves are pointed sharply (as in myocardial infarction), grossly notched (as they sometimes are in children), it indicates some abnormality is present. The height is normally not higher than 5 mm in any standard lead. Usually T waves that are unusually tall suggest myocardial infarction or potassium intoxication.

By following this regular routine with a logical order, arrhythmias will become more meaningful to you. You will automatically recognize abnormalities, defects, and rhythm variations. And as you become more proficient at recognition, you will learn to classify arrhythmias as to their sites of origin and their mechanism, as well as "feeling" whether they are minor, major, or death-producing.

Before looking at the individual arrhythmias, there are still some other factors which will make our understanding more lasting.

## The Spontaneous Discharge Cycle

"Autorhythmicity" is a characteristic of the heart (Fig. 1). Because of this property, the heart of a laboratory animal will continue to beat when isolated from the body under experimental conditions.

Depolarization of the entire myocardium results from the spread of a depolarization wave from fiber to fiber. Normally, depolarization of myocardial fibers can be initiated by a propagated discharge from other myocardial fibers and the spontaneous discharge of a myocardial fiber.

The nature of impulse origin and cardiac rhythmicity has demonstrated that the normal resting muscle cell potential of approximately 90 millivolts falls on electrical stimulation (depolarization) to a critical level, the *threshold* potential (Figs. 2 and 3). Unlike subthreshold stimuli which result in lesser

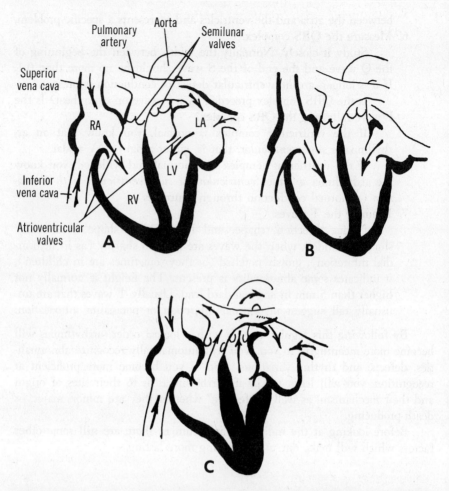

FIG. 1 Stages in the cardiac cycle. A. Heart relaxed; semilunar valves are closed; atrioventricular valves are open. Atria and ventricles are filling with blood. B. Atria are contracting; ventricles are relaxed and filling. Semilunar valves remain closed; atrioventricular valves are open. C. The atria are relaxed as the ventricles contract. The atrioventricular valves are closed; the semilunar valves are open and blood is pumped into the pulmonary artery and the aorta.

depolarization and local responses, adequate stimuli produce self-sustaining depolarization with conduction of the impulse. In pacemaker fibers, however, the resting transmembrane potential is not constant, but falls steadily after depolarization. Spontaneous excitation, accounting for inherent rhythmicity of cardiac pacemakers, occurs when the threshold has been reached. Pacemaker frequency depends on either the rate of spontaneous depolarization or the level of threshold potential. It is also influenced by certain drugs but,

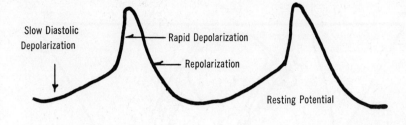

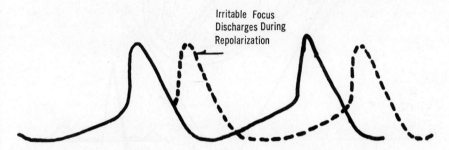

*FIG. 2* The nature of impulse origin and cardiac rhythmicity has demonstrated that the normal resting muscle cell potential of 90 millivolts falls on electrical stimulation (depolarization) to a critical level, the *threshold* potential. Unlike subthreshold stimuli which result in lesser depolarization, and local responses, adequate stimuli produce self-sustaining depolarization with conduction of the impulse. In the pacemaker fibers, however, the resting transmembrane potential is not constant, but falls steadily after repolarization. Spontaneous excitation, accounting for inherent rhythmicity of cardiac pacemakers, occurs when the threshold potential has been reached. Pacemaker frequency depends on either the rate of spontaneous depolarization or the level of threshold potential. It is also influenced by certain drugs, but, more frequently, by vagal nerve influence.

more frequently, by nervous stimuli, namely, the vagus nerve.

Myocardial fibers in the SA node have a spontaneous discharge cycle for one second or less. Moving away from the SA node in the direction in which impulses normally travel, one encounters myocardial fibers with longer and longer cycles, the longest being up to 10 seconds. This part would be in the ventricles, since they are farthest from the SA node.

Immediately after depolarization, a muscle cannot respond to further stimulation. A fraction of a second later, the muscle responds slightly to stimulation, but more slowly than a resting muscle. This whole period is called the "refractory" period. That part of the refractory period during which the muscle does not respond to stimuli is called the "absolute" refractory period. There is a time when it will respond to a greater stimulus than normal;

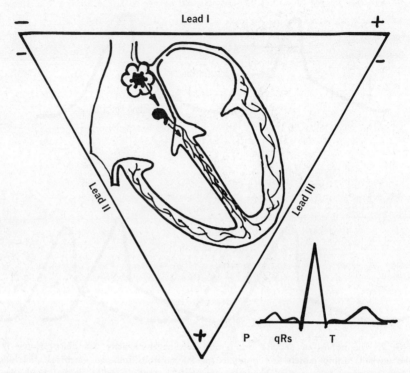

**FIG. 3** The normal cardiac cycle. *The P wave* represents atrial activity and is approximately 0.1 second wide (or 2½ small squares).

*The PR interval*, measured from the beginning of the P wave to the beginning of the q wave is 0.18 second (or 4½ small squares). It is normally not more than 0.20 second long.

*The QRS complex* represents ventricular activity and is approximately 0.1 second or less normally. The tip of the R wave occurs about 0.05 second after the beginning of a q wave. This is intrinsicoid deflection. The intrinsicoid deflection occurs over the right ventricle within 0.02 second or less and over the left ventricle within 0.05 second or less.

*The ST segment* is the state of electrical systole. No electric potential is apparent during this period, and thus, thereafter, the ST segment is on the iso-electric line.

*The T wave* represents the forces active during repolarization, or the return to the resting state. This wave usually moves in the same direction as the QRS complex.

*The horizontal lines* are 1 mm apart and represent 0.1 of a millivolt. The height of the upright deflections is measured from the top of the baseline, and the inverted complexes are measured from the bottom of the baseline.

Normally:

P wave is 1½ mm tall
q wave is 1 mm deep
R wave is 14 mm tall
s wave is 1½ mm deep
T wave is 2 mm tall.

then it is said to be in the "relative" refractory period. The process which occurs during the refractory period is repolarization, that is, a resting period before the muscle is receptive to electrical stimuli.

With these thoughts in mind, let us look briefly at the vagus nerve. You remember that under normal circumstances, the SA node is the cardiac pacemaker. The vagus nerve has a continually maintained "tone," changes in which influence the heart rate. The vagus inhibits the node, or slows the rate. Less vagal tone will speed rate—the neurotransmitter in this case is acetylcholine.

As vagal tone *increases,* cardiac rate *decreases* and the P-P interval increases, or becomes *longer.*

With a *decrease* in vagal tone, the activity of the SA node is enhanced and the heart rate *increases* and the P-P interval decreases, or becomes *shorter.*

You can see that vagal tone may well become variable. It can change with inspiration and expiration, with excitement, or temperature changes. When it is the cause of change of heart rate, there are usually arrhythmias involving changes within the SA node. Thus, an irregular vagal stimulation and depression will cause a corresponding change in sinus rhythm; this is called *sinus arrhythmia.* When the rate is over 100 beats per minute, it is called sinus tachycardia; when the rate is under 60 beats per minute, it is called sinus bradycardia. However, with the latter two, nothing else will be changed except the rate. This will help in your recognition of other bradycardias and tachycardias.

### *Normal Sinus Rhythm*

When electrical conduction is carried along the normal pathway and muscle contractions so stimulated are maintaining efficient blood circulation, the electrocardiograph tracing will reflect this. We say the pattern shows a *normal sinus rhythm,* indicating that the impulses originate in the SA node and follow the normal conduction pattern (Fig. 4).

### Normal Sinus Rhythm

- Atrial rate—60 to 100/minute
- Ventricular rate—60 to 100/minute
- Rhythm—regular
- PR interval—0.12 to 0.20 second
- P wave—upright in leads 1, 2, aVF; inverted in aVR; variable in 3, aVL, and chest leads
- QRS complex—normal
- Conduction mechanism—SA node to atria to bundle of His to left and right bundle-branches to Purkinje fibers to ventricular myocardium
- Treatment considered—none
- Significance—desirable

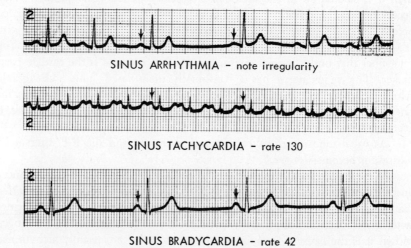

SINUS ARRHYTHMIA – note irregularity

SINUS TACHYCARDIA – rate 130

SINUS BRADYCARDIA – rate 42

**FIG. 4** Sinus rhythms. Normal P wave precedes every QRS.
(Reprinted with permission from Marriott, CCU Nursing Slides, 1967,
Tampa Tracings, Oldsmar, Fla.)

We have used the format for interpretation previously outlined and have added additional factors as to significance and treatment. We will continue to do this with all discussions of arrhythmias and most likely will add anything which will add to your recognition and understanding.

## Sinus Bradycardia

Sinus bradycardia may be a normal variation of sinus rhythm. For instance, through training, athletes normally will have heart rates sometimes as low as 30 while at rest with no great increase during exercise. It is a physiologic reaction to sleep, fright, carotid sinus massage, or ocular pressure; or it may result from such disease processes as jaundice (obstructive), glaucoma, carotid sinus sensitivity, increased intracranial pressure; or it may be seen in convalescence and as a result of digitalis therapy.

### Sinus Bradycardia

- Atrial rate—under 60/minute
- Ventricular rate—under 60/minute
- Rhythm—regular and slow (normal rate of impulse formation slow)
- P-R interval—0.10 to 0.20 second—may be upper limits of normal

- P wave—same as NSR
- QRS complex—normal
- Conduction mechanism—normal in all respects except slowness
- Treatment considered—atropine, Isuprel
- Significance—may presage cardiac arrest and, because of slowness, an irritable focus may take over pacemaking

## Sinus Tachycardia

In adults the rate in sinus tachycardia usually varies between 100 and 160, but in children (and in adults with severe hypermetabolic states) the rate may be higher. Clinically the rhythm is basically regular, but minimal cyclic variations may be present. The ECG will show slight but significant changes in rate if monitored over a period of 5 to 10 minutes. Response to carotid sinus pressure is variable; there is often slight and gradual slowing, but the arrhythmia is not terminated. Sinus tachycardia is frequently a manifestation of congestive heart failure in the CCU setting and will not respond to digitalis administration; indeed, digitalis given to the anoxic, hypovolemic, or septic patient with sinus tachycardia may produce severe ventricular arrhythmias. Therapy is directed at the underlying cause.

### Sinus Tachycardia

- Atrial rate—100 to 180/minute
- Ventricular rate—100 to 180/minute
- Rhythm—regular—rapid
- P-R interval—0.12 to 0.20 second
- P wave—same as NSR
- QRS complex—normal
- Conduction mechanism—rapid formation of stimulus; normal of SA nodes; P wave sometimes rides on end of preceding T.
- Treatment considered—propranolol; treatment of underlying cause, that is, fever, excitement, hypoxia, shock, congestive heart failure
- Significance—frequently innocuous but may be potentially dangerous; propanolol or pacing may be considered.

## Sinus Arrhythmia

In sinus arrhythmia, the pacemaker is in the SA node, but the node forms impulses irregularly. They are influenced (as previously stated) by inspiration and vagal tone; that is, the heart accelerates with inspiration and slows with expiration. However, there is a less common type in which the changes in rate bear no relationship to the phases of respiration. A sinus arrhythmia can be a perfectly normal finding, but on occasion it can be confused with other arrhythmias because of severe irregularity.

## Sinus Arrhythmia

- Atrial rate—60 to 100/minute.
- Ventricular rate—60 to 100/minute.
- Rhythm—irregular R-R should vary at least 0.12 second between longest and shortest. Increase /c inspiration; decrease /c expiration.
- P-R interval—varies 0.12 to 0.20 second.
- P wave—normal, but may vary in configuration.
- QRS complex—normal.
- Conduction mechanism—normal variations due to vagal influence.
- Treatment considered—none; this may be a normal variation.
- Significance—Sinus node forms impulses irregularly. There are two varieties:
  1. One that waxes and wanes with the phases of respiration, the heart accelerates /c inspiration and slows /c expiration.
  2. Less common. Bears no relationship to phases of respiration. May be perfectly normal, but occasionally so irregular that it can be confused clinically with other more important arrhythmias.

## Sinus Block or Sinus Arrest

Sometimes, impulses from the SA node are blocked before they reach the atria. ECG tracing reveals a complete loss of one complete complex. The pause is equal to twice the length of one cycle, and is termed *sinus block* or *sinus arrest*.

## Sinus Block

- Atrial rate—60 to 100/minute.
- Ventricular rate—60 to 100/minute.
- Rhythm—regular except for period of sinus block.
- P-R interval—0.10 to 0.20 second.
- P Wave—normal when preesnt.
- QRS complex—normal.
- Conduction mechanism—complete absence of PQRST complex. The pause is in multiples of the normal P-P interval.
- Treatment considered—atropine. This may suggest digitalis overdose; isoproterenol or pacemaker may be needed at times.

## Sinus Arrest (Fig. 5)

- Atrial rate—60 to 100/minute, toward lower limits.
- Ventricular rate—60 to 100/minute, toward lower limits.
- Rhythm—regular except for period of sinus arrest.
- P-R interval—0.10 to 0.20 second.
- P wave—normal when present.
- QRS complex—normal.
- Conduction mechanism—complete absence of PQRST complex. This pause is not an exact multiple of the P-R interval.
- Treatment considered—atropine. This may suggest digitalis overdose; isoproterenol or pacemaker may be needed at times.

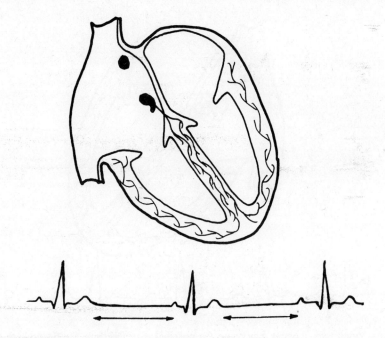

*FIG. 5* Sinus arrest. The SA node refuses to "fire" during pause which may be twice the length of the normal cycle.

## *Wandering Pacemaker*

The pacemaker may shift within the SA node. The ECG may reveal slight changes in the configuration of the P waves. This phenomenon is usually associated with sinus arrhythmia.

Variations in vagal tone may cause a shift of the pacemaker from the SA node to the AV node and back again (Fig. 6). Progressive changes in the size and shape of the P waves will correspond with the shifting of the stimulus.

A continually changing heart rate caused by the shifting of the maker is said to be a *wandering pacemaker*.

### Wandering Pacemaker

- Atrial rate—60 to 100/minute.
- Ventricular rate—60 to 100/minute.

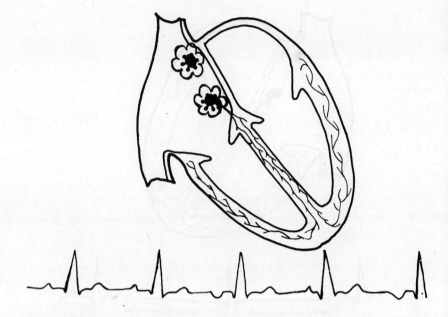

*FIG. 6* Vagal tone changes may cause the pacemaker to shift from the SA node to the AV node and back again.

- Rhythm—irregular.
- P-R interval—variable, from abnormally short to upper limits of normal.
- P wave—varies in configuration; upright diphasic inverted flat.
- QRS complex—normal.
- Conduction mechanism—above the AV node the conduction pathway depends on the site where the impulse originates.
- Treatment considered—usually none; observe for digitalis toxicity; potassium may be given.
- Significance—the site of impulse formation may vary between SA and AV nodes, some arising from one or the other and others arising from the intermediate atrial muscle. This switch of pacemaker is often precipitated by a premature beat.

## *Premature Atrial Contraction (APC) or (PAC)*

If the SA node is depressed by vagal action to the extent that its spontaneous discharge cycle is no longer the shortest in the heart, the ectopic focus with the shortest cycle will take over as the pacemaker. If the SA node is "shielded," or untouchable, or unable to be influenced, by drugs or disease, no atrial or nodal depolarization can reset the spontaneous cycle of the SA node; the atria are still in an absolute refractory state. When this occurs, there may be a lengthened interval between the ectopic beat and the next normal beat. This interval is known as the *compensatory pause*. The interval between a normally occurring beat and a subsequent premature beat is called the *latency interval* (Fig. 7). (Caution: most APCs do not have a compensatory pause as do VPCs.)

The constant latency observation is an important generalization about premature beats and their relationship to the previously occurring beat, that is, for any given ectopic focus the premature beat occurs the same length of time after the previous normal beat. The theory is accepted that when a myocardial fiber outside the SA node fires during its repolarization phase or produces a premature beat, it may be described as having increased "irritability." When an ectopic focus produces a premature beat it may be called an "irritable" focus.

Since constant latency is a characteristic of the firing of an ectopic, or irritable, focus, the early discharge of such a focus must occur at the same point in its repolarization phase. But, for reasons unknown, an irritable focus may discharge either intermittently or in a constant, repetitive fashion. It is possible for an ectopic to produce (1) one isolated beat, (2) two consecutive beats, (3) a series of consecutive beats, or (4) all of these interchangeably.

To sum up, a cardiac cycle will be produced by that cardiac fiber which discharges earlier than any other. In order to initiate a cardiac cycle, an ectopic focus must fire before the SA node completes its cycle. Thus, if the depolarization wave initiated by an ectopic focus reaches the SA node before its spontaneous discharge cycle is completed, the SA node will be discharged by a propagated wave. On the other hand, an ectopic focus can prevent the SA node from firing spontaneously, when the depolarization wave from the ectopic focus reaches the SA node before the SA node has completed its own spontaneous depolarization cycle.

What this all adds up to is this: An ectopic focus outside the SA node may initiate a cardiac cycle (1) when the SA node is depressed and this cardiac cycle will be shorter than the cycle initiated by the SA node, and (2) when a focus other than the SA node fires before the SA node has completed its normal spontaneous discharge cycle. Thus, whether an atrial ectopic focus takes over either as pacemaker sporadically, infrequently, or regularly, we say there has occurred an atrial premature contraction.

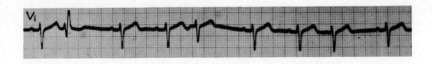

*FIG. 7* Three atrial premature beats with one showing ventricular aberration.
(Reprinted with permission from Marriott, CCU Nursing Slides, 1967,
Tampa Tracings, Oldsmar, Fla.)

## Premature Atrial Contraction

- Atrial rate—usually normal.
- Ventricular rate—usually normal.
- Rhythm—regular except for premature beats.
- P-R interval—0.10 to 0.20 second.
- P wave—normal except for PACs.
- QRS complex—normal.
- Condition mechanism—irritable atrial focus /c rate exceeding that when SA node intiates the impulse.
- Treatment considered—frequently heralds onset of atrial fibrillation on paroxysmal atrial tachycardia, or frequently is manifestation of underlying congestive heart failure, thus digitalis and diuretic therapy considered; propranolol, quinidine, lidocaine sedation (digitalis, if not digitalis-induced).
- Significance—minor if PACs sporadic or less than 6/minute. They foretell a more rapid repetitive rhythm or a more serious atrial arrhythmia.
- Salient features:
  1. Abnormal, often inverted, premature P wave
  2. Normal QRST
  3. Ensuing interval about equal to, or slightly longer than, the normal cardiac cycle

## *Atrial Tachycardia*

A premature beat can disturb the rhythm of the heart. Occasionally, an atrial premature beat appears so early that the AV node is unable to respond; this is a blocked atrial premature contraction, and the QRS complex may be absent. Just as it may block beats, the atrial premature contraction may speed up their firing. Atrial tachycardia may be produced by a repetitive firing of an ectopic focus (Fig. 8). This may be continuous or last for only brief

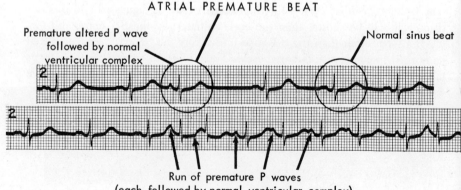

ATRIAL PREMATURE BEAT

Premature altered P wave
followed by normal
ventricular complex

Normal sinus beat

Run of premature P waves
(each followed by normal ventricular complex)
= ATRIAL TACHYCARDIA

*FIG. 8*  Atrial premature beat and atrial tachycardia.
(Reprinted with permission from Marriott, CCU Nursing Slides, 1967,
Tampa .Tracings, Oldsmar, Fla.)

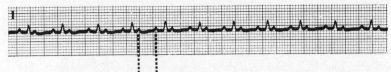

Two P waves for every QRS - only every alternate impulse is
conducted to the ventricles.

*FIG. 9* Atrial tachycardia with 2 to 1 AV block.
(Reprinted with permission from Marriott, CCU Nursing Slides, 1967,
Tampa Tracings, Oldsmar, Fla.)

periods at a time. In the latter instance, the ectopic beats must occur at least
four times in a row at a rate exceeding 100 per minute and more likely somewhere between 160 to 240 per minute. The P waves, when recognizable, show
an abnormal form like that of an atrial premature contraction. The P wave
may be superimposed on the T wave making its identity difficult or impossible. The QRS group in this form of tachycardia may be perfectly normal,
or slightly or markedly different; this is referred to as *aberrant conduction.*
Paroxysmal tachycardia usually begins and stops abruptly.

## Paroxysmal Atrial Tachycardia (Fig. 9)

- Atrial rate—140 to 220, usually 180 to 220/minute.
- Ventricular rate—140 to 220, usually 180 to 220/minute.
- Rhythm—regular.
- P-R interval—not definable.
- P wave—usually fused onto preceding T wave.
- QRS complex—usually normal.
- Conduction mechanism—rapid succession of atrial rhythmic contractions.
- Treatment considered—carotid sinus pressure, Valsalva maneuver, Neo-synephrine (vasopressor),
  edrophonium chloride (short-acting cholinesterase inhibitor), sedation, quinidine, procainamide,
  short-acting digitalis preparation.
- Significance—dangerous if persistent and rates continue high because of reduced cardiac output. Morbidity increases with age and underlying heart disease.
- Salient features:
  1. Rapid, regular, normal QRS complexes
  2. Abnormal P waves preceding QRS (rarely discernible)
  3. ST-T depressions frequently seen

## *Paroxysmal Supraventricular Tachycardia*

This represents a paroxysmal atrial tachycardia (PAT), paroxysmal nodal tachycardia, or a group of arrhythmias in which the course of the ectopic
focus cannot be determined (Fig. 10). The rate varies from 150 to 300 plus,
but most of these arrhythmias are in the 160 to 200 range; the atrial and

ventricular rates are the same. Clinically the rhythm is characterized by a monotonous regularity, often of sudden onset and cessation; a 10–15-minute period of ECG monitoring will show variation of less than three beats per minute. Carotid sinus pressure either abolishes the arrhythmia or produces no effects. The ECG shows a more or less normal QRS complex, but confusion may arise when there is marked aberration or bundle-branch block occurring with more rapid rates; this is particularly common in patients with diseased hearts or the Wolff-Parkinson-White (WPW) syndrome. Supraventricular tachycardias frequently occur in patients with otherwise normal hearts. As a rule they do not constitute severe medical emergencies unless they have precipitated cardiac heart failure, vascular collapse, or pain of coronary insufficiency. In these latter situations the urgency for immediate restoration of sinus rhythm would weigh strongly for cardioversion as the therapy of choice if carotid sinus massage and administration of vasopressors do not abolish the arrhythmias promptly. In less seriously ill patients, the other measures discussed below may be tried. Young healthy patients with supraventricular tachycardias often respond to one or more of the first four measures described, but patients wtih heart disease frequently require digitalis for restoration of sinus rhythm. Sedation and reassurance often will restore normal sinus rhythm.

Many attacks can be terminated by increasing vagal tone. Carotid sinus pressure is usually tried first. The patient must be lying down; the ECG should be monitored constantly. The right carotid sinus should be massaged first, for 10 to 30 seconds, and if this is ineffective, then the left. Both carotid sinuses should *not* be massaged simultaneously since there is danger that asystole or cerebrovascular thrombus may result. Eyeball pressure is not recommended because of occasional retinal detachment. Edrophonium chloride (Tensilon), a short-acting cholinesterase inhibitor, acts by preventing the depolarization of the end plate at the myoneural junction. It aids the accumlation of acetycholine stimulating parasympathetic division of the autonomic nervous system.

Vasopressors are generally used whenever hypotension exists, but in addition, they are frequently effective in normotensive patients, probably by stimulating the carotid sinus and aortic receptors and increasing coronary blood flow. Neo-Synephrine, 0.5–1.0 mg, or metaraminol (Aramine), 0.5–2.0 mg, may be injected intravenously over a 2 to 3-minute period. Ectopic beats and significant rises in blood pressure may occur.

From our discussion so far, rapid digitalization is the most effective and consistent therapy, and is usually tried if simple measures do not terminate the attack promptly. Digoxin may be given orally to those patients in no great distress, but usually intravenous administration is indicated for those whose arrhythmias require rapid termination. Cedilanid, 0.4–0.8 mg, is usu-

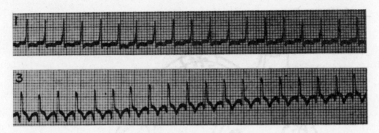

*FIG. 10* Supraventricular tachycardia. So called because there is no sure way to be sure whether they are atrial or AV nodal.

(Reprinted with permission from Marriott, CCU Nursing Slides, 1967, Tampa Tracings, Oldsmar, Fla.)

ally given intravenously over 2 to 3 minutes, followed by another 0.4 mg 60 to 90 minutes later. Equivalent doses of digoxin are sometimes used, 0.75–1.0 mg initially, followed by another 0.25–0.5 mg in 60 to 90 minutes. Recently, Ouabain has come into use but the initial dosage varies, and almost continuous ECG is required. The dosage of 0.25–0.5 mg every 30 to 45 minutes thereafter. Quinidine, procainamide, or diphenylhydantoin may be used in certain situations also. Probability of recurrent attacks is lessened by sedation, avoidance of coffee, tea, tobacco, and overfatigue and, if necessary, the patient is kept on maintenance doses of digitalis and/or quinidine.

## *PAT with Block*

This rhythm (Fig. 11), the "great masquerader," may appear clinically as normal sinus rhythm, atrial flutter, or supraventricular tachycardia. More than 75 percent of cases result from digitalis excess. Cardinal ECG findings include a rapid atrial rate, usually between 150 and 210, rarely faster. (With flutter the atrial rate is greater.) In contrast to flutter the S-T segments are isoelectric, the P waves are upright in leads 2 and 3, and the atrial rate may vary considerably, demonstrating a "ventriculophasic" effect, that is, the P-P interval surrounding a ventricular complex is shorter than the P-P interval not enclosing a QRS. The P waves are often small, bizarre, and spiked in shape; they may be recognizable in only one lead, often $V_1$ or other right-sided leads (precordial). The ventricular rate varies, depending on the degree of AV block, and may be almost regular to grossly irregular. Response to carotid sinus pressure varies, but often there are variations in AV conduction, while changes in atrial rate are rare. It is most necessary to differentiate PAT with block from atrial flutter; the former is frequently a manifestation of digitalis excess, whereas the latter is rarely so.

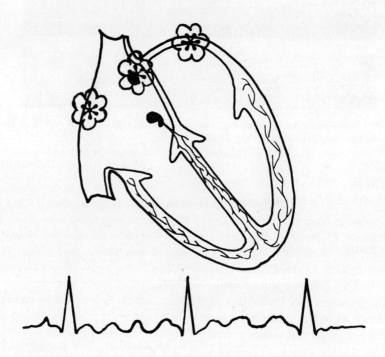

*FIG. 11* Atrial flutter is very similar to atrial fibrillation. The atrial rate generally varies between 240 and 350; but, in certain patients, especially if they are receiving quinidine, it may be 200 or less. The ventricular rate varies with the degree of block.

The treatment usually consists in stopping digitalis immediately if it is being given. If digitalis intoxication is suspected, the physician gives potassium. In urgent situations, potassium is given intravenously 40 mEq KCl in 500 ml 5 percent D/W over 1 to 3 hours. In less serious situations KCl may be given orally; 4–5 g initially, followed by 2 g every 3 to 4 hours as needed. Procainamide, in usual dosage, may be used alone or in addition to potassium salts.

*A point to remember:* When PAT with block is not a reflection of digitalis intoxication, digitalis is usually the drug of choice for therapy.

### PAT with Block

- Atrial rate—180 to 220/minute.
- Ventrical rate—depends on degree of AV block.
- Rhythm—regular.
- P-R interval—lower limits of normal if definable.

- P wave—upright.
- QRS complex—normal.
- Conduction mechanism—ratio block; only intermittent impulses are conducted through the AV node. Same as in atrial tachycardia. Some impulses from atria do not get through to the ventricles and therefore, QRS does not follow these P waves, as high as 5:1 block.
- Treatment considered—stop digitalis; give IV potassium.
- Significance—most usually associated with digitalis toxicity. Potentially dangerous.

## *Atrial Flutter*

This arrhythmia is very similar to atrial fibrillation. The atrial rate generally varies between 240 and 350; in certain patients, especially if they are receiving quinidine, it may be 200 or less; still, in rare cases, it has been known to go as high as 400. The ventricular rate varies with the degree of AV block, which is usually 2:1 in untreated cases. A 1:1 block is rare, but any regular rhythm with a ventricular rate greater than 270 is almost usually flutter with 1:1 conduction and constitutes one of the real cardiac emergencies. Response to carotid sinus pressure, if one occurs, is manifested by a sudden jerky mathematical reduction in rate as the degree of AV block is increased. Physician may be able to make his diagnosis of observing *rapid A waves* in the neck veins. ECG recognition is not always easy: With constant 2:1 block the second F wave (flutter) may not be obvious, but carotid pressure will often make the arrhythmia wave clear. An important point to look for is a characteristic undulating or "saw-toothed" base line (Fig. 12), usually best seen in leads 2, 3, and aVF. F waves may well be seen in the right precordial leads and in any lead where the QRS complex is small. The etiology of flutter is frequently the same as fibrillation, but in almost all cases digitalis intoxication can be excluded as the cause.

The most important differential is from PAT with block as previously discussed, especially since the latter arrhythmia is *secondary* to digitalis excess in more than 75 percent of cases.

Control of flutter may require 2 or 3 times the usual digitalizing dose, even when patients are receiving maintenance digitalis. An important point to remember now is that following administration of digitalis the degree of AV block is increased, and the ventricular rate slows. The rhythm may revert to sinus or to atrial fibrillation. If the latter occurs, quinidine may be given in an attempt to convert to sinus rhythm, but occasionally careful withdrawal of digitalis will be followed by resumption of a sinus mechanism. Atrial flutter almost always responds to cardioversion, and for seriously ill patients with rapid ventricular rates this may be the initial therapy of choice. In less urgent cases drug therapy is usually tried first. Quinidine should not be given to a patient with atrial flutter without first giving digitalis since it can be frequently implicated as a cause for 1:1 conduction in this situation.

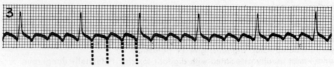

4 "F" waves to each QRS = 4 to 1 A-V conduction.

*FIG. 12* Atrial flutter. "Sawtooth" atrial flutter ("FF") waves in regular relationship to QRS.

(Reprinted with permission from Marriott, CCU Nursing Slides, 1967, Tampa Tracings, Oldsmar, Fla.)

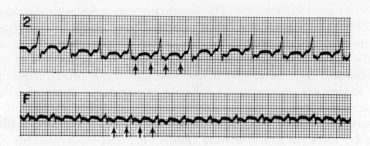

*FIG. 13* Atrial flutter. When the AV ratio is 2 to 1 (as it most often is) the F waves are not always easy to spot (arrows).

(Reprinted with permission from Marriott, CCU Nursing Slides, 1967, Tampa Tracings, Oldsmar, Fla.)

## Atrial Flutter (Fig. 13)

- Atrial rate—250 to 350–400/minute.
- Ventrical rate—depends on degree of AV block, 70 to 150–200/minute as a function of block.
- Rhythm—atrial rhythm 15 regular; ventricular rhythm regular if degree of block 13 consistent.
- P-R interval—not definable.
- P wave—saw-toothed flutter waves.
- QRS complex—normal usually.
- Conduction mechanism—same as PAT /c block ectopic site or "circus mechanism" in atrial muscle produce extremely rapid impulses AV node cannot respond to each impulse and thus some form of block.
- Treatment considered—carotid pressure increases degree of block (diagnostic), digitalis, quinidine (if no spontaneous reversions), cardioversion (start at 20 joules).
- Significance—potentially dangerous because of possible tachycardia. Reduced pumping efficiency may result in lessened cardiac output, congestive heart failure, or coronary insufficiency.
- Salient features:
  1. "Saw-tooth" or undulating base line of "F" waves in lead 2, 3 and aVF.
  2. Normal QRS complexes in 2:1 to 8:1 ratio
  3. T waves swamped by the F wave pattern

## *Atrial Fibrillation*

Atrial fibrillation is characterized by a rapid rate and irregular rhythm (Fig. 14). In undigitalized patients, the ventricular rate is generally over 100 and may even exceed 200. Clinically no jugular A waves are seen; the first heart sound is variable in intensity; a pulse deficit is usually present. Carotid sinus pressure produces gradual and transient slowing of the ventricular rate but no reversion. The ECG shows gross irregularity associated with a QRS complex which is usually normal, but occasionally widened and bizarre due to ventricular aberration or bundle-branch block. No matter how bizarre the QRS, however, a very rapid, grossly irregular rhythm is usually atrial fibrillation or atrial flutter with varying block; these should not be confused with ventricular tachycardia.

Chronic atrial fibrillation is most often associated with rheumatic heart disease (particularly mitral valve disease), ischemic or hypertensive heart disease, and diffuse myocardial disease. Occasionally, it may occur in patients with constrictive pericarditis, thyrotoxicosis, or the WPW syndrome. In some patients no heart disease is demonstrable. Paroxysmal atrial fibrillation may be produced by digitalis intoxication or pulmonary embolus. It may occur in young, healthy persons under increased emotional stress.

Primary treatment consists of digitalization of the patient. If rapid digitalization is necessary, the IV route of administrations is used, but if the patient is not acutely ill, the oral route is more frequently used. Digitalization proceeds until the ventricular rate is controlled in the range of 60–80 beats per minute at rest or 90–110 beats per minute after slight exercise; maintenance doses may then be given. Larger than usual doses of digitalis are frequently necessary to control the ventricular rate.

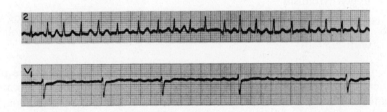

*FIG. 14* Two views of atrial fibrillation: with rapid ventricular response (170 rate); with slow ventricular response (40 rate).
(Reprinted with permission from Marriott, CCU Nursing Slides, 1967, Tampa Tracings, Oldsmar, Fla.)

Special problems may be presented by the patient with atrial fibrillation and slow ventricular response rate (40–60 beats per minute); these patients are often in the older age groups and have vascular disease or disease of the AV node. Generally, if such patients do not develop excessive ventricular rates after exercise or show evidence of congestive heart failure, the physician feels there is no immediate need for digitalis administration. However, these patients have a high inclination of further rhythm disturbances such as sino-atrial standstill, sinoatrial block, slow AV nodal rhythm associated with reversion of atrial fibrillation.

During or after digitalization, conversion to normal sinus rhythm may occur; if it does not, then the controversial problem arises as to whether further measures are to be attempted to restore sinus rhythm.

The dangers of attempting reversion in any given patient, you will remember from our discussion on electrical conversion, must be weighed against the dangers of allowing atrial fibrillation to continue. Some of the guidelines useful in assisting the physician in making this decision are as follows:

- *Indications.* Conversion of atrial fibrillation, according to most cardiologists, should be considered in the following cases:

  1. Those who are incapacitated by their cardiac disease despite intensive therapy; for instance, angina, persistent congestive heart failure
  2. Those patients of any age whose cardiac status has deteriorated following the appearance of atrial fibrillation
  3. Those with episodes of peripheral or pulmonary emboli thought to originate from the atria
  4. Those with atrial fibrillation of less than six months' duration, whether symptomatic or not, especially in the younger age group
  5. Those who have undergone a technically successful mitral valvotomy or valve replacement
  6. Those with atrial fibrillation persisting after successful treatment of hyperthyroidism
  7. Those in whom the awareness of cardiac irregularities is disturbing
  8. Those in whom the ventricular rate cannot be adequately controlled with digitalis

- *Contraindications.* Reversion must be considered in the light of the patient's tolerance of a "maintenance" drug such as quinidine or procainamide since some such drug usually is given to prevent relapse, though this is not "routine." Quinidine is not indicated in patients whose atrial fibrillation has repeatedly recurred after previous successful reversions.

Methods for conversion of atrial fibrillation to sinus rhythm may be by drug or electrical. The use of the cardiovertor and pharmacology of quinidine and procainamide have already been discussed.

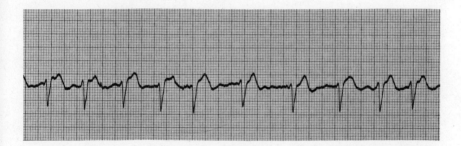

*FIG. 15* Atrial fibrillation strip taken on a 76-year-old male who did not respond to various forms of treatment. Atrial rate at 110. (See also Chap. 18, Figure 17.)

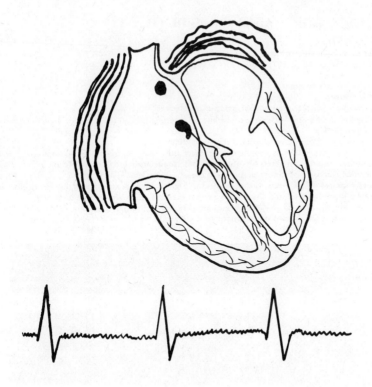

*FIG. 16* Atrial fibrillation is characterized by a very rapid rate of the atrii with intermittent ventricular response.

## Atrial Fibrillation (Figs. 15 and 16)

- Atrial rate—over 400/minute.
- Ventrical rate—variable; random impulses are conducted through the AV node.
- Rhythm—totally irregular.
- P-R interval—nonexistent.
- P wave—fibrillation waves; no true P, rather rapid and chaotic F waves.
- QRS complex—usually normal, may differ in size due to fatigue factor.
- Conduction mechanism—random impulses are conducted through the AV node. Atrial ectopic focus or foci discharge at rates as high as 500/min., producing irregular oscillations rather than P waves. Result is random response of ventricle and irregular QRS rhythm.
- Treatment considered—digitalis; quinidine; propranolol; cardioversion usually converts 90 percent; anticoagulants; hypothermia (if all else fails).
- Significance—particularly dangerous with ventricular responses over 100/min. Digitalis increases AV block which slows ventricles. Occasionally converts to sinus rhythm, especially if secondary to failure.
- Salient features:
  1. Absence of P waves, which are replaced by irregular "F" waves (or no sign at all of atrial activity)
  2. Normal QRS complexes, irregular in time and sometimes varying in amplitude.

## Atrial Standstill (Fig. 17)

- Atrial rate—nonexistent (atrial paralysis)
- Ventricular rate—50 to 80/minute
- Rhythm—regular
- P-R interval—non-existent
- P wave—none
- QRS complex—depends on site of ectopic pacemaker
- Conduction mechanism—ectopic pacemaker originating in the AV node or below /c no retrograde conduction
- Treatment considered—stop digitalis; stop quinidine
- Significance—pacemaker is completely knocked out, and two things can happen: (1) a lower pacemaker, usually in the AV junction but sometimes in the ventricles, takes over, or (2) cardiac standstill continues and patient dies.
- Salient features—If (1) occurs, and ventricles beat independently, nodal or ventricular escape is said to have occurred and the heart's rhythm is called idionodal or idioventricular:
  1. Complete absence of R—QRS—T sequence 1R by a straight and unadorned base line.
  2. Independent QRST complexes appear at a slow rate while P waves remain absent.

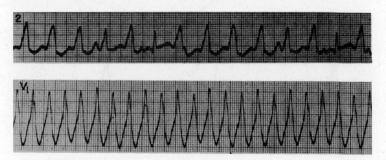

FIG. 17  Ventricular tachycardia; one with independent P waves; one with no atrial activity.  (Reprinted with permission from Marriott, CCU Nursing Slides, 1967, Tampa Tracings, Oldsmar, Fla.)

## *Cardioversion*

External electrical reversion of cardiac arrhythmias became clinically practical with the development by Paul Zoll of an AC (60-cycle alternating current) defibrillator capable of terminating episodes of ventricular fibrillation. It was soon apparent that AC "shock" could terminate other arrhythmias as well, but its use was reserved as a "last resort" measure because of serious drawbacks; the shock was long in duration (160 milliseconds) and could provoke protracted arrhythmias or cardiac standstill; electrical discharge occurring during the ventricular vulnerable period precipitated ventricular fibrillation; and the high energy levels required for reversion occasionally produced myocardial damage as evidenced by ECG changes and enzyme rises. The development of capacitor discharge (DC) by Lowen circumvented these hazards. Capacitor discharge of 2.5 milliseconds and synchronization of shock to avoid the ventricular vulnerable zone (a brief interval of about 30 milliseconds at the ascending limb and apex of the T wave) prevented development of ventricular fibrillation (Fig. 18).

*Cardioversion,* now meaning "DC electrical reversion of arrhythmias through the intact chest wall," was used initially only in patients with atrial fibrillation who were "drug failures" or required rapid reversion of the arrhythmia because of critical clinical status. The incidence of side effects of DC reversion proved low, and the technique became the method of choice of many observers for reverting chronic atrial fibrillation, atrial flutter, ventricular tachycardia, and those cases of supraventricular tachycardia resistant to drug therapy. Unfortunately, cardioversion equipment is not universally available; the cost of equipment is still high; and indications for its use have not been fully defined. Although the response to countershock is immediate and dramatic, availability of this form of therapy will not remove the necessity for administration of antiarrhythmic drugs in a wide variety of clinical circumstances.

Most observers agree that cardioversion, when available, is the initial therapy of choice for ventricular tachycardia accompanied by circulatory col-

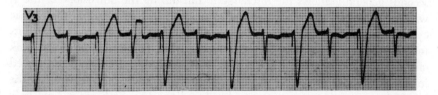

**FIG. 18** Artificial pacemaker beats regularly interpolated between normal (?) sinus beats.

lapse unresponsive to bolus lidocaine. Supraventricular tachycardias with rapid ventricular rates should be treated promptly with DC electrical shock if a response to drug therapy does not occur quickly in patients compromised hemodynamically. Atrial flutter not responsive to full doses of digitalis and a several-day period of quinidine administration can be converted to sinus rhythm with countershock; some physicians recommend a prior dose of quinidine. More than 90 percent of these arrhythmias respond. Atrial fibrillation, even that of long duration or resistant to large doses of quinidine, can be converted to sinus rhythm in a similar percentage of cases, but unfortunately the number of patients who maintain normal sinus rhythm for any length of time, despite quinidine prophylaxis, is considerably less (about 40 percent). In general, patients are chosen for cardioversion of atrial fibrillation by the same criteria used in selecting them for quinidine administration; the incidence of conversion with cardioversion, however, is approximately twice that with quinidine.

Cardioversion is usually not useful in the treatment of recurrent tachycardias, in the treatment of atrial fibrillation associated with rheumatic heart disease, in those patients who cannot tolerate quinidine (since maintenance of normal sinus rhythm is virtually impossible), and in the treatment of drug-induced arrhythmias. Cardioversion should not be used, then, for treatment of arrhythmias resulting from digitalis intoxication since ventricular fibrillation or cardiac standstill may occur.

The technique for cardioversion is well described in Bellet's textbook, *Clinical Disorders of the Heart Beat* (2nd ed., Philadelphia: Lea and Febiger, 1963) and in reports by Low (*New Eng. J. Med.* 269: 325, 1963). Patients with atrial fibrillation are frequently given anticoagulants for 2 to 3 weeks before attempts at cardioversion on the same grounds governing their use prior to attempts at reversion with quinidine. If they are fully digitalized, as a rule it is usual to wait 24 to 48 hours after the last dose; and they are given quinidine 0.3 g every four hours for 24 hours before cardioversion.

The procedure is carried out under light thiopental anesthesia, but cardioversion also seems well tolerated by patients receiving only narcotic sedation. The patient is connected to the apparatus, the synchronizer is adjusted to a setting of zero milliseconds (an intrinsic instrumental delay of about 20 milliseconds generally allows the discharge to fall during the downslope of the R wave or within the S wave), and the accuracy of discharge within the cardiac cycle is checked by discharging the paddles against each other. Adjustments in synchronization are made, if necessary, to avoid the ascending limb or peak of the T wave. The paddles are coated with electrode paste, one being placed in the third right intercostal space at the sternal border, and the other in the left fifth intercostal space in the midaxillary line. The discharge is fired only when a stable base line appears on the oscilloscope (to prevent triggering by artifact) (Fig. 19). In case of failure to revert, energy of successive dis-

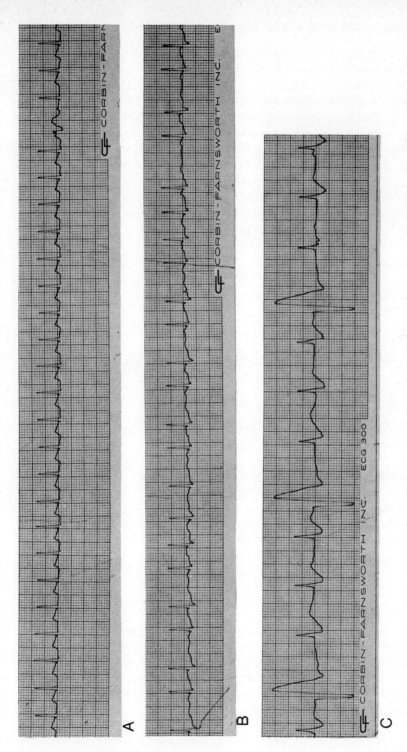

FIG. 19 A. 1:1 conduction or atrial tachycardia with occasional AV block. B. After conversion. C. Same patient—disturbed by noise.

charges is increased by increments of 100 watt-seconds until a final discharge of 400 watt-seconds is reached. After successful conversion, maintenance quinidine dosage is started.

Adverse effects to cardioversion are few. Muscle soreness and irritation of the skin at the electrode sites are not uncommon; burns may be kept at a minimum by applying adequate amounts of electrode paste. Enzyme rises (in LDH and SGOT) occur rarely, and are considered to derive from local muscle trauma. Atrial, nodal, or ventricular ectopic beats and other minor arrhythmias may occur transiently after restoration of sinus rhythm. Reports of serious arrhythmias, such as ventricular tachycardia, are few; fatalities due to ventricular fibrillation or cardiac standstill are very rare, and almost always have occurred in patients with digitalis excess.

*Indications for Artificial Pacing*

- In chronic complete AV block:
  1. Stokes-Adams attack
  2. Inadequate cardiac output
  3. Effort intolerance
  4. Congestive heart failure
- In myocardial infarction:
  1. 2–3-degree AV block
  2. Symptomatic sinus or other bradycardia
  3. "Outpacing" ventricular dysrhythmias
- To suppress tachycardias or "tachy"-arrhythmias

*Artificial Pacing—Special Points*

- In the absence of AV block, atrial pacing is preferable to ventricular
- In the presence of complete AV block, paced rates of 60–90 usually suffice to suppress all ventricular dysrhythmias

# Summary

In this chapter we have discussed some of the important arrhythmias associated with myocardial infarction. Study the illustrations well, because although there seem to be an infinite number of arrhythmias, they are not all that easy to recognize. For this reason, each was summarized in outline form at the end of the discussion individually and by group. You will find further clarification in the review and advance questions.

*Review and Advance*

1. *Does the information obtained from a rhythm strip mean the same as that obtained from an electrocardiogram?*
   It is important to remember that a rhythm strip is only a small segment of an ECG and useful for rhythm analysis, hence, the name "rhythm strip." The 12-lead electrocardiogram is a diagnostic tool for revealing cardiac pathology and designating its source or location.

2. *Literally, what is an arrhythmia?*
   Literally, the word is derived from the Latin prefix "a or ab," meaning from, away from, or absence of, and from the Greek, "rhythmos," meaning rhythm. Thus, taken literally, it can be said to imply "an absence of rhythm, a rhythm away from the normal rhythm, or variation from rhythm," depending upon the interpreter, since all variations in rhythms do not necessarily imply "absence from normal."

3. *What is the most common usage?*
   Loss of rhythm. However, others may disagree with the author on this term.

4. *Is procainamide considered a drug of the past with the advent of lidocaine?*
   Procainamide (Pronestyl), commonly used for treatment of ventricular premature contractions or other arrhythmias, still is used by many physicians who have not been eager to adopt lidocaine. Procainamide may be given to patients who require quinidine but are sensitive to that drug.
   Lidocaine, which many nurses know as Xylocaine, has been useful as a local anesthesic for many years. It has a mechanism of action similar to that of procainamide but, in contrast to it, lidocaine causes no fall in blood pressure or decrease in myocardial contractility. Since it is a myocardial depressant it decreases electrical excitability, conduction, and force of contraction. Its onset of action is rapid but its duration of action is brief. For example, it may be effective within a minute or two and effects are gone within 20 to 30 minutes. It is used to suppress ventricular arrhythmias, much as procainamide, but is ineffective in atrial dysrhythmias.

5. *How is lidocaine administered?*
   Lidocaine is usually administered intravenously by bolus (one single dose) or by intravenous infusion. The usual dosage is 1 mg per kg body weight intravenously every twenty minutes, if necessary, until a maximum of 750 mg has been given. However, if the method preferred is by intravenous infusion without an initial bolus, it may be taken approximately an hour before the drug can produce an effect. Lidocaine is always administered precisely as ordered, and the patient must be observed for possible side effects, such as drowsiness, dizziness, analgesia, blurred or double vision, numbness, and excessive perspiration. More severe symptoms include hypotension, convulsions, and coma. At the first sign of toxic effects the dosage should be decreased, and stopped if toxic symptoms remain, since high doses or prolonged use may precipitate respiratory arrest.

6. *Occasionally, physicians ask for diphenylhydantoin (Dilantin). Isn't that a drug used for convulsions?*
   Yes, Dilantin Sodium is a very efficient drug in the treatment of epilepsy. It is more effective for grand mal seizures than for petit mal. It is also effec-

tive in controlling convulsions due to brain injury or accidents and is used following many brain surgeries. However, indications for Dilantin Sodium in treating cardiac arrhythmias is not well defined, nor established. Reports indicate that a number of arrhythmias may be controlled or terminated. Ventricular arrhythmias, particularly multifocal VPCs and bigeminy, respond well, as do arrhythmias precipitated by digitalis excess. Ventricular tachycardia may be terminated. Observers note that the incidence of ventricular arrhythmias associated with acute myocardial infarction or thoracic surgery may be reduced by prophylactic administration of Dilantin Sodium.

Supraventricular tachycardias and APCs may also cease. Atrial flutter and fibrillation are not converted to a normal rhythm, but the ventricular rate may slow greatly due to the effects of Dilantin Sodium on increasing the degree of heart block. From these indications, the drug should not be given in the presence of marked bradycardia or high degree of AV block.

The drug may be given orally as a maintenance dose in 100–200 mg three or four times a day. For acute arrhythmias 250 mg may be injected over a five-minute interval. Response, if it is to occur, can be seen in five minutes.

The nurse should be aware of certain side effects which may follow intravenous administration: tremors, ataxia, drowsiness, and confusion. However, side effects are relatively rare.

7. *Why are vasopressors given for rapid cardiac arrythmias or tachycardias since the rate is already rapid?*
Rapid cardiac arrhythmias, such as atrial, nodal, and ventricular tachycardias, are often associated with varying degrees of low blood pressure. Restoration of the systemic blood pressure with vasopressor agents (Levophed, Aramine, etc.) may terminate such arrhythmias in a significant number of patients, and administration of such drugs is often the first therapeutic measure used by many physicians.

The antiarrhythmic effects of pressor drugs are most likely related to increased coronary perfusion, effects on the carotid sinus and arch, and, perhaps, a direct myocardial action.

Remember that the patient must be carefully monitored when on any vasopressor drug, for elevation of blood pressure to excessive levels may be complicated by the development of serious ventricular arrhythmias.

8. *What is the "circus rhythm" theory?*
This name may be misleading in that it certainly does not have anything to do with the circus, but rather, refers to a circle. Briefly, it implies that an impulse originated at a site in the atrium, usually around the orifices of the superior and inferior vena cava, continues to go around and around in a circle. According to this theory, the atrial rate is determined by the speed with which the impulse travels the circle circuit, and the speed, in turn, is determined by the conductivity, refraction period, and length of the circus ring of the muscle. Since the impulse is moving outside the conductivity pathway, it is assumed to be traveling in relatively refractory tissue at a lower rate of speed. From the "circus" excitation wave, centrifugal waves are said to flow uniformly and regularly in the various parts of the atrial muscles. This results in weak but distinct atrial contractions.

9. *What is the "repetitive stimuli" theory?*
This theory states that stimuli arising in ectopic foci are responsible for ectopic or premature beats and that repetitive stimuli from such foci produce

paraxysmal atrial tachycardia, atrial flutter or fibrillation, depending upon the rate of firing or impulse formation.

10. *Are some tachycardias normal?*

The question should be reworded to read, "Are there regular tachycardias?" In this way it is better to observe whether the cardiac rhythm is regular or irregular, and whether the rate is unusually rapid (or unusually slow) or normal.

Tachycardias which are regular include:
  a. sinus tachycardia
  b. paroxysmal atrial tachycardia
  c. ventricular tachycardia
  d. atrial flutter with 1:1 response or with unchanging degree of block

Tachycardias which are irregular include:
  a. atrial fibrillation
  b. atrial flutter with varying block
  c. paroxysmal atrial tachycardia with block
  d. sinus tachycardia with numerous premature beats

11. *Are there regular and irregular bradycardias?*

Bradycardias with regular rhythm include:
  a. sinus bradycardia
  b. nodal rhythm
  c. severe partial heart block with constant degree of block
  d. complete heart block

Bradycardias with irregular rhythm include:
  a. sinoatrial bradycardia with marked sinus arrhythmia or frequent premature beats
  b. partial heart block with frequent dropped beats or changing degree of block

By the same token, irregular rhythms with normal heart rate include:
  a. frequent premature beats
  b. atrial fibrillation with ventricular rate slowed by digitalis, sinus arrhythmia, partial heart block with dropped beats and interference dissociation with many captured beats

12. *How is the conduction pathway differentiated from regular muscle tissue?*

The conduction system of the heart is composed of specialized cells which differ from myocardial cells in structural, chemical, and functional properties. The cells of the conduction system are distinguished by their ability to conduct impulses more rapidly than the myocardial cells and their capacity to function as pacemakers which initiate the impulses leading to activation of the myocardium.

13. *What are the fundamental properties of cardiac tissue?*

The fundamental properties of cardiac tissue are automatically (rhythmicity), excitability (irritability), conductivity, and contractility. The most important to the person is rhythmicity, that is, the ability to beat automatically, or rhythmically, without external stimuli.

14. *What is "physiologic" tachycardia?*

Physiologic sinus tachycardia results from emotional stress, exercise, digestion, or other causes. Certain tests may be performed by the physician to study the patient's reaction to exercise. For example, the "Master 2-step" exercise test was evolved in order to safely subject a patient to a reasonable, yet adequate, amount of exercise calculated to produce diagnostic changes in the electro-cardiogram in the presence of underlying disease. The test was standardized to include variables such as weight and age, as well as sex. The results of the test provide a base line for comparisons for physicians no matter in what part of the world the test is performed.

However, it is still well to remember that strenuous exercise may be dangerous to patients with coronary heart disease, and that after the Master 2-step test a normal heart may show ischemic changes in post-exercise electro-cardiogram if the exercise is too strenuous, or overdone.

15.  *What pathologic conditions are associated with tachycardia?*
First, it is well to note that certain drugs such as atropine and amyl nitrite may be used to produce sinus tachycardia. But, among the pathologic condi-tions associated with sinus tachycardia are fever, hyperthyroidism, anemia, acute hemorrhage, shock, congestive heart failure, and cardiac neurosis. It will also occur when the upright position is assumed by some patients with chronic postural hypotension and, occasionally, in cases of pheochromocytoma, tumor of the adrenal medulla.

The clinical significance depends upon the basic cause, and tachycardia may immediately subside as soon as the basic cause is removed.

16.  *Is phasic arrhythmia a new arrhythmia?*
Phasic arrythmia is another name for sinus arrhythmia—as is juvenile ar-rhythmia. This may have arisen because observers noted that with normal sinus rhythm and rates under 80 per minute, there was no absolute regu-larity and that cycle lengths varied slightly, yet definitely. This is assumed probably to be due to physiologic phasic varations in the vagal tone. Sinus or phasic arrhythmia is merely an exaggeration of this normal tendency. A chronotropic inhibitory effect of the vagus nerve may cause a shift of the pacemaker from one position to another of the sinotrial anode.

Sinus arrhythmias are most common in hearts with bradycardia, pre-sumably because there the vagal influence tends to be greatest. It also occurs commonly among children and the aged.

17.  *How is sinus arrhythmia recognized without an electrocardiogram?*
Clinically, sinus arrhythmia is recognizable by the fairly regular alternation of several rapid heart or pulse beats and then several slower beats. The rela-tion of the rapid beats to inspiration and the slow beats to expiration is notice-able. A test the physician may use is to have the patient hold his breath, which may make the arrhythmia disappear. Exercise and atropine may also abolish it.

18.  *Is sinus arrest the same thing as heart failure? Atrial standstill?*
These two should definitely not be confused. Sinus arrest, also referred to as sinoatrial standstill or sinus pause, really is a *pause* in the cardiac rhythm due to momentary failure of the sinus node to initiate an impulse. It is usually of no clinical significance unless the pause is long enough to cause dizziness, faintness, or even fainting. It is recognizable by the omission or "skipping" of a heart or pulse beat. It must be differentiated from the pause of dropped beats in partial heart block and the compensatory pause following an early premature beat.

*Atrial standstill* denotes a pause in atrial contraction, while the ventricle contracts in response to its own pacemaker. Atrial standstill is secondary to either sinus arrest or sinoatrial block. However, the electrocardiogram shows a regular sequence of ventricular complexes, but one or more P waves are absent. In this case, when the sinoatrial node fails to initiate an impulse or the impulse is blocked from reaching the atrium, there is no atrial contraction. However, a pacemaker of lower rhythmicity in the atrioventricular node, bundle, or ventricle activates the ventricle and causes contraction. The cause of atrial standstill is usually digitalis or quinidine toxicity, but organic factors may be involved. When it is due to drugs, it is temporary; when it is due to or associated with myocardial infarction or hyperpotassemia, it is usually terminal. Clinically, the rhythm is regular, but there may be an intense slowing of the heart. An electrocardiogram is essential for diagnosis.

19. *Do soft drinks high in carbohydrates precipitate premature beats?*
According to Harrison and Resnik, a *meal* high in carbohydrate may precipitate premature beats in patients receiving digitalis. This is apparently related to a low level of potassium in the blood. When this is true, the premature beats are abolished when the patient is given potassium chloride, 3 to 6 g daily in divided doses. This means that the diet should be reviewed.

20. *What is the effect of atrial fibrillation?*
Atrial fibrillation has a number of negative effects on the function of the heart. First, fibrillation of muscle renders it ineffective as a source of power. The conduction system is bombarded by impulses. They may be frequent and irregular, yet none may be strong enough to cause contraction. Many of them fail to stimulate contraction because the conducting system of the myocardium is in an absolute refractory period at the time of their arrival. Even so, the myocardium does respond to many of them with the result that the pulse is rapid and totally irregular. Both the strength of contraction and distance between beats vary from one beat to the next.

When the interval between beats is too short, ventricular contractions may be too feeble to force open the aortic semilunar valves and drive blood into the arteries. The energy expended in each ineffective contraction is wasted. This places an additional burden on the heart. It may cause a pulse deficit.

21. *What is the most accurate method of computing the pulse deficit?*
The most accurate method involves the cooperation of two persons. When this is done, one nurse counts the radial pulse and another nurse, using a stethoscope placed over the apex of the heart, counts the heart beats. One nurse should give the signal to begin so that each will be counting for the same period of time. The difference between the radial pulse and the apical pulse is called the pulse deficit. The results are used to evaluate the extent to which the heart is wasteful of its energy and, most importantly, to evaluate the effectiveness of treatment.

22. *Are there other dangers involved in atrial fibrillation?*
When atrial fibrillation continues for any length of time, congestive heart failure is likely to be precipitated. Therefore, treatment is instituted to restore normal rhythm or to lessen the effect of the abnormal one. Stasis of blood in the atria predisposes to mural thrombosis which may be dislodged if effective contraction is restored; thus, correcting the fibrillation may not be possible or desirable. However, when atrial fibrillation is newly established, the danger of mural thrombosis is minimal.

23. *What is the Wolff-Parkinson-White syndrome?*
This is usually seen in young and otherwise healthy persons, especially females. The essential feature in the ECG tracing is a short P-R interval (0.10 second or less) and widening of the QRS complex due to slurring at

the onset of the upstroke of the R wave (so-called *delta wave*). These patients are subject to recurrent attacks of paroxysmal atrial tachycardia or atrial flutter or, on occasion, even atrial fibrillation, which may be considered erroneously a ventricular tachycardia because of aberrant or bizarre QRS pattern.

The condition is usually benign, but sudden death may occur during an attack of paroxysmal tachycardia. Recurrent attacks of tachycardia may be reduced by administration of sedatives, but if this measure is not effective, the physician may choose either quinidine or procainamide. Digitalis is not given, as a rule, since it blocks the spread of the impulse through the atrio-ventricular node and increases normal excitation, with a resultant increase in ventricular rate. However in all fairness to this drug, on rare occasions arrhythmias which do not respond to other antiarrhythmic drugs may respond to digitalis.

# 18 AV NODE AND VENTRICULAR ARRHYTHMIAS

At several points, we have discussed the nurse's responsibility and nursing care of the patient suffering from myocardial infarction and associated complications. However, it must be emphasized that nursing care and responsibilities will vary to fit the particular patient's needs. In arrhythmias, nursing care includes identifying the arrhythmia and documenting it with a lead write-out that best substantiates it. Usually, patients are "hooked up" to lead 2, which may or may not be the best lead to focus on in a particular disorder.

Reassurance of the patient at frequent intervals is an important aspect of lessening his anxiety since any sudden hustle of activity is likely to fill him with alarm. The nurse will check the radial and apical rate, the blood pressure and venous pressure readings, and report these to the physician.

Since anticipation is the best part of prevention, it is a good idea always to have emergency drugs on hand as well as having the defibrillator ready to go.

Although most of the fibers of the cardiac conduction system are specialized for rapid transmission of impulses, one structure in this system conducts more slowly than the rest of the heart. This is the structure from which normal impulses pass directly into the bundle of His, that is, the atrioventricular node, or AV node.

The delay of impulses at the AV node allows the ventricles to fill before ventricular contraction. Since impulses normally pass through the AV node immediately before depolarizing the ventricles, you can reasonably expect to find that portion of the ECG reflecting the conduction of impulses through the AV node immediately preceding the QRS complex. The delay of the depolarization wave at the AV node produces a resultant cardiac vector of zero; the delay of the impulse at the AV node, therefore, is recorded on the ECG as an isoelectric or straight line. This isoelectric line is called the P-R segment.

The distance between the beginning of the P wave and the end of the P-R segment is called the P-R interval.

## Nodal Rhythm

You will remember that it has been stated that the vagus nerve has a continuously maintained tone, changes in which would influence the heart by enhancing or depressing the activity of the pacemaker. An increase in the tone of the vagus depresses the activity of the SA node; the higher the tone of the vagus, the greater the depressant effect on the SA node. If the SA node is depressed, the focus with the next shortest spontanous discharge cycle takes over as pacemaker. This may be an atrial focus; if all the myocardial fibers in the atria were too depressed to function, the pacemaker may move to the AV node (Fig. 1).

When the impulse is initiated in the AV node, it travels up through the atria and down through the ventricles more or less simultaneously. The impulse travels down through the ventricles through the normal conduction pathway, so you can expect the QRST sequence to remain unchanged. However, it is traveling in reverse, or retrograde, through the atria and the P wave will be abnormal. It will be recorded as a negative, or inverted, P wave in leads where it ordinarily would be upright. So, the clue to nodal rhythms is to carefully examine the P wave:

- If the impulse reaches and spreads through the atria first, the abnormal P waves closely precede the QRS complex; the P-R segment is shortened.
- If the impulse reaches the ventricles first, the abnormal P wave will be recorded on the ECG following the QRS complex.
- If the impulse reaches and spreads through the atria and ventricles at the same time, the P wave is lost in the QRS complex.

## Nodal Rhythm (Fig. 2)

- Atrial rate—low normal 40 to 100/minute.
- Ventricular rate—low normal 40 to 100/minute.
- Rhythm—regular.
- P-R interval—same as nodal tachy—variable.
- P wave—same as PNCs.
- QRS complex—same as PNCs regular.
- Conduction mechanism—same as PNCs.
- Treatment considered—stop quinidine, stop Pronestyl, stop lidocaine, stop digitalis.
- Significance—AV node usurps pacemaking function of SA node, atria stimulated in reverse fashion causing inverted P wave. In high nodal rhythm. P leads QRS. In mid-nodal rhythm P is not discernible within the QRS. In low nodal rhythm, P follows QRS.
- Salient features:
  1. Abnormal P waves closely preceding or following QRS, or absent P waves
  2. Normal QRST sequence except ST and T waves may be distorted by P waves

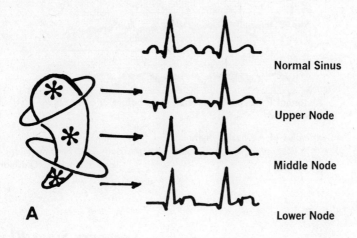

Normal Sinus

Upper Node

Middle Node

Lower Node

A

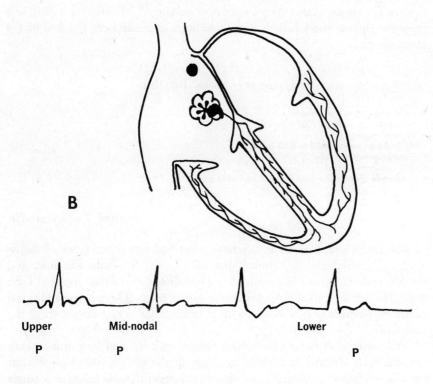

B

Upper     Mid-nodal     Lower

P         P                      P

*FIG. 1* A, atrio-ventricular nodal mechanisms. B, nodal rhythms.

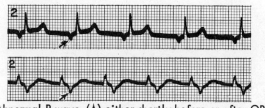

Abnormal P wave (↑) either shortly before or after QRS.

*FIG. 2* Two examples of AV nodal rhythm.
(Reprinted with permission from Marriott, CCU Nursing Slides, 1967,
Tampa Tracings, Oldsmar, Fla.)

## Coronary Sinus Rhythm

When P waves have the same shape and direction as those of AV nodal rhythm *but* are associated with a normal or prolonged P-R interval instead of a short one, investigators believe that these beats originate from the area of the coronary sinus.

### Coronary Sinus Rhythm

- Atrial rate—60 to 100/minute
- Ventricular rate—60 to 100/minute
- Rhythm—regular
- P-R interval—normal 0.10 to 0.20 or more
- P wave—inverted in lead 2
- QRS complex—normal
- Conduction mechanism—both forward and retrograde

## Nodal Tachycardia

So far in our discussion, we have identified two other types of tachycardia: (1) atrial and (2) sinus. Anatomically, the SA node, the atria, and the AV node are above the ventricles. Therefore, tachycardias initiated from these area foci are called supraventricular tachycardias. There is one additional tachycardia which will be touched upon briefly later in our discussion of the ventricles.

You remember that tachycardia is defined as a series of four or more consecutive beats of atrial or ventricular origin at the rate of 100 or more beats per minute. Most tachycardias are due to the repetitive discharge of a single focus; that is, most tachycardias can be considered to be runs of consecutive premature beats from one focus.

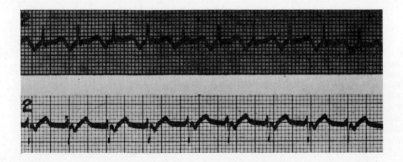

FIG. 3 Two examples of AV nodal tachycardia: upper strip—with retrograde P wave preceding QRS; lower strip—with retrograde P following QRS.

(Reprinted with permission from Marriott, CCU Nursing Slides, 1967, Tampa Tracings, Oldsmar, Fla.)

Like normal and premature beats, tachycardias from the supraventricular foci are transmitted through the atria and through the cardiac conduction system to the rest of the heart. Assuming that the cardiac conduction system transmits every beat or impulse, each P wave will be assocaited with a QRS complex. This type of conduction is expressed as a 1:1 ratio. This will be helpful to you later in your study of AV blocks.

### Nodal Tachycardia (Fig. 3)

- Atrial rate—100 to 250/minute
- Ventrical rate—100 to 250/minute
- Rhythm—regular
- P-R interval—shortened, or P wave may be buried in or following QRS
- P wave—same as PNCs
- QRS complex—same as PNCs regular
- Conduction mechanism—same as PNCs
- Significance—a rapid nodal rhythm greater than 100/minute, often paroxysmal and potentially dangerous because of high rates and reduced cardiac output

## *Premature Nodal Contraction (PNC) or NPC*

A nodal premature contraction is due to an ectopic focus in the AV node. NPC's are associated with retrograde depolarization as has been described previously in this chapter. Therefore, you would expect the P wave to be negative and either to precede, follow, or be lost in the QRS complex. The P-R interval is characteristically less than 0.12 second. Therefore, if the duration of the P-R interval of a premature contraction is less than 0.12 second, the site of origin of the contraction is likely to be the AV node. It will never be longer than the P-R interval of an atrial premature contraction.

## Premature Nodal Contraction (PNC) or NPC

- Atrial rate—60 to 100/minute
- Ventricular rate—60 to 100/minute
- Rhythm—regular except for PNCs
- P-R interval—normal except for PNCs 2
- P wave—normal except PNCs, then inverted in Lead 2, 3, aVF; buried in QRS; following QRS
- QRS complex—normal unless P wave is buried in it
- Conduction mechanism—in the PNCs the conduction is both forward and retrograde
- Treatment considered—quinidine, Pronestyl

## *Atrioventricular Heart Blocks*

A delay in, or absence of, conduction from the atria to the ventricles due to either abnormal refractoriness or to physical interruption of the AV conducting system is defined as atrioventricular block, or more simply, as AV block or heart block. Such alterations may be caused by toxicity, vagal influence, or organic disease.

AV block may be classified as partial or complete, or in terms of degree, such as first-degree, second-degree, or third-degree (Figs. 4, 5 and 6).

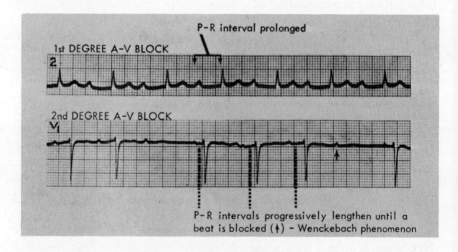

FIG. 4  First- and second-degree AV blocks.
(Reprinted with permission from Marriott, CCU Nursing Slides, 1967, Tampa Tracings, Oldsmar, Fla.)

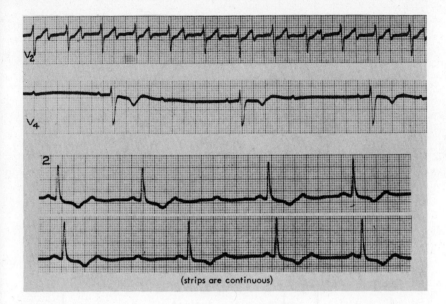

(strips are continuous)

**FIG. 5** Various degrees of AV block: upper strip—first-degree (prolonged P-R interval); middle strip—high grade (2 to 1), lower strip—high grade varying between 2 to and 3 to 1.

(Reprinted with permission from Marriott, CCU Nursing Slides, 1967, Tampa Tracings, Oldsmar, Fla.)

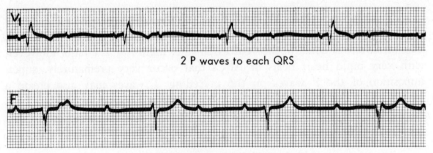

2 P waves to each QRS

Changing P to QRS relationship
Ventricles slow and regular – idioventricular rhythm

**FIG. 6** Top: high grade block (2 to 1); bottom: complete AV block.

(Reprinted with permission from Marriott, CCU Nursing Slides, 1967, Tampa Tracings, Oldsmar, Fla.)

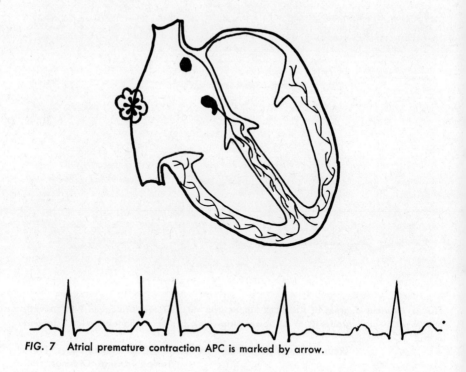

*FIG. 7* Atrial premature contraction APC is marked by arrow.

## FIRST-DEGREE AV BLOCK (Incomplete or Partial)

In first-degree AV block there is only a delay in conduction to the ventricles which is recorded on the ECG as a prolongation of the P-R interval. The atrial rate is equal to the ventricular rate, there is a 1:1 ratio. However, with very rapid heart beats or APCs that occur very prematurely, superimposition of the P waves on the preceding T waves may also create a lengthened P-R interval (Fig. 7). So, for differentiation, remember first-degree block is said to clearly exist when *the P-R interval is prolonged and the P waves follow the T wave of the preceding beat.*

### Arrhythmia—First-Degree AV Block

- Atrial rate—60 to 100/minute
- Ventricular rate—60 to 100/minute
- Rhythm—regular.
- P-R interval—greater than 0.20, sometimes prolonged beyond .22 second because of delay in activation due to abnormality at AV node.
- QRS complex—normal.
- Conduction mechanism—delayed conduction at AV node.

- Treatment considered—Atropine; stop digitalis; give K, stop quinidine, stop Pronestyl.
- Significance—They presage a more dangerous rhythm or a higher degree of block. May indicate myocarditis, digitalis toxicity, or ischemia.
- Salient features, AV block:
  1. Incomplete—impaired AV condition indicated by
     a. Prolonged P-R interval (first-degree block)
     b. Dropped beats—P waves not followed by QRST (second- and third-degree)
  2. Complete—atria and ventricles independent
     a. P waves at sinus rate (60–90)
     b. QRST at idioventricular rate (30–40)
     c. QRS interval normal or prolonged, depending on site of ventricular pacemaker

## SECOND-DEGREE AV BLOCK (Incomplete or Partial)

The P-R intervals in first-degree block are usually of constant duration, although prolonged. Second-degree block is associated with two types of P-R intervals: those of constant length, whether prolonged or normal; and those that progressively lengthen until AV conduction fails entirely and a QRS complex is dropped . . . after which the cycle begins again. This latter type is called the Wenckebach phenomenon (Fig. 8). Several cycles of sinus

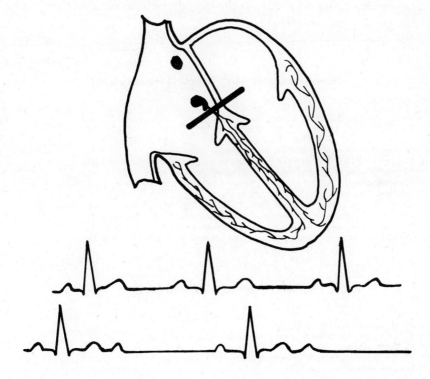

*FIG. 8* Wenckebach phenomenon. P-R interval progressively prolonged until a beat is dropped.

discharge and prolonged conduction are necessary before the P-R interval is so prolonged that the beat is dropped.

The frequency with which failure of conduction occurs in second-degree block is variable. For this reason, absence of the QRS complex occurs with varying frequency in relation to the conducted beats. The frequency with which dropped beats occur in AV block is expressed as a ratio of atrial to ventricular rates. For example, if three ventricular beats are dropped for every four atrial beats, so that there are four atrial beats and one ventricular beat, a 4:1 block exists. The term "simple ratio," as applied to this relationship between atrial and ventricular beats or rates, designates a readily apparent pattern. In other words, when the ventricular rate is dependent upon the atrial rate in AV block, the relationship between the two will form the readily apparent repetitive ECG pattern which can be expressed as a simple ratio. The ventricular rate is dependent upon the atrial rate in cases of first-degree and second-degree AV blocks only. In third-degree AV block, no such constant relationship can be seen.

Upon auscultation, however, the ventricular rhythm will seem regular or irregular depending upon whether the spacings between successive ventricular beats are the same or different.

## Second-Degree AV Block (Incomplete)

- Atrial rate—upper limits of normal, 60–100/min.
- Ventricular rate—depends on ratio of nonconducted to
                    (35–50/ min. /c 2:1 block)
  conducted impulses   (20–33/min. /c 3:1 block).
- Rhythm—regular if ratio of block consistent, or irregular due to dropped beats.
- P-R interval—normal or prolonged on conducted beats.
- P wave—normal.
- QRS complex—normal.
- Conduction mechanism—only intermittent impulses pass through the AV node. Every other beat is blocked. Conduction beats may have normal or prolonged P-R interval.
- Treatment considered—Stop digitalis, give atropine, or Isuprel. Pacemaker.
- Significance—same as 1st-degree block; may progress to complete heart block.

## Arrhythmia—Wenckebach

- Atrial rate—normal, 60 to 100/minute.
- Ventrical rate—variable; follows a cyclic pattern.
- Rhythm—ventricular rhythm, irregular.
- P-R interval—progressively prolonged until a beat is dropped.
- P wave—normal.
- QRS complex—normal.
- Conduction mechanism—P-R interval progressively prolonged until a beat is not conducted. This cycle repeats itself.
- Treatment considered—stop digitalis.

independent P waves

pacemaker impulses followed
immediately by stimulated ventricular complexes

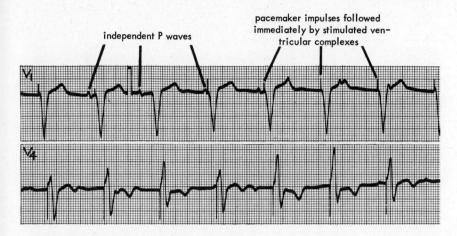

**FIG. 9** Dangerous ventricular beats land on the T waves (R-on-T phenomenon)—in the "vulnerable" period; from a patient with inferior infarction (acute).

(Reprinted with permission from Marriott, CCU Nursing Slides, 1967, Tampa Tracings, Oldsmar, Fla.)

In atrial flutter, just as in supraventricular tachycardias, supraventricular impulses may depolarize the ventricles or conducting fibers during their relative refractory period. This depolarization, called *aberrant conduction,* produces QRS complexes of abnormal configuration.

When this occurs intermittently, the aberrant beats may be confused with VPCs. The clinical significance of the two conditions, however, is very different:

VCPs are an indication of ventricular irritability and in certain circumstances may be followed by ventricular tachycardia or even ventricular fibrillation (Fig. 9).

Every sinus beat is followed by a ventricular premature beat.

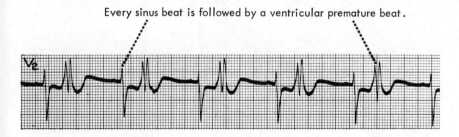

**FIG. 10** Ventricular bigeminy.

(Reprinted with permission from Marriott, CCU Nursing Slides, 1967, Tampa Tracings, Oldsmar, Fla.)

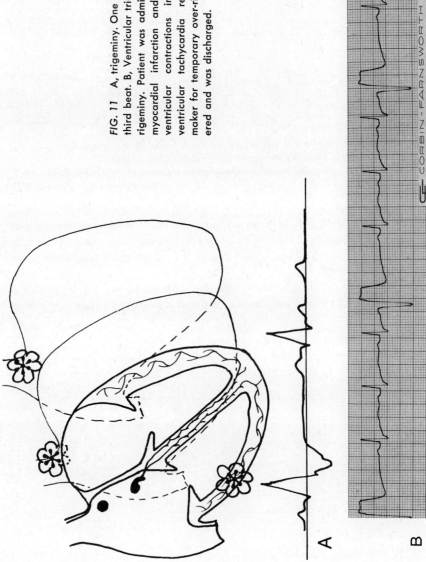

FIG. 11 A, trigeminy. One ectopic beat every third beat. B, Ventricular trigeminy and quadrigeminy. Patient was admitted with possible myocardial infarction and rare premature ventricular contractions increased. Finally, ventricular tachycardia required a pacemaker for temporary over-ride. Patient recovered and was discharged.

A

B

Aberrant conduction, on the other hand, has little clinical significance. It occurs when there is inadequate time for complete repolarization of the ventricles or conducting system before the next depolarization wave arrives.

The term "unifocal" is applied to premature ventricular contractions when they are discharged from a single ectopic focus, and "multifocal" when they are fired from numerous ectopic foci.

When an irritable focus in the atria or ventricles fires in such a way that one ectopic beat follows every normal beat, the condition is called *bigeminy* (Fig. 10). In *trigeminy*, an ectopic beat occurs regularly after every two normal beats (Fig. 11). In *quadrigeminy*, an ectopic beat follows regularly after every three normal beats.

An ectopic beat occurring between two normal beats that are separated by a normal P-P interval is called an "interpolated" beat. The occurrence of an interpolated beat requires:

1. A slow heart rate
2. An ectopic beat occurring early enough so that the myocardium is no longer in its absolute refractory period at the next sinus discharge
3. Retrograde block

When complete failure of conduction to the ventricles occurs, as in third-degree AV block, the ventricles will start beating spontaneously at a rate which is slower than that of the atria. This is because ventricular myocardial fibers have spontaneous discharge cycles which are longer than those of atrial fibers. An impulse which arises within the ventricles is called "idioventricular" (Fig. 12).

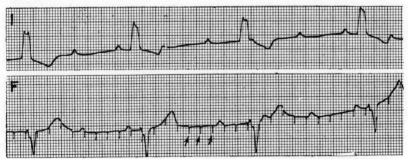

Pacemaker 'blips' (↟) at rate 350 (fortunately ineffective).
Note that pacemaker activity is not visible in lead 1.

*FIG. 12* Runaway pacemaker. Complete AV block with idioventricular rhythm.
(Reprinted with permission from Marriott, CCU Nursing Slides, 1967,
Tampa Tracings, Oldsmar, Fla.)

The pacemaker for the atria is usually in the SA node and for the ventricles somewhere below the blocked AV node. The lower the ventricular pacemaker is situated, the slower will be its rhythm. For this reason, the ventricular rate is usually less than the atrial rate.

Since some characteristics are shared by both second- and third-degree AV block, the diagnosis may be difficult at times. When the ventricular rhythm is regular, it is the dependence of the ventricular rate upon the atrial rate as seen on the ECG that suggests the origin is supraventricular though "hooking" may occur, meaning there may be long periods of time where there are two P waves associated with one QRS in third-degree AV node.

When conductions are such that an idioventricular pacemaker becomes effective because of the absence of the supraventricular impulses, "ventricular escape" is said to occur (Figs. 13 and 14). Thus, ventricular escape beats may occur occasionally in second-degree block but are responsible for all ventricular activity in third-degree block.

*Since ventricular escape beats originate from an idioventricular focus, the QRS complex would usually be abnormal in configuration and wider than normal.*

The presence of an idioventricular pacemaker represents an escape phenomenon; that is, it occurs when a ventricular myocardial fiber is able to complete its own spontaneous discharge cycle. The source of the discharge is not an "irritable" focus in the ventricles, but the freeing of a fiber so that its own discharge cycle can proceed to completion.

Therefore, when ventricular escape beats occur only occasionally, as they do in second-degree block, the QRS complexes of the escape beats will be late in relation to the basic ventricular rhythm.

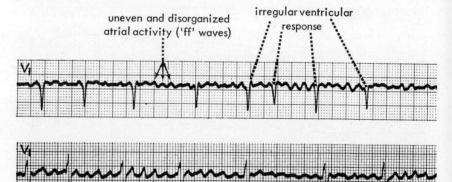

FIG. 13   Two examples of atrial fibrillation.
(Reprinted with permission from Marriott, CCU Nursing Slides, 1967, Tampa Tracings, Oldsmar, Fla.)

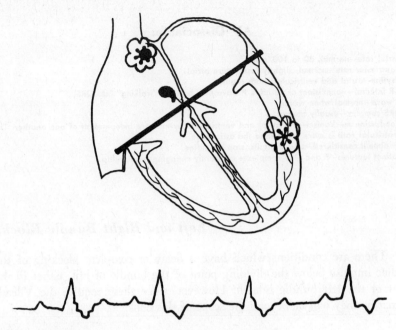

*FIG. 14* Complete heart block and ventricular escape beats.

## Third-Degree AV Heart Block

* Atrial rate—normal, 60 to 100/min.
* Ventricular rate—slow, usually under 40 (25 to 40/min.).
* Rhythm—atrial and ventricular, both regular.
* P-R interval—irrelevant.
* P wave—normal (in dependent rhythm rather than with QRS).
* QRS complex—configuration depends on site of secondary pacemaker (independent of P).
* Conduction mechanism—Atrial and ventricular rhythms are independent of one another.
* Treatment considered—atropine and Isuprel. Pacemaker.
* Significance—conduction: P-R interval widely variable as atria and ventricles have independent formation of impulses and act quite independently of each other. P waves appear normal and QRS complexes are sometimes bizarre. Particularly dangerous with potential onset of ventricular standstill or ventricular fibrillation.

## *AV Dissociation*

If a supraventricular (from above ventricles) impulse reaches the ventricles just after ventricular escape occurs, normal refractoriness rather than AV block, may prevent ventricular response. Thus, ventricular escape further increases the dependence of the ventricles on the supraventricular response.

## AV Dissociation

- Atrial rate—normal, 60 to 100/min.
- Ventricular rate—normal, slightly faster than atrial.
- Rhythm—atrial and ventricular, both regular.
- P-R interval—nonexistent or variable P wave may be seen "walking" into QRS.
- P wave—normal when visible.
- QRS complex—usually normal.
- Conduction mechanism—the atrial and ventricular rhythms are independent of one another. The ventricular rate is more rapid than the atrial rate.
- Treatment considered—stop digitalis; stop quinidine.
- Salient features—P and QRS complexes constantly changing relationship.

## Left and Right Bundle Blocks

There are conditions which have a delay or complete blocking of the cardiac impulse below the dividing point of the bundle of His, either in the right or the left bundle branch. However, since these require the V leads primarily, they will be beyond the scope of this book.

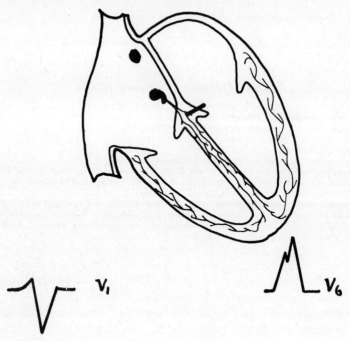

FIG. 15  Left bundle-branch block.

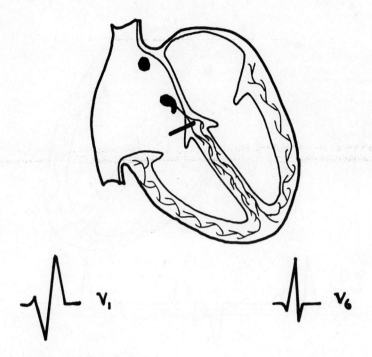

*FIG. 16* Right bundle-branch block.

*Arrhythmia—Left Bundle-Branch Block* (Fig. 15)

- QRS complex—QRS + 0.12 sec. or more No. g, wide R in lead 1 and V₆ Wide QS or rS in lead V₁

*Arrhythmia—Right Bundle-Branch Block* (Fig. 16)

- QRS complex—wide S in leads 1 and V₆M shaped QRS complex in V (sometimes wide R or gR) QRS interval = 0.11 or more

## *Ventricular Premature Contractions*

When an impulse from the ectopic focus in the ventricles cannot reach the SA node, for whatever reason, *retrograde block* is said to be present.

An ectopic focus may arise anywhere in the ventricles, usually in the Purkinje network. However, impulses arising from ectopic ventricular foci are propagated (spread) through ordinary ventricular myocardium rather than

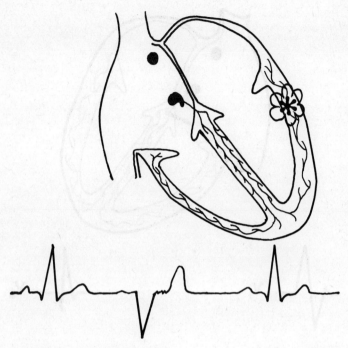

*FIG. 17* Ventricular premature contraction.

through the Purkinje system. From this, one would expect the speed with which ectopic ventricular impulses is propagated through the ventricles to be slower than the normal impulses which travel through the normal conduction pathway.

Thus, a widened QRS complex is characteristic of all PVCs because of the slow conduction rate of ordinary ventricular myocardium and occurs during the relative refractory period.

Remember: Both atrial and ventricular depolarization are usually produced by PNCs (premature nodal contractions); but atrial depolarization is not usually produced by a VPC due to a "shielding" process.

### Ventricular Premature Contractions (Fig. 17)

- Atrial rate—normal, 60 to 100/min.
- Ventricular rate—normal, 60 to 100/min.
- Rhythm—regular except for VPC.
- P-R interval—normal except for VPC.
- P wave—normal except for VPC; sometimes no preceding P wave.
- QRS complex—normal except for VPC, then it is widened, bizarre, thus irregular due to VPCs and differs markedly in appearance as a function of site of origin.

- Conduction mechanism—an irritable focus in the ventricle discharges before the normal SA nodal discharge. The R-R interval is equal to two normal R-R intervals due to compensatory pause.
- Treatment considered—Pronestyl, lidocaine, quinidine.
- Significance—ominous if frequent, danger increases as frequency of VPCs exceeds 6/min. May foretell development of ventricular tachycardia or ventricular fibrillation.

## *Parasystole and Fusion Beats*

In earlier discussions you learned that every myocardial fiber has its own spontaneous discharge cycle; the fibers with the longest spontaneous discharge cycles are in the ventricles. However, ventricular fibers do not discharge spontaneously because they are all depolarized by every depolarization wave initiated by the SA node.

The phenomenon of resetting can apply to the spontaneous discharge cycle of any focus, not just that of the SA node. For instance, if a ventricular focus were shielded from regular depolarization by a drug or by disease, this shielded ventricular focus would be able to depolarize spontaneously, but it *would not* be reset by SA nodal depolarization waves.

This condition in which an ectopic myocardial focus, locally shielded from regular depolarization, discharges spontaneously according to its own spontaneous discharge cycle is called *parasystole*. Although parasystoles occur in both atria and ventricles, it occurs more frequently in the ventricles.

To fully understand this phenomenon, let us review once again. Immediately after depolarization, a myocardial fiber cannot respond to further stimulation; a fraction of a second later, the fiber responds to stimulation, but more slowly than a resting fiber. The former is said to be in the absolute refractory period; the latter, in relative refractory period. For instance, suppose that, in a case of parasystole, the spontaneous depolarization of a shielded fiber were to occur immediately after a normal QRS complex had just been recorded. The myocardium would be unable to respond to the parasystolic discharge because it would be in the absolute refractory period, and there would be no indication of it on the ECG.

On the other hand, if the firing of the shielded focus occurred slightly before the arrival of the depolarization wave was initiated by the normal SA discharge, only the parasystolic beat would appear on the ECG. Since it has its own spontaneous discharge cycle, it will appear again and again on the ECG tracing. The cycles of parasystoles may vary less than 0.01 second, in contrast with sinus impulses which are more variable. *However*, when a parasystolic beat does *not appear* in rhythm with the rest of the parasystolic beats, the missing beat is called an "interfered beat." In other words, once the repetitive pattern of parasystolic beats begins, and occasionally one is missing, it is interfered with and unable to penetrate through the absolute refractory period of the myocardium.

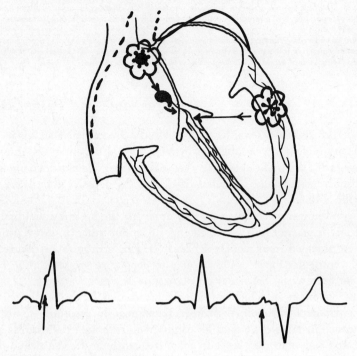

*FIG. 18* Fusion beat and parasystole.

There are more mechanisms governing parasystoles than other forms of premature beats. In APCs, PNCs, and VPCs, the interval between the ectopic beat and the previous normal beat is always about the same; this is called the latency period or interval. The constant latency period has been explained by the theory that an irritable focus, after having been reset by the preceding sinus beat, will occasionally fire at a certain point in its own repolarization. Because of this resetting of the SA node, the latency interval of impulses arising from an unshielded ectopic focus is *dependent* upon the previous beat, or the irritable focus is reset by the preceding sinus discharge. A parasystolic focus, on the other hand, is said to discharge independently of the SA node because its spontaneous discharge cycle is shielded from resetting by the sinus discharge. Thus, the latency interval from the previous normal beat will not be constant for a parasystolic focus, and the interval between successive discharges of the parasystolic focus is variable.

When a normal sinus discharge and a parasystolic discharge meet in the ventricles, the ECG records a single beat which has a normal P wave and a QRS complex "intermediate in form," or a mixture, between the QRS and the parasystolic QRS. Such beats are called "fusion beats," that is, beats which

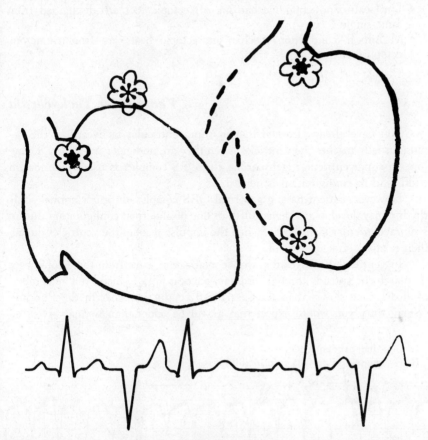

*FIG. 19* An ectopic beat occurring between two normal beats that are separated by a normal P-P interval is called an *interpolated beat.*

result from the combined depolarization of the ventricles by two different pacemakers (Fig. 18).

To briefly categorize these various kinds of ventricular aberrancy:

- Bigeminy—conduction mechanism; every other beat is a VPC; usually digitalis toxicity.
- Trigeminy—conduction mechanism; every third beat is a VPC.
- Interpolated—conduction mechanism; VPC between two normal beats with no break in regular rhythm (Fig. 19).
- Parasystole—an ectopic focus, locally shielded from regular depolarization, discharges spontaneously according to its own spontaneous cycle.
- Fusion beat—conduction mechanism; meeting of a single beat between a sinus beat and VPC.

- Unifocal—conduction mechanism; all ectopic foci are discharged from same single focus.
- Multifocal—conduction mechanism; ectopic beats are from numerous ectopic foci.

## *Ventricular Tachycardia*

You have already learned that in supraventricular tachycardias, the impulse usually reaches the ventricles when they are no longer refractory. Therefore, in supraventricular tachycardias the QRS complex is usually normal in width and its configuration is normal.

However, patient having a normal QRS complex during a normal sinus rhythm may develop a widened QRS or one of abnormal configuration during a supraventricular tachycardia, when the impulse reaches the ventricles during their relative refractory period.

In ventricular tachycardia, the depolarization wave from the ectopic ventricular focus spreads through ordinary myocardium, which, you remember, conducts more slowly than the specialized conduction fiber in the Purkinje system; thus, you would expect that it will be wider than normal (Figs. 20

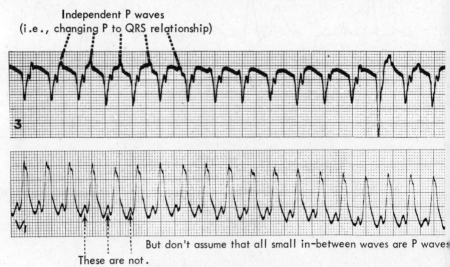

Independent P waves
(i.e., changing P to QRS relationship)

But don't assume that all small in-between waves are P waves
These are not.

If they move along independently, as they do in the top strip
you know they're P waves. If they don't you often can't be s

FIG. 20  Two examples of ventricular tachycardia.
(Reprinted with permission from Marriott, CCU Nursing Slides, 1967,
Tampa Tracings, Oldsmar, Fla.)

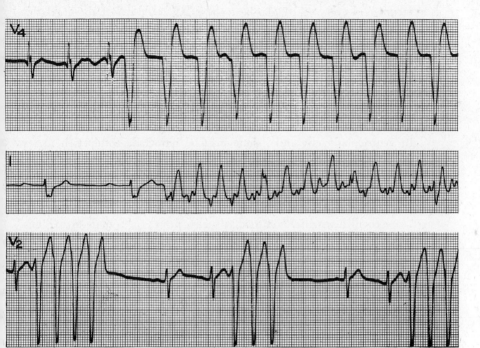

*FIG. 21* Three more examples of ventricular tachycardia.
(Reprinted with permission from Marriott, CCU Nursing Slides, 1967,
Tampa Tracings, Oldsmar, Fla.)

and 21). This is the second time we have mentioned conditions in which the QRS will be widened—the other being in VPCs. In VPCs and ventricular tachycardias, the depolarization waves spread out in all directions from the ectopic focus. The configuration of the QRS complex, therefore, is usually abnormal. (Occasionally, VPCs and ventricular tachycardias arise from foci in or near the bundle of His and spread through the cardiac conduction system to the ventricles. On these occasions, the QRS complex will be normal.) Because of these exceptions, the form of the QRS complex is not always a useful method of differentiating supraventricular and ventricular tachycardias.

As discussed in the previous paragraph, the QRS complexes in supraventricular tachycardia may occasionally be widened and abnormal in configuration; this phenomenon is called "aberrant conduction." Aberrant conduction occurs when a supraventricular impulse reaches the ventricles during their relative refractory period. Thus, if aberrant conduction occurs when the ventricular rhythm is regular in supraventricular tachycardia, repolarization is interrupted in every ventricular beat; the ECG would reflect abnormality in the QRS complex in every beat. When ventricular rhythm is irregular, aberrant conduction might occur either occasionally or with every beat.

Remember, QRS complexes with aberrant conduction occur in conjunction with P waves and appear in constant relation to the P wave with each aberrant beat. QRS complexes of ventricular parasystole have no relation to the P wave, have no constant latency interval, and exhibit a basic rhythm of their own.

In ventricular tachycardia, there may be retrograde conduction in less than 25 percent of the cases. Therefore, the atria are likely to be depolarized as usual by the SA node. Thus, in ventricular tachycardia, the ventricular rate is *always* faster than the atrial rate. The ventricles are independent of atrial action, and their rhythm may be regular or irregular. The P waves are difficult to recognize usually. Ventricular tachycardia is a serious arrhythmia. It may occur on occasions, or paroxysms. To differentiate between ventricular tachycardia and supraventricular, some physicians apply carotid sinus pressure; if the paroxysm is supraventricular in origin, it slows the heart. It will have no effect in ventricular tachycardia.

### Ventricular Tachycardia

- Atrial rate—usually normal; no relation to ventricular.
- Ventricular rate—140 to 200 (greater than 100/min.).
- Rhythm—slightly irregular, usually not visible in atria.
- P-R interval—nonexistent.
- P wave—only occasionally identified.
- QRS complex—widened and bizarre, seemingly regular rapid; all are not necessarily identical; amplitudes greater than normal.
- Conduction mechanism—Than the atria respond to an SA nodal pacemaker. The ventricles respond to a rapid irritable ventricular stimulus.
- Treatment considered—Lidocaine, Pronestyl, quinidine; diphenylhydantoin (Dilantin), especially with digitalis-induced ventricular tachycardia. Countershock if urgent—cardioversion. (Start with 100–200 joules.)
- Significance—extremely dangerous and requires emergency action.

## *Ventricular Fibrillation*

Ventricular fibrillation is often called a terminal rhythm of a dying heart (Figs. 22, 23, and 24). Irregular wide oscillations of the base line form the typical ECG picture. Atrial activity is absent. The patient is pulseless, the blood pressure zero, and no heart sounds can be heard by ear. The patient presents the signs of clinical death. *While the fibrillation waves can be seen on the ECG or oscilloscope monitor,* there is no ventricular contraction, and blood circulation has ceased.

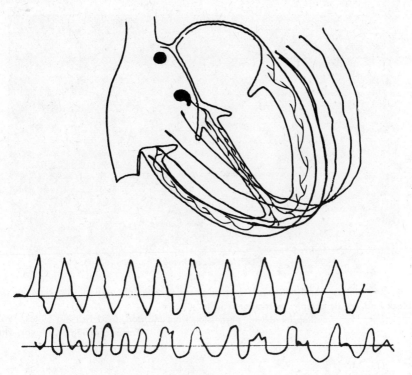

FIG. 22 Ventricular fibrillation is often called a terminal rhythm or a dying heart. Irregular wide oscillations of the base line is typical. Atrial activity is absent. The patient presents a picture of clinical death.

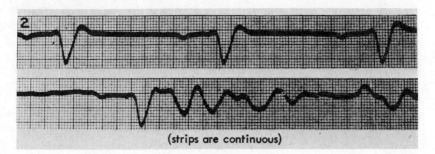

(strips are continuous)

FIG. 23 Dying heart. All complexes and intervals spread-eagled in upper strip, giving place to ventricular fibrillation in lower.

(Reprinted with permission from Marriott, CCU Nursing Slides, 1967, Tampa Tracings, Oldsmar, Fla.)

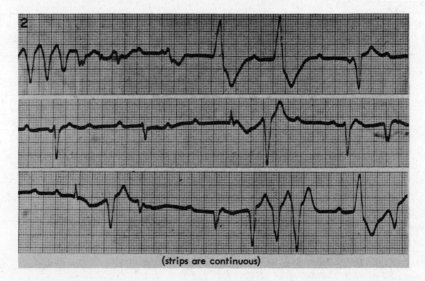

(strips are continuous)

*FIG. 24* Sinister combination of ventricular tachycardia alternating with complete AV block and erratic ectopic ventricular activity.

(Reprinted with permission from Marriott, CCU Nursing Slides, 1967, Tampa Tracings, Oldsmar, Fla.)

In the past, ventricular fibrillation has always been fatal, but in recent years, cardiac massage and electric defibrillation sometimes have been successful in terminating the ventricular fibrillation and saving the patient's life.

*Here lies the major purpose of the coronary care unit: That nursing personnel anticipate this catastrophe and be prepared to prevent it, or, should it occur, be prepared to act quickly to save a heart that is too good to die* (Fig. 25).

## Ventricular Fibrillation

- Atrial rate—not visible.
- Ventricular rate—not determinable; wild, not defined.
- Rhythm—chaotic and irregular.
- P-R interval—nonexistent.
- P wave—not visible.
- QRS complex—bizarre and totally irregular.
- Conduction mechanism—ineffectual twitchings of individual ventricular muscle fibers.
- Treatment considered—immediate defibrillation after oxygen (High shock—400 joules).
- Significance—chaotic undulation, wildly indifferent contractions (fib. movements) of ventricles gives rise to grossly chaotic ECG patterns of wide, slurred, and bizarre configurations of varying amplitudes and durations. Tantamount to cardiac standtstill or arrest.

### Ventricular Asystole

- Atrial rate—usually not identifiable.
- Ventricular rate—none.
- Rhythm—nonexistent.
- P-R interval—nonexistent.
- P wave—sometimes visible.
- QRS complex—not present.
- Conduction mechanism—no ventricular activity.
- Treatment considered—Adrenalin, Isuprel, calcium, pacemaker.
- Significance—biological death.

### *Indications for Countershock*

- *Emergency*—400 joules:
  1. Ventricular fibrillation
  2. Cardiac arrest—if mechanism is known
  3. Any tachycardia complicated by pulmonary edema, shock, etc.

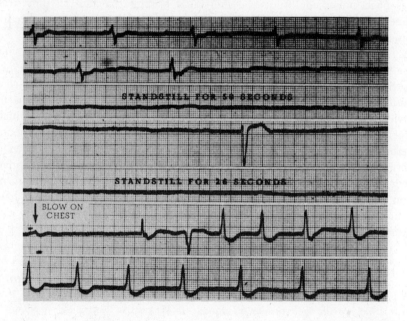

*FIG. 25* Complete AV block and idioventricular rhythm; then ventricular standstill temporarily restored by a thump on the chest.

(Reprinted with permission from Marriott, CCU Nursing Slides, 1967, Tampa Tracings, Oldsmar, Fla.)

- *Urgent*—start with 20–100 joules:
  1. Potentially dangerous tachycardias or tachyarrhythmias (ventricular tachycardia, any tachycardia in presence of heart disease, atrial flutter with 1:1 conduction, etc.)

- *Elective*—start with 20–100 joules:
  1. Any tachyarrhythmia resistant to other forms of therapy
  2. Atrial fibrillation or flutter regardless of ventricular rate—if conversion indicated

- *Anticipated results:*

    Electrical current discharges through the heart and stops the heart momentarily, allowing the sinoatrial node to reestablish its own pacing eliminating the ectopic foci causing the abnormal pattern.

## Summary

In this chapter a discussion of variations in nodal and ventricular rhythms has been presented. Study the individual electrocardiogram rhythm strips closely. It is suggested that the student start a card file of her own, collecting variations with appropriate interpretations.

In many cases no definite policies can be stated in a text of this size since the policies governing the coronary care unit must, of necessity, be governed by hospital policies and the appropriate coronary care or medical staff committee. However, the nurse should have a pretty clear idea of what the individual hospital policies are in regard to nurses being allowed to initiate emergency treatment. In some cases, oxygen is the only emergency action permitted; however, more and more hospitals have widened their policies to permit the nurse to defibrillate, take blood gases, and administer appropriate actions until the physician arrives. Hospital policies concerning administration of intravenous medications and initial nursing history-taking can have definite effects upon the effectiveness of the operations of the coronary care nursing team.

## Review and Advance

1. *What are the arrhythmias most likely to progress to ventricular fibrillation?*
   The arrhythmias may be listed as:
   - increasing ventricular premature contractions
   - multifocal ventricular premature contractions
   - ventricular premature contraction on T wave
   - VPCs occurring more than six per minute

- runs of VPCs, or ventricular tachycardia
- ventricular tachycardia
- complete, or third-degree, heart block

2. *In what condition would the physician insert an internal pacemaker as a preventive measure?*
If the physician suspects or fears that ventricular standstill may occur, he may insert an internal pacing electrode through a peripheral vein. An increasing P-R interval may be such an example to lead him to suspect that preventive action must be in readiness.

3. *Why would you expect the S-T segment and the T wave to be abnormal in tracings of ventricular permature contractions?*
They would be abnormal because abnormal depolarization is followed by abnormal repolarization. If the QRS complex is missing in an APC and PNC, by the same token, the S-T segment and T wave are missing also.

4. *How does depolarization occur?*
Autorhythmicity is a characteristic of the heart. Because of this property, the heart of a laboratory animal can continue to beat when removed from the body under experimental conditions. Depolarization of the myocardium is initiated by spontaneous discharge, usually at the sinoatrial node. Depolarization of the entire myocardium results from the spread of a depolarization wave from fiber to fiber. Thus, we may say that normally, depolarization of myocardial fibers can be initiated by the spontaneous discharge of a myocardial fiber. We know, too, that nervous stimuli influence depolarization, bringing changes in the heart rate. The occurrence of rapid depolarization defines the onset of systole; the slow depolarization phase occurs during diastole.

5. *Do myocardial fibers have different discharge cycles?*
Myocardial fibers in the SA node normally have spontaneous discharge cycles of one second or less. Moving away from the SA node, in the direction in which impulses normally travel, myocardial fibers are longer, thus have longer cycles—the longest, up to ten seconds, located in the ventricles. Myocardial fibers with spontaneous discharge cycles of intermediate length would be found in the AV node, or high in the ventricles. If a myocardial fiber at some focus outside the SA node were to develop a spontaneous discharge cycle shorter than that of the SA node, the pacemaker of the heart would be the former, commonly referred to as an ectopic focus.

6. *Why is the patient with VPCs considered critically ill?*
The greatest danger of VPCs lies in their tendenry to initiate ventricular tachycardia and ventricular fibrillation. Thus, the nurse must recognize that the patient with VPCs must have 24-hour observation. There can be no compromise. The significance of VPCs lies upon their frequency of occurrence; an occasional VPC does not usually change the patient's vital signs and may be controlled through rest by sedation and continuous lidocaine drip. However, if premature contractions occur more than six times per minute and are multifocal (initiated from more than one focus), the patient is considered critical and bears vigilant watching.

7. *How does the vagus nerve affect the activity of the myocardial pacemaker?*
The vagus nerve has a continuously maintained tone, changes in which influence the heart by enhancing or depressing the activity of the pacemaker. In the absence of vagal innervation the SA node would continue to fire. An

increase in the tone of the vagus depresses the activity of the SA node. In other words, the higher the tone of the vagus, the greater the depressant effect on the SA node. As vagal tone increases, the cardiac rate decreases and the P-P interval increases. A decrease in the tone of the vagus enhances the activity of the SA node. The lower the tone of the vagus, the more the activity of the SA node is enhanced. Thus, a decrease in vagal tone enhancing the activity of the SA node would increase the heart rate and decrease the P-P interval.

8. *What is the theory of reentry in relation to ectopic or premature beats?*
According to Friedburg (1967), the fact that premature beats often follow the preceding normal beat at exactly the same intervals (referred to as fixed coupling) suggests that the normal contraction in some way controls the ectopic beat which follows. Another observer suggests that the theory of reentry could explain this exact coupling: according to this concept, the sinus impulse preceding the premature beat activates the heart, but the activation wave is delayed in an area of diminished irritability. Eventually, the impulse activates this abnormal area, but by this time the remainder of the heart has recovered from its response to the sinus impulse. The impulse now reenters the ventricular muscle from the previously depressed zone and elicits another (the premature) contraction. A similar reentry mechanism involving more than one depressed area and multiple reentries has been invoked to account for ectopic tachycardias.

9. *Are premature beats caused by any special etiology?*
The clinical causes of premature beats are uncertain since there are no mechanisms identical with those which induce premature beats in experimental animals. It may be that they follow reflex stimulation of the vagus and sympathetic nerves; for example, the premature beats occasionally induced by painful stimuli, carotid sinus pressure, breath holding or forced respiration. A majority of patients with premature beats are not found to have organic heart disease. However, the presence of heart disease has the tendency to increase the occurrence and frequency of premature beats.

Atrial premature beats are likely to occur in association with disease or enlargement of the atria, such as occurs in cor pulmonale or mitral stenosis, and also in hyperthyroidism and in coronary heart disease. They may also be precursors to atrial tachycardia or fibrillation.

In noncardiac patients, premature beats usually appear without any apparent cause, but may sometimes seem to be related to emotional stress, mental and physical fatigue, irregular dietary habits, particularly when these are combined with excessive smoking and drinking of alcohol or coffee. But the relationship is not clear in that only certain individuals are susceptible to premature beats when exposed to these conditions, and the same individual does not always respond in the same way to the same stimuli. Premature beats may be due to drugs: excesses of digitalis, Dexedrine, isoproterenol, and others. On the other hand, premature beats have been noted in patients with biliary and renal colic as well as in cases of chronic disease of the biliary tract. Infections, particularly those associated with fever, have been said to precipitate premature beats. They have been at times related to cerebral lesions; they have been seen to occur frequently during cardiac catheterization. In short, the occurrence of premature beats is so frequent that a causal relationship to any given factor is often difficult to prove or exclude.

10. *What is atrioventricular block?*

    Atrioventricular block, or AV block or heart block, is the cardiac mechanism resulting from defective conduction of the impulse from the atrium to the ventricle. There may be merely an abnormal delay in transmission of the impulse through the atrioventricular node and bundle of His, or there may be a complete interruption of occasional or of all impulses. Accordingly, AV block is classified as:

    a. prolonged AV conduction time (first-degree block)
    b. partial heart block (second-degree block)
    c. complete heart block (third-degree block)

    Its incidence is uncertain since lesser degrees of heart block are mostly overlooked. It is probable that heart block is exceeded in frequency only by premature beats, atrial fibrillation and paroxysmal atrial tachycardia. The order of frequency in the incidence of heart block is as listed above: first, second, and third.

# 19  CARDIAC ARREST

The principal modes of death from myocardial infarction are cardiogenic shock, congestive heart failure, and arrhythmias. These may appear alone or together, since one may precipitate another. Research has shown that in advanced cases of congestive heart failure and cardiogenic shock, death cannot always be averted; however, the situation is different in cases of cardiac arrest and arrhythmias of certain types. Here, the tremendous life-saving potential of the newer knowledge and methods for early detection and intervention is brought to bear.

## Review of the Term "Sudden Death"

Sudden death is the sudden and unexpected cessation of respirations and functional circulation. The term "sudden death" is synonymous with cardio-pulmonary arrest or heart-lung arrest. A person who dies gradually of an organic disease such as cancer, or is under treatment for a coronary thrombosis and has progressive but gradual loss of cardiac function, is not dying from "sudden death." In short, not everyone who dies is to be considered for emergency life-saving measures.

If the last sentence is studied, the reader will recogize the rationale behind it. Think of your individual hospital policies concerning candidates for "Code 99," "Code Blue," or whatever name is used for emergency cardiac arrest or cardiopulmonary resuscitation. Most hospitals request the patient's physician to note in his orders whether life-saving measures are to be employed on certain patients; other hospitals have been reluctant to do so. Thus, the American Heart Association has recommended that physicians be aware that certain patients suffering from terminal or progressive diseases should not be candidates for emergency measures or cardiopulmonary resuscitation.

312

The lack of respiration and the absence of effective circulation are the two areas to be considered in the problem of sudden death. While the absence of respiration is usually obvious, the absence of functional circulation may not be. It is always possible that the heart may be beating feebly but with minimal cardiac output. In such a situation, functional circulation is usually not adequate to maintain the viability of the vital centers of the body.

## Physiology of Sudden Death

In discussing the physiology of death, the difference between clinical death and biologic death should be recognized. Clinical death occurs at the moment when a person's heart stops beating and he ceases to breathe. At this time the physician might legally sign the death certificate.

The vital higher centers of the central nervous system of the body remain viable, however, for a further period of four to six minutes.[1] In fact, much of the body seems to be alive biologically for much longer periods of time. The most important and sensitive tissue of the body is in the brain. Irreversible changes occur at the cellular level in the human brain at somewhere between four and six minutes. Resuscitation in the treatment of sudden death, or cardiac arrest, is dependent upon this grace period of four to six minutes. After that period, even though the heart might yet be started again, the possible return to a normal functional existence would have been preempted. Thus, the urgency of reestablishment of the oxygenation system of the body must occur between this four- to six-minute grace period and cannot be over-emphasized.

## History of Treatment of Cardiac Arrest [2]

Many individuals are of the opinion that cardiac arrest treatment is of fairly recent origin, yet we read in Elisha, II Kings ". . . And he lay upon the child and put his mouth upon his mouth, his eyes upon his eyes, and his hands upon his hands, and the breath of the child waxed warm."

This biblical passage is probably the first description ever to be written of mouth-to-mouth artificial respiration. In 1543 Vesalius described a form of artificial respiration which consisted of placing a reed into the trachea of an experimental animal and inflating the lungs. Vesalius also carried out the first tracheotomy and left detailed sketches of the circulatory system as well as the respiratory system.

1. "Emergency Measures in Cardiopulmonary Resuscitation," American Heart Association in cooperation with The Heart Association of Maryland, 1965.
2. Adapted from "Emergency Measures in Cardiopulmonary Resuscitation," American Heart Association in cooperation with The Heart Association of Maryland, 1965.

Open-chest cardiac massage was first performed by Schiff in Florence, Italy, in the latter half of the nineteenth century while carrying out experimental work on resuscitation from sudden death under chloroform anesthesia. By 1874, the technique of open-chest direct cardiac massage was established.

In 1878 Boehm in Germany carried out experiments on cats using a form of external heart compression by rhythmically compressing the sides of the cat's thorax with good results. In 1881 Niehaus attempted to resuscitate a human being from cardiac arrest occurring under anesthesia by use of the open-chest direct cardiac massage but was unsuccessful. In 1890, Maas, working in Koenig's Clinic in Goettingen, Germany, resuscitated a child and a young lady from sudden death under anesthesia by using the closed-chest cardiac compression technique. These were the first and second recorded resuscitations of human beings from cardiac arrest. Thus, the progress of closed-chest cardiac massage advanced slowly and cautiously over the years.

It was not until 1901 that Igelsrud in Norway described and recorded the resuscitation of a forty-year-old woman who, undergoing a hysterectomy, had had a cardiac arrest. He used the open-chest direct cardiac massage technique. One year later, Starling and Lane reported similar succesess in England. In 1904, George Crile, Sr., introduced the use of intravenous or intracardiac epinephrine into the procedure of resuscitation from cardiac arrest. He also used a form of external cardiac compression in successful resuscitation of at least one patient.

In the following decades the technique of closed-chest cardiac compression was used only sporadically, and then, the results went unrecorded. The open-chest direct massage procedure seemed to gain favor and saved many lives, with reported percentage rates sometimes as high as 65 percent but averaging from 25 to 35 percent. Tournade did some experimental work in France in the 1930's on closed-chest cardiac compression and the Russians, in the 1940's, did similar work. The latter use was associated with external electrical defibrillation of the heart from ventricular fibrillation but was not employed in human beings. Closed-chest cardiac compression was put on a firm physiologic basis and employed on large numbers of clinical cases in 1960 by Kouwenhoven and associates at Johns Hopkins Hospital, Baltimore, Maryland.

Prevost and Batelli are credited with doing the basic work in 1898–99 on reverting the heart from the nonfunctional state of ventricular fibrillation. Between 1929 and 1933 Hooker, Langworthy, and Kouwenhoven also carried out studies in electrical conversion of ventricular fibrillation, using both the open-chest and closed-chest techniques. From their work evolved a technique successfully applied on the first human being by Claude Beck in 1947. This was on a young boy who went into ventricular fibrillation suddenly during an operation. He remains alive today after electrical fibrillation applied directly to the heart. In 1955, Paul Zoll reported the first human being to be resuscitated from ventricular fibrillation by external electric countershock and shortly following this similar reports were made independently by Kouwenhoven and associates.

Evolvement of expired air artificial respiration of mouth-to-mouth, mouth-to-nose, or mouth-to-airway and closed-chest cardiac compression allowed simplified means of preventing biologic death by properly trained individuals, both lay and professional.

## *The Nurse's Responsibility*

It is important to remember that arrhythmias and cardiac arrests do not occur only in the severely ill patient, but occur just as frequently in the so-called milder forms of heart disease. The myocardial damage need not be great and the immediate cause of a fatality may be only a transient disturbance. If this disturbance is successfully interrupted, or reversed, satisfactory cardiac activity can resume.

Thus the coronary care unit has been organized around a central theme: the major life-saving potential of the unit requires that all nursing personnel understand the one-lead electrocardiogram pattern so that they can recognize arrhythmias immediately. Identifying and calling the physician's attention immediately to those monitored irregularities which may be precursors of more serious arrhythmias may provide the physician with sufficient time to use therapeutic measures and drugs to prevent arrest (Figs. 1 and 2).

### VENTRICULAR FLUTTER

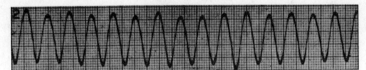

Semi-formed complexes - regular zigzag

### VENTRICULAR FIBRILLATION

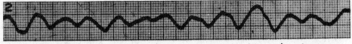

Completely unformed complexes - disorganized irregular zigzag

*FIG. 1* The dying heart.

(Reprinted with permission from Marriott, CCU Nursing Slides, 1967, Tampa Tracings, Oldsmar, Fla.)

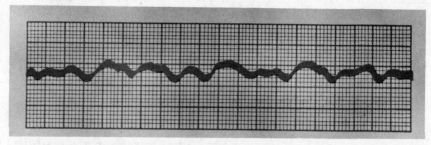

*FIG. 2* Ventricular arrhythmia preceding cardiac arrest.
(Reprinted with permission from Marriott, CCU Nursing Slides, 1967,
Tampa Tracings, Oldsmar, Fla.)

But, sometimes, recognition is not enough. For therapy, the nurse will have atropine in readiness for a patient observed to be in bradycardia; for the patient whom she observes developing premature ventricular contractions, she will have lidocaine or propranolol ready for intravenous use; for a patient with conduction defects, she will have a pacemaker and the specially prepared intrathoracic pacemaker wires ready in anticipation of the physician's actions.[2] The coronary care nurse may, in some hospitals, deliver DC countershock when she recognizes ventricular fibrillation. She may also be permitted to give the above drugs.

During a cardiac arrest, the nurse administers sodium bicarbonate intravenously and prepares epinephrine, calcium, and other drugs in anticipation of the physician's needs. She runs "rhythm" electrocardiogram strips, performs twelve-lead electrocardiograms, and operates trend recorders when such documentation is required.

It is not unusual for one or more of the nurses from the coronary care unit to respond to emergency calls "Code 99" throughout the hospital (Fig. 3). In addition, these nurses serve as nursing consultants on problems occurring in the general medical units.

So far in this text, you have been given information to enable you to acquire skill in recognizing various cardiac arrhythmias and how to differentiate between those which closely resemble each other. This information has been arranged mostly in outline form where possible to provide simplified reference.

This chapter presents the standard procedure for cardiac resuscitation, as well as other conditions in which the state of the patient resembles cardiac arrest. It will be broken down into the barest amount of words in final summary.

2. Donna Zschoche and Lillian Brown. Intensive Care Nursing, Specialism, Junior Doctoring, or Just Nursing. *A.J.N.,* Nov., 1969.

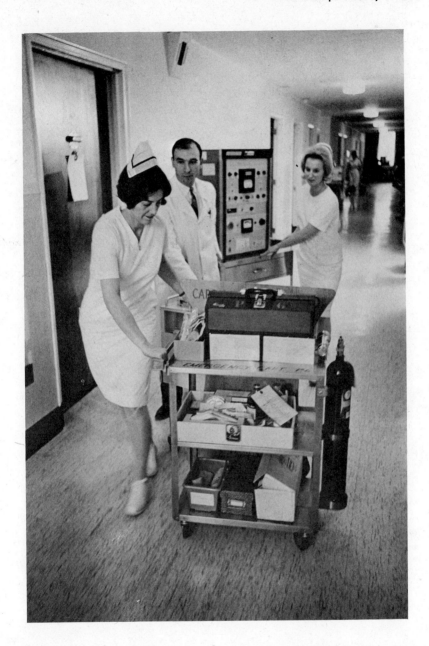

FIG. 3 Cart will be brought to the scene. One is usually standard part of coronary care unit. If arrest occurs outside the unit, or cart is not on the unit, the Emergency Room personnel bring their cart to the scene.

(Courtesy of Tufts-New England Medical Center, Boston, Mass.)

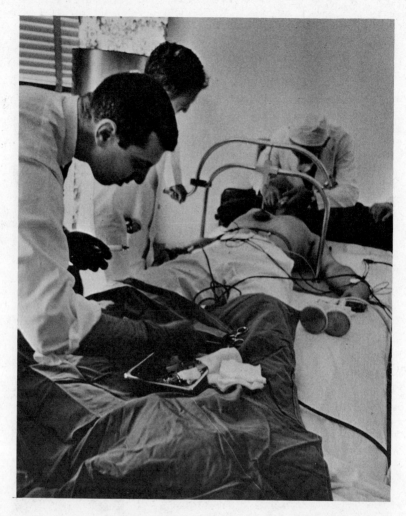

*FIG. 4* A physician performs a venous cutdown to insert a catheter into the vein for administration of intravenous fluids.

(Courtesy of Tufts-New England Medical Center, Boston, Mass.)

## Cardiac Arrest

Cardiac arrest may be secondary to ventricular fibrillation and asystole. For this reason, it is discussed here. External resuscitation should be applied until the mechanism for the arrest is found. If ventricular fibrillation is present, external defibrillation should be carried out. The American Cardiologists' Association urges that all nurses on duty in the coronary care unit be equipped to carry out this procedure. Although most nursing personnel are familiar with the procedure of external cardiac resuscitation, the following approach is usually followed:

- Obtain ECG or monitor patient to determine type of cardiac arrest (asystole or ventricular fibrillation).
- If indicated by presence of ventricular fibrillation, apply external defibrillator.

These two procedures are usually done immediately following the check for criteria of arrest:

- Absent pulse
- Dilated pupils
- Respirations down or absent

If confirmed, the patient will be unconscious or becoming so with abnormal rhythm on scope, skin cool, moist, or cyanotic. At times, the patient may convulse. At this point, the procedure may differ according to whether the patient is in asystole, ventricular fibrillation or tachycardia.

## Asystole

- Strike chest; if not immediately effective, then
- Place board under chest
- Remove pillow
- External pacemaker, if available
  Set rate at 75; voltage up p.r.n., chest wall contraction.
  Check for pulse: if present, check blood pressure; if absent, continue.
- Circulate and ventilate
  Apply cardiac compressions at approximately 60/minute.
  Open airway: ventilate 12/minute with mouth-to-mouth, bag and mask, O2.
- Sodium bicarbonate 3.75 g q. 5–10 minutes IV or IV drip 5 percent in 500 cc
- Isuprel (isoproterenol hydrochloride) 1 mg in drip 500 cc 5 percent D/W
- Vasopressors in IV drip to maintain blood pressure (Fig. 4):
  Isuprel (isoproterenol 1 mg in 500 cc 5 percent D/W
  Aramine (metaraminol bitartrate) 200 mg-500 cc 5 percent D/W
  Levophed (arterenol) 16 mg-500 cc 5 percent D/W
- Calcium chloride intracardiac, 5 cc of 10 percent solution
- Pacemaker
- Epinephrine intracardiac, 0.5 cc, 1:1000 (Fig. 5)
- Idioventricular rate 40:
  Atropine 1mg in 10 cc NS, IV
    or
  Isuprel 1 mg in 500 cc 5 percent D/W
- Pacemaker
- Cardiac electrode

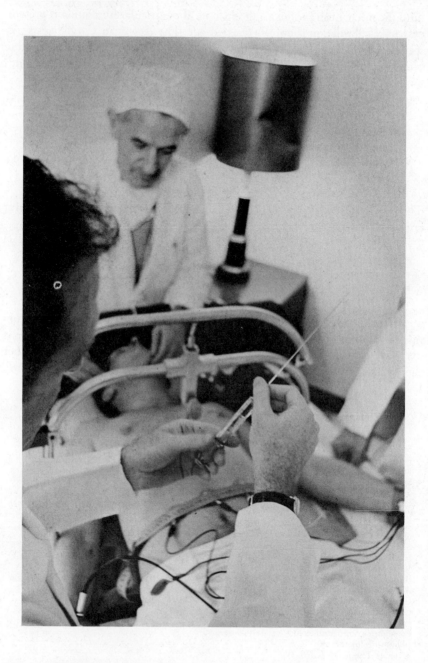

*FIG. 5* The anesthesiologist has taken over artificial ventilation, while another physician prepares to administer an intracardiac injection.

(Courtesy of Tufts-New England Medical Center, Boston, Mass.)

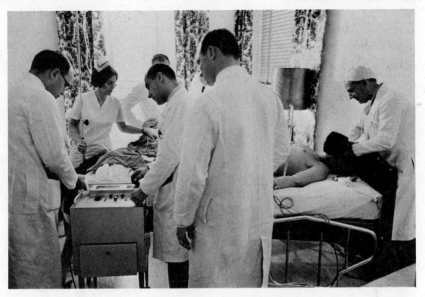

*FIG. 6*  ECG pattern is observed for signs of restored circulation.
(Courtesy of Tufts-New England Medical Center, Boston, Mass.)

The nurse is usually the person to initiate treatment and call for help by calling the operator to announce "Code 99" (or whatever code name is used in the hospital). She may proceed through the first five steps before assistance arrives then, as the physician assumes control, she acts as his assitant. She assembles drugs, airways, oxygen, bedboard, etc., initiates record sheet, and relates events to the physician. If an anesthesiologist answers the call, he assumes control of cardiopulmonary resuscitation.

The physician assumes general control and performs ECG analysis (Fig. 6), drug therapy, defibrillation (Fig. 7), pacing, etc.

### Ventricular Fibrillation or Ventricular Tachycardia

- Strike chest; if not immediately effective, then
- DC shock: 400 watt/sec. within 30 sec. of cardiac arrest
- DC shock: repeat singly and in series within another 15–20 sec.
- Circulate and ventilate
  Apply cardiac compression at approximately 60/minute.
  Open airway: ventilate 12/min., mouth-to-mouth, bag and mask, O2
- Sodium bicarbonate 3.75 g q. 5–10 min. IV or IV drip 5 percent in 500 cc.
- Lidocaine 100 mg IV
- DC shock
- Aramine 200 mg in 500 cc 5 percent D/W
- DC Shock

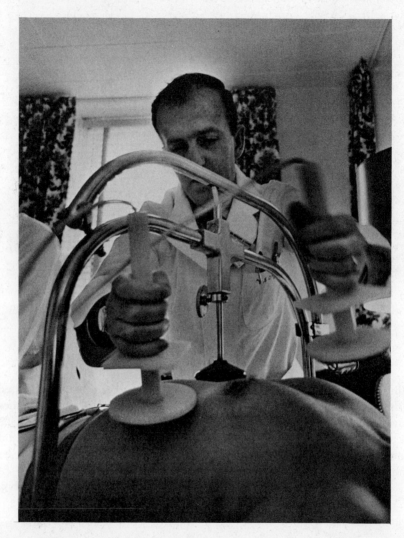

*FIG. 7* The mechanical cardiac massage equipment is momentarily stopped while the physician applies electrical shock.

(Courtesy of Tufts-New England Medical Center, Boston, Mass.)

- Epinephrine intracardiac, 0.5 cc, 1:1,000
- DC Shock
- Calcium chloride intracardiac, 5 cc of 10 percent solution
- DC Shock

The method described here is the technique basically as outlined by Kouwenhoven and associates.

## Adams-Stokes Attacks

This term refers to attacks of acute cerebral ischemia with or without unconsciousness and convulsions following sudden changes in cardiac rhythm which markedly decrease cardiac output. These may occur during bursts of ventricular tachycardia or fibrillation and during prolonged asystole with transition from sinus rhythm to complete heart block, or during shifts between complete and incomplete block. Symptoms of impaired consciousness begin about 3 to 10 seconds after transient circulatory arrest, and complete loss of consciousness occurs after 10 to 20 seconds. In the majority of cases no precipitating factors are demonstrable. The attacks begin suddenly, seldom last longer than 1 to 2 minutes, and are *not followed* by postictal confusion as common in seizures of epilepsy. During the attack pallor is often marked, pulse and heart sounds are absent of asystole or ventricular fibrillation is the mechanism.

Treatment during repeated attacks should sound familiar now. During the last year, more and more frequently we have been advised that the first thing to do upon discovery of cardiac arrest is "to direct one vigorous thump on the precordium in an effort to initiate cardiac contraction." One can understand why anyone finding the patient in an attack of Adams-Stokes deduces "cardiac arrest" for momentarily, the patient, for all appearances, is in that state. A vigorous thump, or a few rapid direct thumpings on the precordium may reactivate the pacemaker.

Transistorized electrical pacemakers attached to an electrode catheter placed in the right ventricle may maintain heart rate temporarily. Catheter pacemakers with a subcutaneous power-pack are now being used on a permanent basis and have largely replaced transthoracic myocardial implantations. Many cardiologists recommend early installation of such artificial pacemakers in patients with recurrent Adams-Stokes attacks and feel that drug therapy has little place in the continuing therapy in this situation.

Isoproterenol (Isuprel) and epinephrine are the drugs most effective in acute attacks, but Isuprel is preferred by many because its activity is largely restricted to the higher cardiac pacemakers (sinus and AV nodes); it is five times as potent as epinephrine in increasing rhythmicity of the ventricular pacemakers; it has much less tendency to produce ventricular fibrillation in the presence of previous damage, and it has essentially no vasoconstrictor action.

Epinephrine may cause striking elevation of the blood pressure and may precipitate ventricular tachycardia or fibrillation; it generally is not used unless it is certain that asystole is present. Both drugs may be given by intracardiac injection for the treatment of cardiac arrest, as has been discussed before. However, both drugs are much less effective if acidosis is present. Suggested routine for these drugs is as follows:

- Isuprel IV infusion: 1–2 mg diluted in 200 cc 5 percent D.W. administer at rate of 0.5–0.10 cc/minute.
  Subcutaneously: 0.2 mg q.3.h.
  Sublingually: 10–20 mg q.2–4.h.
- Epinephrine IV infusion: 3.0 cc, 1:1,000 solution diluted in 300 cc 5 percent D/W, administration rate dictated by adequacy of heart rate.
  Subcutaneously: 0.2–0.3 cc, 1:1,000 solution q.1–2.h.
  Intramuscularly: 0.5–1.0 cc, 1:1,000 epinephrine in oil q.6–12 h.

Other measures used for less urgent situations include:

- Sympathomimetic drugs for maintenance
  a. Isuprel, sublingually, 10–20 mg, q. 3–4 h.
  b. Ephedrine, 10–20 mg, q.3–4 h.
  c. Amphetamine, 5–10 mg. q.i.d.
- Atropine, 0.5–1.0 mg subcutaneously, t.i.d. or q.i.d. as useful adjunct to improve AV conduction.
- Corticosteroids may be useful in heart block associated with acute myocardial infarction, according to some physicians. The reasoning here is that steroids decrease inflammation and edema in the area of the conducting system, thereby accelerating AV conduction. Large doses (e.g., prednisone 40–60 mg daily) are usually given for several days.
- Thiazides in large doses (e.g., hydrochlorothiazide, 500–1,000 mg daily) have been reported to be beneficial in certain patients, probably inducing mild hypokalemia. This mechanism is still under continuing research.

## Adams-Stokes Syndrome

- Atrial rate—usually normal.
- Ventricular rate—variable.
- Rhythm—ventricular tachycardia, fibrillation, asystole.
- P-R interval—noncontributory.
- P wave—may or may not be present.
- QRS complex—may be bizarre, irregular or absent.
- Conduction mechanism—usually due to failure of ventricular pacemaker in the presence of complete heart block.
- Treatment considered—Isuprel, pacemaker, thumping on precordium may initiate cardiac contraction.

## Summary

The nurse's role is not easily identified in every situation, and, at times, it is difficult to delineate where the nurse's role ends and the physician's role begins. For this reason, the team concept of patient care becomes a very real thing in the coronary care unit. Hospital policies play a large part in deciding whether the nurse is free to apply DC countershock after recognizing a death-dealing arrhythmia, or must sound the alarm and immediately commence to ventilate and circulate when she is faced with a patient in suddent arrest. In any case, the role of the nurse as an astute observer and recorder throughout the procedure never ceases. She will anticipate the physician's needs and attempt to assist every step of the way. On the other hand, the nurse in a small hospital may find that hospital administration in conjunction with the medical committee has laid down broad guidelines within which she may operate. If she feels she is competent and can safely act within those guidelines, making full use of her knowledge and skills, then she must act accordingly.

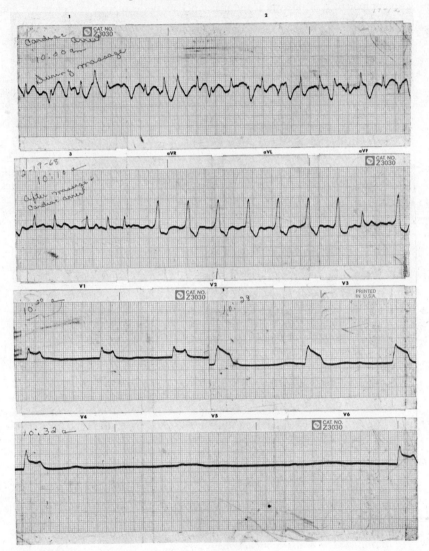

*FIG. 8* Strips run during cardiac massage manually, and after a brief activity, cardiac arrest ensues.

*Review and Advance*

1. *What factors contribute most to the success of cardiopulmonary resuscitation?*
   The two factors contributing to a successful attempt to cardiopulmonary resuscitation are the organization of equipment and the training of personnel.
   The latter is by far the more important since all the latest and most modern
   equipment is of no avail if the personnel are not equipped to understand and
   use it properly.

2. *What are the identifiable signs of cardiac arrest?* (See Figure 8.)
   Immediate recognition is essential:
   a. Erratic or no tracing on ECG monitor, if patient is on monitor.
   b. Loss of consciousness.
   c. Absence of pulses—carotid or femoral. If the patient is on the cardiac
      monitor, there will always be a pattern of ventricular fibrillation or
      standstill; this is adequate for diagnosis.
   d. Absence of respirations.

3. *Is it possible for a cardiac arrest victim to have pinpoint pupils?*
   Yes, it is. This may be one of several unreliable signs. The pupils may be
   constricted because of the effects of drugs which have been previously given,
   such as morphine; they may remain constricted for as long as 5 to 6 minutes
   after arrest. Other unreliable signs are pulses of smaller arteries as well as
   auscultation; and finally, the alarm of the monitoring system may activate for
   reasons other than cardiac arrest.

4. *What is the "A-B-C-D" system of cardiopulmonary resuscitation?*
   This is simply an easy code to remind the nurse that there are certain priority
   steps that she may perform before assistance arrives. However, many hospitals
   use this system in standard "Code 99" procedures as follows:

   A = Airway must be patent
   B = Breathing must be done for the patient
   C = Circulation must be kept going
   D = Definitive treatment by drugs, ECG, pacemaker, defibrillator, etc.

   The last, incidentally, may run through the entire alphabet, and helps to
   prevent panic.

5. *Is the "S-tube" really more effective than mouth-to-mouth breathing?*
   This technique is more difficult to apply but is more acceptable to some
   rescuers. However, experienced rescuers using several methods and airway
   devices had the least delay and best tidal volume with the tube identified as
   "the flanged tube with bite block," called the *rescue breather* (available from
   Medical Supply Company, Rockford, Illinois). However, mouth-to-mouth
   breathing is the best way to provide ventilation during the emergency phase.
   Once additional assistance is available, an experienced rescuer may elect to
   use a bag and mask. A bag and mask or endotracheal tube allow the addition
   to the ventilation system. The problem of retching and laryngospasm in the
   patient is lessened somewhat.

6. *Can the patient be attached to an automatic cycling machine or respirator
   during cardiac arrest resuscitation?*
   Ordinary pressure-cycled intermittent positive pressure breathing machines

(IPPB) are not helpful in cardiopulmonary resuscitation because external cardiac compression triggers cessation of the inspiratory phase, and the flow rate is too slow to give adequate ventilation without an excessively long pause. However, certain volume-cycled apparatus may be of use after the emergency phase, this with careful evaluation of your equipment. The author is familiar with one such ventilator assistance apparatus which spaces inspiration at a one to five ratio with chest compressions. In fact, there are several such mechanical aids providing both ventilation and external cardiac compression simultaneously. Although they spare manpower during prolonged resuscitation (and relieve exhausted rescuers), their disadvantage includes their high cost and the human tendency to delay the essentials of maintaining a patent airway, breathing, and circulation while setting up the equipment.

7. *Are complications common to cardiopulmonary resuscitation?*
Surely, there are complications to this procedure just as there are to almost any emergency technique. Certainly any complications can be minimized by proper technique; however, one can never be certain as to how or when they may occur. The most common complications include fractured ribs, separated costochondral junctions and fractured sternum. Occasionally, pneumothorax or injury to the heart, liver, and spleen occur. Although they are all undesirable, they are to be preferred to no resuscitation attempt at all.

8. *What is meant by "definitive" therapy?*
Definitive therapy of cardiac arrest is directed toward the cause of the cardiac arrest and its effects.

9. *Differentiate between ventricular standstill, ventricular fibrillation, and cardiovascular collapse.*
Ventricular standstill indicates no visible rhythm of either atria or ventricles, thus cardiac arrest. Ventricular fibrillation is a death-dealing arrhythmia. The time from its onset to its termination in physical or biologic death is no longer than six minutes. When the usual rhythm of the myocardial fibers acting as a unit begins to behave erratically, producing a wriggling twitching organ (one physician describes it as a wriggling bag of worms), the quivering heart cannot contract to force the blood into the circulation in response to the body's needs. The patient becomes pulseless, cyanotic and convulsed.

Cardiovascular collapse resembles a "power failure." The circulatory failure is of central origin, that is, heart failure rather than peripheral or blood vessel origin. In short, the patient is suffering from cardiogenic shock: failure of the cardiac pumping mechanism results in cardiogenic shock. The effects of such cardiac failure are the same as for hematogenic shock: a deficiency of cellular nutrition and oxygenation, and a deficiency in the removal of cellular wastes. It may occur with anaphylaxis, hypokalemia, drug toxicity, e.g., quinidine, digitalis, procaine). The treatment is directed toward the underlying causes, if known.

10. *When should attempts at cardiopulmonary resuscitation cease?*
The American Heart Association offers the following criteria in determining when resuscitative efforts should cease:
   a. Cardiac death—when there has been no evidence of electrical activity on the oscilloscope for at least 30 minutes; inability to maintain satisfactory rhythm; persistent ventricular fibrillation despite all forms of therapy.

    b. Brain death—as shown by fixed dilated or "box-car" pupils and absence of spontaneous respirations.

    c. Patient's history—where there has been a known delay of ten minutes or more before resuscitation was initiated, or presence of irreversible or terminal disease with no chance of return to functional existence.

    d. No improvement—of any kind after 60 minutes of intensive resuscitation.

11. *What is the nurse's responsibility in postresuscitative care?*
The nurse becomes the patient monitor. She not only observes the ECG monitor but, by her astute observations, will recognize and treat arrhythmias as ordered. She will monitor vital signs and neurologic signs and record these accurately and frequently, as well as maintain adequate intake and output records and support ventilation and circulation as required. She has an obligation to reassure the patient and his family, as well as provide supportive nursing care to the patient.

12. *How is metabolic acidosis corrected during cardiac arrest?*
In the presence of circulatory collapse, profound metabolic acidosis occurs and persists in spite of cardiopulmonary resuscitation which perfuses body tissues, at a markedly reduced level. Sodium bicarbonate, 3.75 g, should be promptly administered and repeated each ten minutes of cardiac compression. The maintenance of an approximately normal pH through such efforts renders the myocardium more responsive to innate and administered cathecholamines. Where readily available, the determination of blood pH may be a useful guide.

13. *What is the effect of external cardiac compression on blood pH?*
Experimentally in the dog, a rapid fall in blood pH during ventricular fibrillation is apparent in spite of effective external cardiac compression. Administration of sodium bicarbonate in doses of 0.63 mEq/Kg of body weight at frequent intervals readily restores the blood pH to normal. In human adults, 44.6 mEq (3.75 g) should be used every ten minutes without regard for weight. With profound depression of pH, hyperventilation is common and often necessary as a compensatory respiratory mechanism following resuscitation.

14. *What is the principle of electric countershock?*
The basic principle of electric countershock is the simultaneous complete depolarization of the entire myocardium. This allows spontaneous depolarization and synchronous discharge from the sinoatrial node.

# III   Appendices

# A TERMINOLOGY COMMON TO CARDIOVASCULAR DISEASE

**ADRENALIN**

One of the secretions of two small glands, called adrenal glands, located just above the kidneys. This secretion, also called epinephrine, and sometimes prepared synthetically, constricts the small blood vessels (arterioles), increases the rate of heart beat, and raises blood pressure. It is called a vasoconstrictor or vasopressor substance.

**AMINE**

An organic compound that may be derived from ammonia by the replacement of one or more of the hydrogen atoms by hydrocarbon radicals.

**ANASARCA**

Generalized edema.

**ANEURYSM**

Localized weakening of the elasticity of the aortic membrane resulting in a localized "bulge" of the vessel.

**ANGINA PECTORIS**

Paroxysmal pain characterized by a sense of oppression and severe constriction about the chest. The pain radiates from the precordium to the left shoulder and down the arm to the ulnar nerve; associated with it is a sense of apprehension of impending death. The pain is caused by myocardial ischemia and occurs suddenly because of emotional stress or physical exertion.

**ANGIOCARDIOGRAM**

A procedure used to determine cardiac defects. An opaque fluid which shows up as a shadow on x-ray is injected rapidly into a large vein. Its course of travel through the heart, to the lungs, back to the heart, and out through the aorta is followed in a rapid series of x-ray pictures. The individual chambers of the heart are visualized, anomalous pathways for the blood stream are demonstrated, and chamber enlargement can be determined.

## ANOREXIA

Lack or loss of appetite for food.

## ANOXIA

Hypoxia: absence of oxygen. Failure of tissue to either receive or to utilize an adequate amount of oxygen.

## ANTICOAGULANT

A drug which delays clotting of blood. (Heparin, Dicumarol, warfarin.)

## ANTIHYPERTENSIVE AGENTS

Drugs which are used to lower blood pressure. Rauwolfia, resperpine, Veratrum, hydralazine (Hemamethonium-chloride).

## ANXIETY

A feeling of apprehension, the source of which is unrecognized.

## AORTA

The large vessel arising from the left ventricle and distributing, through its branches, arterial blood to every part of the body except the lungs.

## AORTIC ARCH

The part of the aorta, or large artery leaving the heart, that curves up over the top of the heart like the handle of a cane.

## AORTIC INSUFFICIENCY

Incompetent valve action between the aorta and the lower left chamber of the heart, admitting a back flow of blood. Symptoms: diastolic murmur and "waterhammer" pulse.

## AORTIC STENOSIS

A narrowing of the valve opening between the lower left chamber of the heart and the large artery called the aorta. The narrowing may occur at the valve itself or slightly above or below the valve. Aortic stenosis may be the result of scar tissue forming after a rheumatic fever infection, or may have other causes.

## AORTIC VALVE

Valve at the junction of the aorta, or large artery, and the lower left chamber of the heart. Formed by three cup-shaped membranes called semilunar valves, it allows the blood to flow from the heart into the artery and prevents a back flow.

**AORTITIS**

Inflammation of the aorta.

**AORTOGRAPHY**

X-ray examination of the aorta (main artery conducting blood from the lower left chamber of the heart to the body) and its main branches. This is made possible by the injection of a dye which is opaque to x-rays.

**APEX**

The blunt rounded end of the heart, directed downward, forward, and to the left.

**APNEA**

Temporary cessation of breathing (as in Cheyne-Stokes respiration).

**APOPLEXY**

Frequently called apoplectic stroke or simply stroke. A sudden interruption of the blood supply to a part of the brain caused by the obstruction or rupture of an artery. Initially may be manifested by a loss of consciousness, sensation, or voluntary motion, and may leave a part of the body (frequently one side) temporarily or permanently paralyzed.

**ARRHYTHMIA**

A disturbance in cardiac rate or rhythm.

**ARRHYTHMIA (Fatal)**

Demands immediate resuscitation (defibrillation) in order to prevent death.

**ARRHYTHMIA (Major)**

Reduces efficiency of the heart and warns of impending danger.

**ARTERIAL BLOOD**

Oxygenated blood. The blood is oxygenated in the lungs, passes from the lungs to the left side of the heart via the pulmonary veins. It is then pumped by the left side of the heart into the arteries which carry it to all parts of the body.

**ARTERIOGRAM**

X-ray examination of a peripheral artery after injection of radiopaque dye. Test used to confirm diagnosis of occlusive disease of the peripheral arteries.

**ARTERIOLES**

The smallest arterial vessels (about 0.2 mm or 1/125 inch in diameter), resulting from repeated branching of the arteries. They conduct the blood from the arteries to the capillaries.

## ARTERIOSCLEROSIS

Degenerative changes in arteries resulting in thickening of walls, loss of elasticity, and sometimes calcium deposits.

## ARTERY

A blood vessel that carries blood away from the heart to the various parts of the body. The arteries usually carry oxygenated blood, except for the pulmonary artery which carries unoxygenated blood from the heart to the lungs for oxygenation.

## ASCHOFF BODIES

Spindle-shaped nodules, occurring most frequently in the tissue of the heart, often formed during attacks of rheumatic fever. Named after Ludwig Aschoff (1866–1942), the German pathologist who described them.

## ATHEROMA

Deposits in the intimal layer of an artery.

## ATHEROSCLEROSIS

Lipid or fatty deposits or plaques within and beneath the intima of an artery.

## ATRIAL SEPTAL DEFECT

A communication (or opening) between the left and right atria.

## ATRIAL SEPTUM

Sometimes called interatrial septum or interauricular septum. Muscular wall dividing left and right upper chambers of the heart which are called atria.

## ATRIOVENTRICULAR BUNDLE

Also called *bundle of His, auriculoventricular bundle,* or *AV bundle.* A bundle of specialized muscle fibers running from a small mass of muscular fibers (atrioventricular node) between the upper chambers of the heart, down to the lower chambers. It is the only known direct muscular connection between the upper and lower heart chambers, and serves to conduct impulses for the rhythmic heart beat from the atrioventricular node to the heart muscle.

## ATRIOVENTRICULAR HEART BLOCK

Condition wherein conduction of the impulse between the atria and ventricles is slowed or impeded. Three forms occur:

First-Degree: AV block—prolonged AV conduction.
Second-Degree: Partial AV block—beats are dropped.
Third-Degree: Complete AV block—ventricular contractions are independent of the atria and assume their own rhythm, about thirty to forty beats per minute.

## ATRIOVENTRICULAR (AV) NODE

A small mass of special muscular fibers at the base of the wall between the two upper chambers of the heart. It forms the beginning of the bundle of His.

## ATRIOVENTRICULAR VALVES

The two valves, one in each side of the heart, between the upper and lower chamber. The one in the right atrium is called the *tricuspid valve,* and the one in the left side is called the *mitral valve.*

## ATRIUM

One of the two upper chambers of the heart. Also called auricle, although this is now generally used to describe only the very tip of the atrium. Right atrium receives unoxygenated blood from the body. Left atrium receives oxygenated blood from the lungs. Capacity in adult is about 57 cc.

## AUENBRUGGER, LEOPOLD JOSEPH (1722–1809)

Austrian physician who invented the technique of tapping the surface of the body to determine the condition of organs beneath. The technique is called percussion.

## AURICLE

The upper chamber in each side of the heart. "Atrium" is another term commonly used for this chamber.

## AURICULAR FIBRILLATION

The auricles (atria) quiver ineffectually, and do not contract or propel blood into the ventricles. The ventricles continue to contract but usually at a very rapid rate, creating a *pulse deficit* because not every ventricular contraction is strong enough to come down as far as the wrist pulse. Apex rate exceeds pulse rate.

## AURICULAR SEPTUM

Sometimes called interauricular septum or, more properly, interatrial septum. Muscular wall dividing left and right upper chambers of the heart which are called atria.

## AUSCULTATION

The act of listening to sounds within the body, usually with a stethoscope.

## AUTONOMIC NERVOUS SYSTEM

Sometimes called involuntary nervous system or vegetative nervous system, it controls tissues not under voluntary control, e.g., glands, heart, and smooth muscles.

## BACTERIAL ENDOCARDITIS

An inflammation of the inner layer of heart caused by bacteria. The lining of the heart valves is most frequently affected. It is most commonly a complication of an infectious disease, operation, or injury.

### BALLISTOCARDIOGRAM

A tracing of the movements of the body caused by the beating of the heart. The instrument which records these movements is called a ballisto-cardiograph.

### BALLISTOCARDIOGRAPH

An apparatus for recording the movements of the body caused by the beating of the heart.

### BARBITURATE

A class of drugs that produce a calming effect. A sedative.

### BENZOTHIADIAZINE

A drug used to increase the output of urine by the kidney. A diuretic.

### BICUSPID VALVE

Usually called mitral valve. A valve of two cusps or triangular segments, located between the upper and lower chamber in the left side of the heart.

### BIGEMINY

A premature beat coupled with each normal beat.

### BLOOD PRESSURE

Measurement of arterial blood pressure, or the amount of pressure exerted by the blood against the walls of arteries. It is usually measured at the brachial artery, in millimeters of mercury, by indirect auscultation (stethoscope).

### BLUE BABIES

Babies having a blueness of skin (cyanosis) caused by insufficient oxygen in the arterial blood. This often indicates a heart defect, but may have other causes such as premature birth or impaired respiration.

### BRADYCARDIA

Abnormally slow heart rate. Generally, anything below 60 beats per minute is considered bradycardia.

### BRIGHT, RICHARD (1789–1858)

English physician who demonstrated the association of heart disease with kidney disease.

### BROMIDE

Any one of several drugs that produce a calming effect. A sedative.

### BUNDLE-BRANCH BLOCK

When only one branch of the bundle of His is affected. Rate is normal, but timing is off. There are no symptoms and can be found only through electrocardiagram.

## BUNDLE OF HIS

A bundle of specialized muscle fibers which run down through the septum. It is a direct muscular connection between the upper and lower heart chambers, and serves to conduct the rhythmic heart beat from the atrioventricular (AV) node to the heart muscle. It has two branches, one for each side of the heart.

## CAESALPINUS, ANDREAS

First to use the term "circulation" in connection with the movement of the blood. However, he still believed in many of the classical theories taught by Galen.

## CALORIE

Sometimes called large or kilocalorie. Unit used to express food energy. The amount of heat required to raise the temperature of one kilogram of water one degree Centigrade.

A high caloric diet has a prescribed caloric value above the total daily energy requirement. A low caloric diet has a prescribed caloric value below the total energy requirements.

## CAPILLARIES

Extremely narrow tubes forming a network between the arterioles and the veins. The walls are composed of a single layer of cells through which oxygen and nutritive materials pass out to the tissues, and carbon dioxide and waste products are admitted from the tissues into the blood stream.

## CARDIAC

Pertaining to the heart. Sometimes refers to a person who has heart disease.

## CARDIAC CYCLE

One total heart beat, i.e., one complete contraction and relaxation of the heart. In man, this normally occupies about 0.85 second.

## CARDIAC OUTPUT

The amount of blood pumped per minute according to the demands of the body, and the heart's ability to meet the demand.

## CARDIAC TAMPONADE

Compression of the heart due to an acute or chronic collection of fluid in the pericardial sac.

## CARDIOCENTESIS

The placing of intracardiac electrodes or the injection by insertion of a cardiac needle into the heart.

## CARDIOGENIC DRUGS

Cedilanid-D is used when rapid digitalization is required due to its short latent period. It is useful in cases of paroxysmal tachycardia, auricular fibrillation, and auricular flutter. The same precautions should be observed for Cedilanid-D as for digitalis preparations. Nausea, vomiting, and *extrasystoles* are signs of overdosage and must be reported to the doctor.

## CARDIOGRAM (EKG)

A graphic record of the heart's pulsation taken through the chest wall.

## CARDIOLOGIC FLUOROSCOPE

X-ray device used to

1. Examine the configuration, size, and shape of the heart, and aorta and pulmonary vessels.
2. Look for abnormal pulsations in the heart or great vessels.
3. Determine whether there is congestion or consolidation of the lungs.
4. Find pleural or pericardial effusions.
5. Locate abnormal calcifications in the heart, great vessels, or pericardium.
6. Show any displacement of the esophagus or bronchi.
7. Reveal any tumors or masses in the chest.

## CARDIOPTOSIS

Prolapse of the heart. A downward displacement.

## CARDIOSCOPE (Oscilloscope)

Electrocardiogram which can be visualized immediately for a few seconds' time on a rotating fluorescent belt.

## CARDIOTONIC

A drug that increases the tone of cardiac muscle, e.g., digitalis.

## CARDIOVASCULAR

Pertaining to the heart and blood vessels.

## CARDIOVASCULAR-RENAL DISEASE

Disease involving the heart, blood vessels, and kidneys.

## CARDITIS

Inflammation of the heart.

## CAROTID ARTERIES

The left and right common carotid arteries are the principal arteries supplying the head and neck. Each has two main branches, external carotid artery and internal carotid artery.

## CAROTID BODY

A small oval mass of cells and nerve endings about 5 mm or 1/5 inch long located in the carotid sinus, that is, at the branching point in the arteries supplying blood to the head and neck. The cells respond to chemical changes in the blood by causing changes in the rate of breathing, and certain other body changes. When the oxygen content of the blood is reduced, the carotid body causes an increase in respiration rate.

## CAROTID SINUS

A slight dilation at the point where the internal carotid artery branches from the common carotid artery. The carotid arteries are those arteries which supply blood to the head and neck. The carotid sinus contains special nerve end organs which respond to a change in blood pressure by causing a change in the rate of heart beat. External pressure on the carotid sinus by stimulating some of the nerves in the sinus can also cause a drop in blood pressure and faintness.

## CATHETER

A thin tube of woven plastic or other material to which blood will not adhere, which is inserted in a vein or artery, usually in the arm, and threaded into the heart. The catheter is guided by the physician who watches the progress by means of x-rays falling on a fluorescent screen. A catheter is used as a diagnostic device for taking samples of blood, or pressure readings within the heart chambers, which might reveal defects in the heart.

## CATHETERIZATION (Cardiac)

The passage of a thin, soft catheter through a large vein into the chambers of the heart. Measurements of the venous pressure in the various portions are made, samples of blood are taken, and oxygen content is determined by chemical analysis. The information obtained from this procedure is used to determine the position of certain congenital defects, the degree of mixture of blood of the right and left sides of the heart, and the extent of certain forms of valvular damage.

## CEREBRAL VASCULAR ACCIDENT (VA)

Sometimes called cerebrovascular accident, apoplectic stroke, or simply stroke. An impeded blood supply to some part of the brain, generally caused by one of the following four conditions:

1. A blood clot forming in the vessel (cerebral thrombosis).
2. A rupture of the blood vessel wall (cerebral hemorrhage).
3. A piece of clot or other material from another part of the vascular system which flows to the brain and obstructs a cerebral vessel (cerebral embolism).
4. Pressure on a blood vessel as by a tumor.

**CEREBROVASCULAR**

Pertaining to the blood vessels in the brain.

**CESSATION OF HEART ACTION**

Syn: 1. Ventricular standstill
2. Ventricular asystole
3. Cardiac standstill
4. Cardiac arrest

**CHAGAS' HEART DISEASE**

A form of heart disease resulting from an infection by a microscopic parasite found in South America.

**CHEMOTHERAPY**

The treatment of disease by administering chemicals. Frequently used in the phrase "chemotherapy of hypertension," i.e., the treatment of high blood pressure by the use of drugs.

**CHEYNE-STOKES RESPIRATIONS**

Periods of stertorous respiration interrupted by periods of apnea.

**CHLORAL HYDRATE**

A drug that has a calming action, used to induce sleep. A sedative.

**CHLOROTHIAZIDE**

A chemical compound that increases the output of urine. One of the diuretics sometimes used in the treatment of edema, or water-logged tissues.

**CHOLESTEROL**

A fat-like substance found in animal tissue. In blood tests the normal level for Americans is assumed to be between 180 and 230 milligrams per 100 cc. A higher level is often associated with high risk of coronary atherosclerosis.

**CHORDAE TENDINEAE**

Fibrous chords that serve as guy ropes to hold the valves between the upper and lower chambers of the heart secure when forced closed by pressure of blood in the lower chambers. They stretch from the cusps of the valves to muscles called papillary muscles in the walls of the lower heart chambers.

**CHOREA**

Involuntary, irregular twitching of the muscles, sometimes associated with rheumatic fever. Also called St. Vitus' dance or Sydenham's chorea.

**CIRCULATORY**

Pertaining to the heart, blood vessels, and the circulation of the blood.

**CIRCULATORY DEFICIT**

Congestive failure or the heart's inability to meet the demands and needs of the body.

**CLAUDICATION**

Cramplike pains and weakness of legs, particularly of the calves. Associated with excessive smoking, vascular spasm, and arteriosclerosis.

**CLUBBED FINGERS**

Fingers with a short broad tip and overhanging nail, somewhat resembling a drumstick. This condition is sometimes seen in children born with certain kinds of heart defects.

**COAGULATION**

Process of changing from a liquid to a thickened or solid state. The formation of a clot.

**COARCTATION OF THE AORTA**

A narrowing or constricture of the aortic lining. It causes an obstruction to the flow of blood through the aorta causing an increased workload pressure in the left ventricle.

**COLLATERAL CIRCULATION**

Circulation of the blood through nearby smaller vessels when a main vessel has been blocked.

**COMMISSURE**

The point of union of strands of fibers uniting structures such as cardiac valves.

**COMMISSUROTOMY**

An operation for the relief of mitral stenosis—valvulotomy.

**COMPENSATION**

A change in the circulatory system made to compensate for some abnormality. An adjustment of size of heart or rate of heart beat made to counterbalance a defect in structure or function. Often used specifically to describe the maintenance of adequate circulation in spite of the presence of heart disease.

**CONGENITAL ANOMALY**

An abnormality present at birth.

**CONGENITAL HEART DISEASE**

Present at birth, due to improper development during fetal life.

**CONGESTIVE HEART FAILURE**

When the heart is unable adequately to pump out all the blood that returns to it, there is a backing up of blood in the veins leading to the heart. A congestion or accumulation of fluid in various parts of the body (lungs, legs, abdomen, etc.) may result from the heart's failure to maintain a satisfactory circulation.

## CONSTRICTION

Narrowing, as in the term "vasoconstriction," which is a narrowing of the internal diameter of the blood vessels, caused by a contraction of the muscular coat of the vessels.

## CONSTRICTIVE PERICARDITIS

A shrinking and thickening of the outer sac of the heart which prevents the heart muscle from expanding and contracting normally.

## CONTRACTILE PROTEINS

The protein substance within the heart muscle fibers responsible for heart contraction by shortening the muscle fibers.

## CORONARY ARTERIES

Two arteries, arising from the aorta, arching down over the top of the heart, and conducting blood to the heart muscle.

## CORONARY ATHEROSCLEROSIS

Commonly called coronary heart disease. An irregular thickening of the inner layer of the walls of the arteries that conduct blood to the heart muscle. The internal channel of these arteries (the coronaries) becomes narrowed and the blood supply to the heart muscle is reduced.

## CORONARY OCCLUSION

An obstruction (generally a blood clot) in a branch of one of the coronary arteries which hinders the flow of blood to some part of the heart muscle. This part of the heart muscle then dies because of lack of blood supply. Sometimes called a coronary heart attack, or simply a heart attack.

## CORONARY THROMBOSIS

Formation of a clot in a branch of one of the arteries which conduct blood to the heart muscle (coronary arteries). A form of coronary occlusion.

## COR PULMONALE (due to massive or extensive Pulmonary Embolism)

A state of hypertension in the pulmonary artery due to an obstruction in the *pulmonary* circulation. As a result, the capacity of the lungs to oxygenate blood is reduced, which causes right ventricular strain and eventually right ventricular hypertrophy.

## COUMARIN

A class of chemical substances that delay clotting of the blood. An anticoagulant.

**CYANOSIS**

Blueness of skin caused by insufficient oxygen in the blood. Oxygen is carried in the blood by hemoglobin, which is bright red when saturated with oxygen. When hemoglobin is not carrying oxygen, it is purple and is called reduced hemoglobin. The blueness of the skin occurs when the amount of reduced hemoglobin exceeds 5 grams per 100 cc of blood.

**CYTOLOGIC**

Pertaining to cells, their anatomy, physiology, pathology, and chemistry.

**DECOMPENSATION**

Inability of the heart to maintain adequate circulation, usually resulting in a water-logging of tissues. A person whose heart is failing to maintain normal circulation is said to be "decompensated."

**DEFIBRILLATOR**

Any agent or measure, such as an electric shock, that stops an incoordinate contraction of the heart muscle and restores a normal heart beat.

**DEPRESSANT**

Any drug that decreases functional activity.

**DEXTROCARDIA**

Two different types of congenital phenomena are often described as dextrocardia. The first is a condition in which the heart is slightly rotated and lies almost entirely in the right (instead of the left) side of the chest. The second is a condition in which there is a complete transposition, the left chambers of the heart being on the right side, and the right chambers on the left side, so that the heart presents a mirror image of the normal heart.

**DIASTOLE**

In each heart beat, the period of the relaxation of the heart; auricular diastole is the period of relaxation of the atria, or upper heart chambers. Ventricular diastole is the period of relaxation of the ventricles, or lower heart chambers.

**DIGITALIS**

A drug prepared from leaves of foxglove plant which strengthens the contractions of the heart muscle, slows the rate of contraction of the heart, and by improving the efficiency of the heart, may promote the elimination of fluid from body tissues.

**DILATION**

A stretching or enlargement of the heart or blood vessels beyond the norm.

**DISORDERS OF IMPULSE CONDUCTION**

Difficulties in the transmission of impulses from the auricle to the ventricle occurring within the bundle of His. The conducting ability of the bundle may be merely depressed if only a branch is involved, or it may be completely blocked if both branches are involved.

## DIURESIS

Increased excretion of urine.

## DIURETIC

A medicine which promotes the excretion of urine. Several types of drugs may be used, such as mercurials, chlorothiazide, xanthine, and benzo-thiadiazine derivatives.

## DUCTUS ARTERIOSUS

A small duct in the heart of the fetus between the artery leaving the left side of the heart (aorta) and the artery leaving the right side of the heart (pulmonary artery). Normally this duct closes soon after birth. If it does not close, the condition is known as patent or open ductus arteriosus.

## DYSPNEA

Difficult or labored breathing.

## ECTOPIC

A heart beat or impulse beginning at a point other than the sinoauricular (SA) node.

## EDEMA

Swelling due to abnormally large amounts of fluid in the tissues of the body.
   1. Peripheral: Fluid accumulates in dependent parts such as, ankles, sacral area, etc. It occurs in cardiac failure and is due to increased venous pressure.
   2. Pulmonary: Fluid in the air sacs and interstitial tissue of the lungs.

## EFFORT SYNDROME

A group of symptoms (quick fatigue, rapid heart beat, sighing breaths, dizziness) that do not result from disease of organs or tissues and that are out of proportion to the amount of exertion required.

## ELECTRIC CARDIAC PACEMAKER

An electric device that can control the beating of the heart by a rhythmic discharge of electrical impulses.

## ELECTROCARDIOGRAM

A graphic record used to assess rhythmic patterns or disturbances of the heart.

## ELECTROLYTE

Any substance that, in solution, is capable of conducting electricity by means of its atoms or groups of atoms, and in the process is broken down into positively and negatively charged particles. Examples, sodium or potassium.

## EMBOLISM

The blocking of a blood vessel by a clot or other substance carried in the blood stream.

## EMBOLUS

Any foreign substance that enters the blood stream and obstructs a blood vessel; air bubble, fat globule, pyemic or purulent matter.

## EMPATHY

An instanteous sensing and responding to other people's feelings. The acceptance of the total person.

## ENDARTERIUM

Also called intima. The innermost layer of an artery.

## ENDOCARDITIS

Inflammation of the inner layer of the heart (endocardium), usually associated with acute rheumatic fever or some infectious agents.

## ENDOCARDIUM

A thin, smooth membrane forming the inner surface of the heart.

## ENDOTHELIUM

The thin lining of the blood vessels.

## ENZYME

A complex organic substance which is capable of speeding up specific biochemical processes in the body. Enzymes are universally present in living organisms.

## EPICARDIUM

The outer layer of the heart wall. Also called the visceral pericardium.

## EPIDEMIOLOGY

The science dealing with the factors that determine the frequency and distribution of a disease in a human community.

## EPINEPHRINE

One of the secretions of two small glands, called adrenal glands, located just above the kidneys. This secretion, also called adrenalin, and sometimes prepared synthetically, constricts the small blood vessels (arterioles), increases the rate of heart beat, and raises blood pressure. It is called a vasoconstrictor or vasopressor substance.

## ERYTHROCYTE

Red blood cell.

## ESSENTIAL HYPERTENSION

Sometimes called primary hypertension, and commonly known as high blood pressure. An elevated blood pressure not caused by kidney or other evident disease.

## EXTRACORPOREAL CIRCULATION

The circulation of the blood outside the body as by a mechanical *pump-oxygenator*. This is often done while surgery is being performed inside the heart.

## EXTRASYSTOLE

A contraction of the heart which occurs prematurely and interrupts the normal rhythm.

## EYEGROUND

The inside of the back part of the eye seen by looking through the pupil. Examining the eyeground is one means of assessing changes in the blood vessels. Also called the fundus of the eye.

## FEMORAL ARTERY

Main blood vessel supplying blood to the leg.

## FIBRILLATION

a. Atrial fibrillation: Arrhythmia whereby the atria quiver ineffectually. They do not *contract* or *propel* blood into the ventricles. The ventricles continue to contract but at a very rapid and irregular rate creating a *pulse deficit* because not every ventricular contraction is strong enough to come through at the radial pulse, i.e., apex rate exceeds pulse rate.
b. Ventricular fibrillation: (Fatal arrhythmia)
The ventricles stop contracting and start twitching or quivering. No blood is expelled from either ventricle, and death is instantaneous.

The exact cause of fibrillation is unknown, but it is felt that in coronary heart disease, the oxygen concentration between the injured (ischemic) and uninjured area of the myocardium causes uneven electrical impulses that accelerate the muscle tissue. Other precipitating factors might be attributed to certain cardiac drugs, or anesthetic agents.

## FIBRINOGEN

A soluble protein in the blood that, by the action of certain enzymes, is converted into the insoluble protein of a blood clot.

## FIBRINOLYSIN

An enzyme that can cause coagulated blood to return to a liquid state.

## FLUOROSCOPE

An instrument for observing structures deep inside the body. X-rays are passed through the body onto a fluorescent screen where the shadow of deep-lying organs can be seen.

## FLUOROSCOPY

The examination of a structure deep in the body by means of observing the fluorescence of a screen caused by x-rays transmitted through the body.

## FORAMEN OVALE

An oval hole between the left and right upper chambers of the heart which normally closes shortly after birth. Its failure to close is one of the congenital defects of the heart, called a patent foramen ovale.

## GALLOP RHYTHM

An extra, clearly heard heart sound which, when the heart rate is fast, resembles a horse's gallop. It may or may not be significant.

## GANGLION

A mass of nerve cells, which serves as a center of nervous influence.

## GANGLIONIC BLOCKING AGENTS

A drug that blocks the transmission of a nerve impulse at the nerve centers (ganglia). Some of these drugs, such as hexamethonium and mecamylamine hydrochloride, may be used in the treatment of high blood pressure.

## HEART BLOCK

*First-Degree:* When conduction progresses normally from the SA node to the AV node where the impulse is *delayed* before passing through the bundle of His. This delayed beat is considered a *dropped beat.* It differs from a premature contraction which occurs *before* a beat in normal rhythm. On the oscilloscope or electrocardiograph it is expressed as a prolonged PR wave. The normal PR wave is 0.2 second.

*Second-Degree* (2 to 1 or 3 to 1): When the AV node blocks every second or third impulse from reaching the bundle of His. There is only one ventricular beat for every two or three atrial impulses.

*Third-Degree:* The AV node blocks all impulses from reaching the bundle of His. *Bradycardia* usually (35–49 per min.) is characteristic. *Stokes-Adams syndrome* may be manifested due to the reduced flow of blood to the brain. The electrical external pacemaker is an invaluable therapeutic measure here.

*Complete:* A condition whereby the bundle of His can no longer conduct the impulse from the auricles (atria) to the ventricles. Ventricles are on their own . . . disassociated from the auricles, or else not contract at all.

## HEART-LUNG MACHINE

A machine through which the blood stream is diverted for pumping and oxygenation while the heart is opened for surgery.

## HEMIPLEGIA

Paralysis of one side of the body caused by damage to the opposite side of the brain. The paralyzed arm and leg are opposite to the side of the brain damage because the nerves cross in the brain, and one side of the brain controls the opposite side of the body. Such paralysis is sometimes caused by a blood clot or hemorrhage in a blood vessel in the brain. (See Stroke)

### HEMOGLOBIN

The oxygen-carrying red pigment of the red blood corpuscles. When it has absorbed oxygen in the lungs, it is bright red and called oxyhemoglobin. After it has given up its oxygen load in the tissues, it is purple in color, and is called reduced hemoglobin.

### HEPARIN

A chemical substance that tends to prevent blood from clotting. Sometimes used in cases of an existing clot in an artery or vein to prevent enlargement of the clot or the formation of new clots. An anticoagulant.

### HYPERCAPNIA

Undue amount of $CO_2$ in the blood, causing overactivity in the respiratory center.

### HYPERCHOLESTEREMIA

An excess of a fatty substance called cholesterol in the blood. Sometimes called hypercholesterolemia or hypercholesterinemia. (See Cholesterol)

### HYPERLIPEMIA

An excess of fat or lipids in the blood.

### HYPERTENSION

Commonly called high blood pressure. An unstable or persistent elevation of blood pressure above the normal range, which may eventually lead to increased heart size and kidney damage.

### HYPERTROPHY

The enlargement of a tissue or organ due to increase in the size of its constituent cells. This may result from a demand for increased work.

### HYPERVOLEMIA

Blood volume greater than normal.

### HYPOTENSION

Commonly called low blood pressure. Blood pressure below the normal range. Most commonly used to describe an acute fall in blood pressure, as occurs in shock.

### HYPOTHERMIA

Also called hypothermy. The lowering of the body temperature (usually to 86–88 degrees F) in order to slow the metabolic processes during heart surgery. In this cooled state, body tissues require less oxygen.

**HYPOVOLEMIA**

Decreased blood volume.

**HYPOXIA**

Less than normal content of oxygen in the organs and tissues of the body. At very high altitudes a healthy person suffers from hypoxia because of insufficient oxygen in the air that is breathed.

**IATROGENIC**

Induced by a physician; referring to the effects of a physician's words or actions upon the patient.

**IDIOVENTRICULAR RHYTHM**

Also known as *aurioventricular* (AV). *Disassociation* or *complete heart block*. The rhythm established is usually *bradycardia* . . . as low as 30–40.

**INCOMPETENT VALVE**

Any valve that does not close tight and leaks blood back in the wrong direction. Also called valvular insufficiency.

**INFARCT**

a. Myocardial: A necrotic area of myocardial tissue due to an obstruction in one or both of the coronary arteries which supply the myocardium.
b. Pulmonary: A necrotic area in the lung resulting from an embolus due to phlebothrombosis of the deep vessels of the leg or a thrombosis in a dilated right atrium.

**INNOMINATE ARTERY**

One of the largest branches of the aorta. It arises from the arch of the aorta and divides to form the right common carotid artery and the right subclavian artery.

**INSUFFICIENCY**

Incompetency. In the term "valvular insufficiency," an improper closing of the valves which admits a back flow of blood in the wrong direction. In the term "myocardial insufficiency," inability of the heart muscle to do a normal pumping job.

**INTERATRIAL SEPTUM**

Sometimes called auricular septum or interauricular septum or atrial septum. Muscular wall dividing left and right upper chambers of the heart which are called atria.

**INTERAURICULAR SEPTUM**

Septal defects are openings in the wall of the heart that separate the two auricles (atria). These defects are produced when the foramen ovale fails to close.

### INTERVENTRICULAR SEPTUM

Sometimes called ventricular septum. Muscular wall, thinner at the top, dividing the left and right lower chambers of the heart which are called ventricles.

### INTIMA

The innermost lining of a blood vessel.

### ISCHEMIA

Local anemia due to diminished blood supply, caused by a constriction or an obstruction in the blood vessel supplying that part.

### LINOLEIC ACID

An important component of many of the unsaturated fats. It is found widely in oils from plants. A diet with a high linoleic acid content tends to lower the amount of cholesterol in the blood.

### LIPID

Fat.

### LIPOPROTEIN

A complex of fat and protein molecules.

### LUMEN

The passageway inside a tubular organ. Vascular lumen is the passageway inside a blood vessel.

### MALIGNANT HYPERTENSION

Severe high blood pressure that runs a rapid course and causes damage to the blood vessel walls in the kidney, eye, etc.

### MERCURIAL DIURETIC

Various organic compounds of mercury commonly used to promote the elimination of water and sodium from the body through increased excretion of urine. Sometimes used in congestive heart failure when tissues are waterlogged. Mercury in several different organic forms is used as a diuretic.

### METABOLISM

A general term to designate all chemical changes that occur to substances within the body.

### MITRAL INSUFFICIENCY

An improper closing of the mitral valve between the upper and lower chamber in the left side of the heart which admits a back flow of blood in the wrong direction. Sometimes the result of scar tissue forming after a rheumatic fever infection.

**MITRAL STENOSIS**

A narrowing of the valve (called bicuspid or mitral valve) opening between the upper and lower chamber in the left side of the heart. Sometimes the result of scar tissue forming after a rheumatic fever infection.

**MITRAL VALVE**

Sometimes called bicuspid valve. A valve of two cusps or triangular segments, located between the upper and lower chamber in the left side of the heart.

**MITRAL VALVULOTOMY**

An operation to widen the opening in the valve between the upper and lower chambers in the left side of the heart (mitral valve). Usually performed when the valve opening is so narrowed as to obstruct blood flow, which sometimes happens as a result of rheumatic fever.

**MURAL THROMBUS**

Located on or originating from a diseased area of the endocardium.

**MURMUR**

An abnormal heart sound, sounding like fluid passing an obstruction, heard between the normal lub-dub heart sounds.

**MYOCARDIAL INFARCTION**

The damaging or death of an area of the heart muscle (myocardium) resulting from a reduction in the blood supply reaching that area.

**MYOCARDIAL INSUFFICIENCY**

An inability of the heart muscle (myocardium) to maintain normal circulation. (See Congestive Heart Failure)

**MYOCARDITIS**

Inflammation of the heart muscle (myocardium).

**MYOCARDIUM**

The muscular wall of the heart. The thickest of the three layers of the heart wall, it lies between the inner layer (endocardium) and the outer layer (epicardium).

**NECROSIS (Ischemic)**

Death of tissue due to occlusion of an artery supplying the region.

**NEUROCIRCULATORY ASTHENIA**

Sometimes called soldier's heart or effort syndrome. A complex of nervous and circulatory symptoms, often involving a sense of fatigue, dizziness, shortness of breath, rapid heart beat, and nervousness.

**NEUROGENIC**

Originating in the nervous system.

### NORMAL PACEMAKER

The sinus node (SA) lies high on the right side of the right auricle and is the site of origin of the impulses which drive the heart. It is under control of the *sympathetic* and *parasympathetic (vagus) nerves.*

### NORMOTENSIVE

Characterized by normal blood pressure.

### OCCLUSION

A blood vessel plugged or infiltrated by foreign particles or engorgement.

### OPEN-HEART SURGERY

Surgery performed on the opened heart while the blood stream is diverted through a heart-lung machine. This machine pumps and oxygenates the blood in lieu of the action of the heart and lungs during the operation.

### ORGANIC HEART DISEASE

Heart disease caused by some structural abnormality in the heart or circulatory system.

### ORTHOPNEA

Condition in which there is need to sit up in order to breathe more easily.

### PACEMAKER

The term "pacemaker," or more exactly, "electric cardiac pacemaker" or "electrical pacemaker," is applied to an electrical device which can substitute for a defective natural pacemaker and control the beating of the heart by a series of rhythmic electrical discharges. If the electrodes which deliver the discharges to the heart are placed on the outside of the chest, it is called an "external pacemaker." If the electrodes are placed within the chest wall, it is called an "internal pacemaker."

a. Normal: That portion of the right atrium of the heart, normally the sinoatrial node (SA) where the stimulus for the heart beat originates.
b. Octopicatrial: An impulse originating outside the normal pacemaker, but in the atria.
c. Idioventricular: An impulse originating in the ventricles.
d. Wandering: The subendocardium has hundreds of "extra" or "reserve" pacemakers scattered throughout. Any one of these bits of specialized myocardial tissue is capable of starting a beat.
Hence "wandering pacemaker" is a phenomenon in which the pacemaker shifts away from the SA node but remains within the atrium or atrioventricular (AV) node.

### PALPITATION

A fluttering of the heart or abnormal rate or rhythm of the heart experienced by the person himself.

**PANCARDITIS**

      Inflammation of the whole heart including inner layer (endocardium), heart muscle (myocardium), and outer sac (pericardium).

**PAPILLARY MUSCLES**

      Small bundles of muscles in the wall of the lower chambers of the heart to which the cords leading to the cusps of the valves (chordae tendineae) are attached. When the valves are closed, these muscles contract and tighten the cords which hold the valve firmly shut.

**PAROXYSMAL TACHYCARDIA**

      A period of rapid heart beats which begins and ends suddenly.

**PARASYMPATHETIC (VAGUS) NERVE**

      Slows the heart action.

**PATENCY**

      A state of being freely open.

**PATENT DUCTUS ARTERIOSUS**

      A permanent connection between the aorta and the pulmonary artery. (In fetal life this is a normal opening, but it should normally close soon after birth.)

**PATENT FORAMEN OVALE**

      An abnormal opening between the right and left atria. Left-to-right shunting of blood occurs in this defect.

**PATHOGENESIS**

      The chain of events leading to the development of a disease.

**PERICARDITIS**

      Inflammation of the thin membrane sac (pericardium) which surrounds the heart.

**PERICARDIUM**

      A thin membrane sac which surrounds the heart and roots of the great vessels.

**PERIPHERAL RESISTANCE**

      The resistance offered by the arterioles and capillaries to the flow of blood from the arteries to the veins. An increase in peripheral resistance causes a rise in blood pressure.

**PHLEBITIS**

      Inflammation of a vein.

**PLICATION**

      The procedure of stitching a fold in a vessel wall to reduce its size. Frequently used to prevent thrombus from lower extremities from entering or reaching pulmonary arteries.

## POLYCYTHEMIA

An abnormal condition of the blood characterized by an excessive number of red blood cells.

## PREMATURE CONTRACTION

A systole resulting from a premature impulse discharged by the sinus mode. Patient may complain of palpitations or an occasional "flip" sensation.

## PRESSOR

A substance which raises the blood pressure and accelerates the heart beat. Also denotes certain nerve fibers which produce a rise in blood pressure when stimulated.

## PRIMARY HYPERTENSION

Sometimes called essential hypertension, and commonly known as high blood pressure. An elevated blood pressure not caused by kidney or other evident disease.

## PROCAINAMIDE

A drug sometimes used to treat abnormal rhythms of the heart beat.

## PULMONARY ARTERY

The large artery which conveys unoxygenated (venous) blood from the lower right chamber of the heart to the lungs. This is the only artery in the body which carries unoxygenated blood, all others carrying oxygenated blood to the body.

## PULMONARY CIRCULATION

In this *lesser* circulation blood returns from the entire venous system via the inferior and superior vena cavae to the right atrium. From the right atrium blood passes to the right ventricle where it is pumped through the pulmonary artery to the lungs, where carbon dioxide is removed and oxygen added. This oxygenated blood returns by way of the pulmonary veins to the left side of the heart, and into the aorta which supplies the systemic circulation.

## PULMONARY STENOSIS

Condition whereby the opening of the pulmonary valve is congenitally narrowed.

## PULMONARY VALVE

Valve formed by three cup-shaped membranes at the junction of the pulmonary artery and the right lower chamber of the heart (right ventricle). When the right lower chamber contracts, the pulmonary valve opens and the blood is forced into the artery leading to the lungs. When the chamber relaxes, the valve is closed and prevents a back-flow of the blood.

## PULMONARY VEINS

Four veins (two from each lung) that conduct oxygenated blood from the lungs into the left upper chamber of the heart (left atrium).

## PULSE

The expansion and contraction of an artery which may be felt with the finger.

## PULSE DEFICIT

The difference between apex rhythm and radial pulse.

## PULSE PRESSURE

The difference between systolic and diastolic reading: i.e., 120/80 . . . pulse pressure 40.

## PULSUS ALTERNANS

A pulse in which there is regular alternation of weak and strong beats.

## PURKINJE FIBERS

Specialized fibers scattered throughout the subendocardium of the ventricles which conduct impulses to the muscular wall of the two lower chambers and are the last link in the chain of excitation.

## PURPOSE OF MEASURING VENOUS PRESSURE

1. To prevent or correct inadequate blood replacement. *Hypovolemia*, which reduces *cardiac output.*
2. To prevent overloading of the circulatory system. Hypervolemia, which increases the workload of the heart.
3. To detect early signs of complications.
4. To use as a guide in maintaining normal circulation.

## QUADRIGEMINAL PULSE

A pulse in which a pause occurs after every fourth beat.

## QUINIDINE

A drug sometimes used to treat abnormal rhythms of the heart beat.

## RAUWOLFIA

A drug consisting of powdered whole root of a plant (Rauwolfia serpentina) which lowers blood pressure and slows the heart rate. Sometimes used in treatment of high blood pressure. An antihypertensive agent.

## REGURGITATION

The backward flow of blood through a defective valve.

## RENAL CIRCULATION

The circulation of the blood through the kidneys. Important in heart disease because of its function in the elimination of water, certain chemical elements, and waste products from the body.

## RENAL HYPERTENSION

High blood pressure caused by damage to or disease of the kidneys.

## RESERPINE

One of the organic substances found in the root of the plant, Rauwolfia serpentina, which lowers blood pressure, slows the heart rate, and has a sedative effect. One of the antihypertensive agents.

## RHEUMATIC FEVER

A disease, usually occurring in childhood, which may follow a few weeks after a streptococcal infection. It is sometimes characterized by one or more of the following: fever; sore, swollen joints; a skin rash; occasionally by involuntary twitching of the muscles (called chorea or St. Vitus' dance); and small nodes under the skin. In some cases, the infection affects the heart and may result in scarring the valves, weakening the heart muscle, or damaging the sac enclosing the heart.

## RHYTHMIC DISORDERS

May arise from a disturbance in the following:

1. The normal pacemaker (SA node)
2. Irritable foci (ischemic area) impulse formation
3. Conduction of impulses
4. Digitalis toxicity—drug intoxications
5. Arteriosclerosis
6. Congenital defects
7. Acquired defects

## SA NODE

A small mass of specialized cells in the right upper chamber of the heart which gives rise to the electrical impulses that initiate contractions of the heart. Also called sinoatrial node or *pacemaker*.

## SCLEROSIS

Hardening, usually due to an accumulation of fibrous tissue.

## SECONDARY HYPERTENSION

An elevated blood pressure caused by (i.e., secondary to) certain specific diseases or infections.

## SEMILUNAR VALVES

Cup-shaped valves. The aortic valve at the entrance to the aorta, and the pulmonary valve at the entrance to the pulmonary artery are semilunar valves. They consist of three cup-shaped flaps which prevent the backflow of blood.

## SEPTUM

A dividing wall.

1. Atrial or interatrial septum. Muscular wall dividing left and right upper chambers (the atria) of the heart.
2. Ventricular or interventricular septum. Muscular wall, thinner at the top dividing the left and right lower chambers (the ventricles) of the heart.

## SHOCK

a. Cardiogenic: Caused by inadequate pumping of blood into the arterial tree owing to left ventricular failure, tamponade, or pulmonary embolism.
b. Irreversible: A late state of shock from which recovery cannot be achieved by any known form of therapy.

## SHUNT

A passage between two blood vessels or between the two sides of the heart, as in cases where an opening exists in the wall which normally separates them. In surgery, the operation of forming a passage between blood vessels to divert blood from one part of the body to another.

## SINOATRIAL NODE

A small mass of specialized cells in the right upper chamber of the heart which give rise to the electrical impulses that initiate contractions of the heart. Also called SA node or pacemaker.

## SINUSES OF VALSALVA

Three pouches on the wall of the aorta (main artery leading from left lower chamber of the heart) behind the three cup-shaped membranes of the aortic valve.

## STASIS

A stoppage or slackening of the blood flow.

## STENOSIS

A narrowing or stricture of an opening. Mitral stenosis, aortic stenosis, etc., means that the valve indicated has become narrowed so that it does not function normally.

## STOKES-ADAMS SYNDROME

A result of serious disease of the heart, characterized by a sudden failure of the ventricles to contract. Patient suddenly loses consciousness and frequently convulses. These attacks appear suddenly and without warning. Application of an external electric pacemaker has been found to be of great therapeutic value in this syndrome. *Bradycardia* is a characteristic.

### STROKE

Also called apoplectic stroke, cerebrovascular accident, or cerebral vascular accident. An impeded blood supply to some part of the brain, generally caused by

1. A blood clot forming in the vessel (cerebral thrombosis)
2. A rupture of the blood vessel wall (cerebral hemorrhage)
3. A piece of clot or other material from another part of the vascular system which flows to the brain and obstructs a cerebral vessel (cerebral embolism).

### STROKE VOLUME

The amount of blood which is pumped out of the heart at each contraction of the heart.

### SUBINTIMAL HEMORRHAGE

Bleeding beneath an atherosclerotic plaque dislodging deposits and causing emboli.

### SYMPATHETIC NERVE

Accelerates heart action.

### SYSTEMIC CIRCULATION

In this *greater* circulation, oxygenated blood enters the left atrium and passes to the left ventricle. The left ventricle contracts and propels the blood into the aorta which through its branches supplies all the organs and tissues of the body with oxygen, enzymes, etc.

### SYMPTOM

Subjective sensations of the patient.

### SYNCOPE

Faintness, giddiness, momentary unconsciousness—due to cerebral anemia.

### SYNDROME

A set of symptoms which occur together and are thereby given a name to indicate the particular combination.

### TACHYCARDIA

Sympathetic nerve reflex can stimulate and accelerate heart action and rate in excess of 100.

### TETRALOGY OF FALLOT

A quadruple malformation of the heart consisting of

1. pulmonary stenosis
2. ventricular septal defects
3. overriding aorta
4. hypertrophy of right ventricle

It is the most common defect causing cyanosis in patients beyond two years of age.

**THROMBECTOMY**

An operation to remove a blood clot from a blood vessel.

**THROMBOPHLEBITIS**

Inflammation of a vein with a clot.

**THROMBOSIS**

The formation or presence of a blood clot (thrombus) inside a blood vessel or cavity of the heart.

**THROMBUS**

The formation of a clot. Syn. thrombosis.

**TRICUSPID VALVE**

A valve consisting of three cusps or triangular segments located between the upper and lower chamber in the right side of the heart. Its position corresponds to the bicuspid or mitral valve in the left side of the heart.

**TRIGEMINY**

Grouping of arterial pulse beats in groups of three.

**UREMIA**

An excess in the blood of certain waste substances normally excreted by the kidneys.

**VAGUS NERVES**

Two of the nerves of the parasympathetic nervous system which extend from the brain, through the neck and thorax, into the abdomen. Known as the inhibitory nerves of the heart, they slow the heart rate when stimulated.

**VALVULAR INSUFFICIENCY**

Valves that close improperly and admit a back-flow of blood in the wrong direction.

**VASOCONSTRICTOR**

The vasoconstrictor nerves are one part of the involuntary nervous system. When these nerves are stimulated they cause the muscles of the arterioles to contract, thus narrowing the arteriole passage, increasing the resistance to the flow of blood, and raising the blood pressure. Chemical substances that stimulate the muscles of the arterioles to contract are called vasoconstrictor agents or vasopressors. An example is adrenalin or epinephrine.

**VASODILATOR**

Vasodilator nerves are certain nerve fibrs of the involuntary nervous system which cause the muscles of the arterioles to relax, thus enlarging the arteriole passage, reducing resistance to the flow of blood, and lowering blood pressure. Vasodilator agents are chemical compounds that cause a relaxation of the muscles of the arterioles. Examples of this type of drug are nitroglycerine, nitrites, thiocyanate, and many others.

## VASO-INHIBITOR

An agent or drug that inhibits the action of the vasomotor nerves. When these involuntary nerves are inhibited, the muscles of the arterioles relax, the passage inside the arteriole is enlarged, and the blood pressure is lowered. Examples of this type of drug are compounds of nitrite.

## VASOPRESSOR

A chemical substance that causes the muscles of the arterioles to contract, narrowing the arteriole passage, and thus raising the blood pressure. Such substances are also called vasoconstrictors. An example is adrenalin or epinephrine.

## VENA CAVA

Superior vena cava is a large vein conducting blood from the upper part of the body (head, neck, and thorax) to the right upper chamber of the heart. Inferior vena cava is a large vein conducting blood from the lower part of the body to the right upper chamber of the heart.

## VENOUS BLOOD

Unoxygenated blood. The blood, with hemoglobin in the reduced state, is carried by the veins from all parts of the body back to the heart and then pumped by the right side of the heart to the lungs where it is oxygenated.

## VENOUS PRESSURE

Reflects output of the venous side of the left ventricles, shows pressure in RA, intrathoracic pressure, blood volume.

## VENTRICLE

One of the two lower chambers of the heart. Left ventricle pumps oxygenated blood through arteries to the body. Right ventricle pumps unoxygenated blood through pulmonary artery to lungs. Capacity about 85 cc.

## VENTRICULAR SEPTAL DEFECTS

An abnormal opening between the right and left ventricles. Ventricular defects vary in size and may occur in either the membranous or muscular portion of the ventricular septum.

## VENTRICULAR SEPTUM

Sometimes called interventricular septum. Muscular wall, thinner at the top, dividing the left and right lower chambers of the heart which are called ventricles.

## WANDERING PACEMAKER

*Electrical Pacemaker:* An electric device which can substitute for a defective natural pacemaker and control the beating of the heart by a series of rhythmic electric discharges. If the electrodes which deliver the discharges to the heart are placed on the outside of the chest, it is called an "external pacemaker." If the electrodes are placed within the chest wall, it is called an "internal pacemaker."

# B BIBLIOGRAPHY

*Books*

Abbott Laboratories. *Fluid and Electrolytes.* Abbott Laboratories, North Chicago, Ill., 1960.

Abbott Laboratories. *Parenteral Administration.* Abbott Laboratories, North Chicago, Ill., 1959.

Allen, Edgar, Barker, Nelson, and Hines, Edgar. *Peripheral Vascular Diseases,* 3rd edition. W. B. Saunders Company, Phila., 1962.

American Heart Association. *A Guide to Anticoagulant Therapy.* A.H.A. New York, N.Y., 1961.

American Heart Association. *Emergency Measures in Cardiopulmonary Resuscitation.* Published by A.H.A. in cooperation with The Heart Association of Maryland, 1965.

Andreoli, Kathleen et al. *Comprehensive Cardiac Care: A Handbook for Nurses and Other Paramedical Personnel.* The C. V. Mosby Co., St. Louis, 1968.

Anthony, C. *Textbook of Anatomy and Physiology,* 5th edition. The C. V. Mosby Co., St. Louis, 1959.

Ayres, Stephen and Giannelli, Stanley. *Care of the Critically Ill.* Appleton-Century-Crofts, New York, 1967.

Banyai, A. and Levine, E. R. *Dyspnea, Diagnosis and Treatment.* F. A. Davis Co., Phila., 1963.

Beland, Irene L. *Clinical Nursing: Pathophysiological and Psychosocial Approaches.* The Macmillan Co., New York, 1967.

Bernreiter, Michael. *Electrocardiography,* 2nd edition. J. B. Lippincott Co., Phila., 1958.

Bishop, Louis F. *A Programmed Course in Electrocardiology.* Basic Systems, Inc., Warner-Chilcott Laboratories, Morris Plains, N.J., 1967.

Blake, Thomas M. *An Introduction to Electrocardiography.* Appleton-Century-Crofts, New York, 1964.

Bordicks, Katherine J. *Patterns of Shock: Implications for Nursing Care.* The Macmillan Co., New York, 1968.

Boyd, William. *A Textbook of Pathology,* 7th edition. Lea & Febiger, Phila., 1961.

Brams, William A. *Managing Your Coronary,* 3rd edition. J. B. Lippincott Co., Phila., 1966.

Braun, Harold A. and Diettert, Gerald A. *Coronary Care Unit Nursing, Part I: A Programmed Text in Electrocardiography.* Western Montana Clinic Foundation, Missoula, Mont., 1968.

Braun, Harold; Diettert, Gerald A.; and Wills, Vera E. *Coronary Care Unit Nursing, Part II: A Workbook in Clinical Aspects.* Western Montana Clinic Foundation, Missoula, Mont., 1969.

Brigance, William Norwood. *Speech Communication: A Brief Textbook.* Appleton-Century-Crofts, New York, 1947.

Brooks, Stewart. *Basic Facts of Body Water and Ions.* Springer Publishing Company, Inc., New York, 1960.

Cannon, Walter B. *The Wisdom of the Body.* W. W. Norton Co., Inc., New York, 1939.

Collins, R. Douglas. *Illustrated Manual of Laboratory Diagnosis.* J. B. Lippincott Co., Phila., 1968.

Cooper, Philip. *Ward Procedures and Techniques.* Appleton-Century-Crofts, New York, 1967.

Dean, W. B., Ferrar, Jr., G. E., and Zoldos, A. J. *Basic Concepts of Anatomy and Physiology: A Programmed Study.* J. B. Lippincott Co., Phila., 1966.

Dutcher, I., and Fielo, S. *Water and Electrolytes: Implications for Nursing Care.* The Macmillan Co., New York, 1967.

Fordham, Mary E. *Cardiovascular Surgical Nursing.* The Macmillan Company, New York, 1962.

Friedberg, Charles K. *Diseases of the Heart,* 3rd edition. W. B. Saunders Co., Phila., 1967.

Goldman, Mervin J. *Principles of Clinical Electrocardiography,* 6th edition. Lange Medical Publications, Los Altos, Cal., 1967.

Goldschmidt, Walter. *Exploring the Ways of Mankind.* Holt, Rinehart and Winston, Inc., Chicago, Ill., 1961.

Guyton, Arthur C. *Textbook of Medical Physiology,* 3rd edition. W. S. Saunders Co., Phila., 1968.

Heimlich, H. *Postoperative Care in Thoracic Surgery.* Charles C Thomas, Publisher, Springfield, Ill., 1962.

Hewlett-Packard. *Technician's Guide to Electrocardiography.* Hewlett-Packard Company, Waltham Division, Waltham, Mass., 1966.

Hurst, W. and Logue, B. *The Heart.* McGraw-Hill Book Company, New York, 1966.

Hopps, Howard C. *Principles of Pathology,* 2nd edition. Appleton-Century-Crofts, Inc., New York, 1964.

Krause, Marie V. *Food, Nutrition and Diet Therapy,* 3rd edition. W. B. Saunders Company, Phila., 1961.

Krug, Elsie E. *Pharmacology in Nursing,* 9th edition. The C. V. Mosby Co., St. Louis, 1963.

Levine, Samuel A. *Clinical Heart Diseases,* 5th edition, W. B. Saunders Company, Phila., 1958.

Little, Dolores E. and Carnevali, Doris L. *Nursing Care Planning.* J. B. Lippincott Co., Phila., 1969.

Lockerby, Florence K. *Communication for Nurses,* 3rd edition. The C. V. Mosby Co., St. Louis, 1968.

Luisada, Aldo A., editor. *Cardiology: An Encyclopedia of the Cardiovascular System.* Vol. I: Normal Heart and Vessels; Vol. II: Methods; Vol. III: Clinical

Cardiology; Vol. IV: Clinical Cardiology Therapy; Vol. V: Related Specialty Fields. The Blakiston Division, McGraw-Hill Book Company, Inc., New York (Vol. V) 1961.

MacBride, C. et al. *Signs and Symptoms,* 4th edition. J. B. Lippincott Co., Phila., 1964.

Marriott, Henry L. *Practical Electrocardiography,* 4th edition. The Williams and Wilkins Co., Baltimore, Md., 1968.

Meltzer, L. et al. *Intensive Coronary Care: A Manual for Nurses.* Philadelphia Presbyterian Hospital, Phila., 1965.

Menkin, Valy. *Biochemical Mechanisms in Inflammation,* 2nd edition, Charles C Thomas, Springfield, Ill., 1956.

Metheny, Norma Milligan and Snively, Jr., William D. *Nurses' Handbook of Fluid Balance.* J. B. Lippincott Co., Phila., 1967.

Modell, Walter et al. *Handbook of Cardiology for Nurses,* 5th edition. Springer Publishing Co., New York, 1966.

Netter, F. H. *The Ciba Collection of Medical Illustrations.* Vol. I: Nervous System. Ciba Pharmaceutical Co., Summit, N.J., 1953.

Netter, Frank H. and Walton, J. Harold, editor. *The Electrocardiogram in Myocardial Infarction.* Ciba Pharmaceutical Co., Summit, N.J., 1968.

Nite, Gladys and Willis, Frank N. *The Coronary Patient.* The Macmillan Company, New York, 1964.

Nordmark, M. and Rohweder, A. *Science Principles Applied to Nursing.* J. B. Lippincott Co., Phila., 1959.

Packman, Robert C., editor. *Manual of Medical Therapeutics.* Department of Medicine, Washington University School of Medicine. Little, Brown and Co., 18th edition, Boston, 1966.

Peddie, George H. and Brush, Frances E. *Cardio-Vascular Surgery: A Manual for Nurses.* G. P. Putnam's Sons, New York, 1961.

Powers, M. and Storlie, F. *The Cardiac Surgical Patient: Pathophysiologic Considerations and Nursing Care.* The Macmillan Co., New York, 1969.

Segal, M. S. and Herschefus, J. A. *Oxygen Therapy: Description of a New Face Tent. Bull. New England Medical Center* 13:244, 1951.

Shafer, Kathleen et al. *Medical-Surgical Nursing,* 2nd edition. The C. V. Mosby Co., St. Louis, 1961.

Snively, Jr., W. D. *Profile of a Manager.* J. B. Lippincott Co., Phila., 1966.

Snively, Jr., W. D. *Sea Within.* J. B. Lippincott Co., Phila., 1960.

Squire, Jessie E. *Basic Pharmacology for Nurses,* 4th edition. The C. V. Mosby Co., St. Louis, 1969.

Statland, Harry. *Fluid and Electrolytes in Practice,* 2nd edition. J. B. Lippincott Co., Phila., 1957.

Storlie, Frances. *Principles of Intensive Nursing Care.* Appleton-Century-Crofts, New York, 1969.

Sutton, Audrey Latshaw. *Bedside Techniques in Medicine and Surgery.* W. B. Saunders Co., Phila., 1964.

Uhley, H. N. *Vector Electrocardiography,* J. B. Lippincott Co., Phila., 1962.

White, Paul et al., editors. *Cardiovascular Rehabilitation.* McGraw-Hill Book Company, New York, 1967.

Wintrobe, Maxwell M. *Clinical Hematology,* 5th edition. Lea & Febiger, Phila., 1961.

Wolff, Lu Verne and Fuerst, Elinor V. *Fundamentals of Nursing: The Humanities and the Sciences in Nursing,* 2nd edition. J. B. Lippincott Co., Phila., 1959.

*Articles*

Anderson, Milton W. The Management of Acute Myocardial Infarction. *Medical Clinics of North America,* XLII, No. 4, July, 1958, pp. 849–58.

Aviado, Domingo and Schmidt, Carl F. Physiologic Bases for the Treatment of Pulmonary Edema. *Journal of Chronic Diseases,* IX, No. 5, May, 1959, pp. 495–507.

Beck, C. S. Operations for Coronary Artery Disease. *Amer. J. Nurs.* 54:1076–1079, Sept., 1954.

Bellet, Samuel. Treatment of Cardiac Arrhythmias. *Geriatrics,* XVI, No. 1, Jan., 1961, pp. 1–12.

Berge, Kenneth G. Usefulness and Limitations of Determinations of Serum Transaminase in the Diagnosis of Acute Myocardial Infarction. *Medical Clinics of North America,* XLII, No. 4, July, 1958, pp. 859–60.

Bernstein, Harold et al. Evaluation of Coronary Vasodilators by New Experimental Technics. Abstracts of 36th Scientific Sessions. *Circulation* 28:690, Oct., 1963, Part II.

Bing, Richard, editor. Heart Disease—Selected Aspects of Pathophysiology, Evaluation and Treatment. *Medical Clinics of North America,* XLVI, No. 6, Nov., 1962.

Blalock, Alfred. External Cardiac Massage. *Journal of the American Medical Association,* CLXXVI, No. 7, May 20, 1961, p. 609.

Borg, Joseph F. Long-term Anticoagulant Therapy in Coronary Artery Disease. *Geriatrics,* XVII, June, 1962, pp. 372–78.

Coe, Myrtle. Some Roles of Nursing in Cardiac Disease. *Nursing World,* CXXX, No. 2, Feb., 1956, pp. 7–9.

Coston, Harriet M. Myocardial Infarction: Stages of Recovery and Patient Care. *Nurs. Res.* 9:178–182, Fall 1960.

Creighton, Helen. The Nurse's Role in Cardiac Catheterization. *Nursing World,* CXXXIII, No. 2, Feb., 1959, pp. 25–28.

Hammond, G. et al. Experimental Evaluation of Myocardial Revascularization Procedures. *Ann. Surg.,* 1964, pp. 164–66.

Hoffman, B. F. and Cranefield, P. F. The Physiologic Basis of Cardiac Arrhythmias. *American Journal of Medicine,* Vol. 37, p. 670, 1964.

Hughes, W. L. et al. Myocardial Infarction Prognosis by Discriminant Analysis. *Arch. Intern. Med.* 111:338–345, March, 1963.

Johnson, W. L. Longitudinal Study of Family Adjustment to Myocardial Infarction. *Nurs. Res.* 12:242–247, Fall 1963.

Paul, O. et al. Longitudinal Study of Coronary Heart Disease. *Circulation* 28:20–31, July, 1963.

Spencer, F. C. et al. Experimental Coronary Arterial Surgery with Hypothermia and Cardiopulmonary Bypass. *Circulation* 29:140–144, April, 1964 (Supplement).

Zschoche, Donna and Brown, Lillian E. Intensive Care Nursing: Specialization, Junior Doctoring, or Just Nursing. *Amer. Journal of Nursing,* 1969, pp. 2370–2374.

# C   CASE STUDY OF L. H.

Case Study edited and included by permission of American Heart Association from "Diagnosis and Treatment of Arrhythmias."

### Case Data

A 70-year-old male was admitted to the hospital with his first episode of severe anterior chest pain radiating into the left arm. This was accompanied by nausea, vomiting, and profuse sweating. He had a history of hypertension of 20 years' duration, discovered while he was in the Air Force during World War II. His only previous ECG, in 1938, was said to be normal.

Physical evidence on examination revealed his blood pressure initially to be 150/80 when examined in the emergency room, decreasing to 120/70 by the time he arrived on the nursing unit. There were no other significant positive physical findings.

Admission laboratory studies revealed both the complete blood count and urinalysis to be within normal limits. The chest x-ray and ECG are illustrated (Fig. 1).

### Discussion

The chest x-ray shows some abnormality, with moderate cardiomegaly. The ECG shows typical findings of acute anterolateral myocardial infarction. There is a single ventricular premature beat in lead $V_6$ occurring near the apex of the T wave of the preceding normal beat.

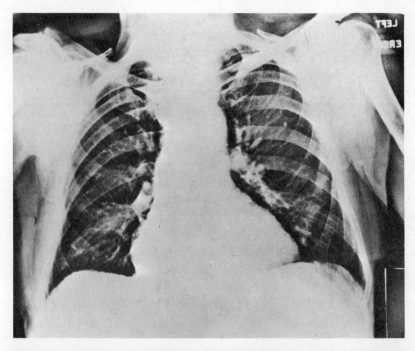

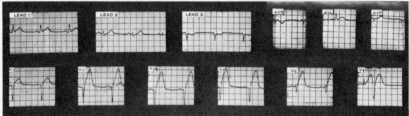

*FIG. 1* Patient L. H.: 70-year-old male with severe anterior chest pain, nausea, vomiting, and profuse sweating.

(From Diagnostic Aids. Courtesy of American Heart Association.)

The patient should be monitored and watched: closely observed. Even a single premature ventricular beat occurring near the vulnerable phase of the cardiac cycle may be the forerunner of life-threatening ventricular arrhythmias. Progressive or serial ECGs show ventricular premature beats increasing and presence of bigeminy, ventricular tachycardia, and fibrillation.

Treatment of choice will be administration of lidocaine; however, cardiac massage should be started immediately if there is delay in giving electric countershock. Patient should be maintained on oral quinidine after rhythm has been stabilized.

The admission ECG, which is shown, showed typical findings of *acute anterolateral myocardial infarction*. The electrocardiographer noted that the *single* ventricular premature beat that was recorded in this tracing in lead V$_6$ occurred near the apex of the T wave of the preceding normal beat. The admitting physician was immediately called and told that the premature beat suggested the possibility of the development of more serious ventricular arrhythmia. This concern over the premature beat probably saved this man's life.

Because no coronary care unit was available in this small hospital, an oscilloscopic monitor was immediately attached to the patient and intermittent representative ECG strips recorded on a direct writing machine. The first tracing showed that ventricular premature beats had increased to eight per minute and were superimposed on the preceding T waves, occasionally occurring as brief bigeminal rhythm. Immediately thereafter, a brief run of ventricular tachycardia was noted. After about 30 seconds, this was followed by ventricular fibrillation. This was treated with brief, closed-chest cardiac massage and ended spontaneously before precordial shock could be delivered.

The patient was then given lidocaine, 50 mg intravenously, and a continuous intravenous drip of lidocaine at a rate of 2 mg per minute was started. Fifteen minutes later, a second 50 mg dose of lidocaine was given intravenously because frequent ventricular premature beats continued. Shortly thereafter, the ventricular premature beats became very infrequent and by the third hospital day had disappeared completely. The intravenous infusion was stopped on the fifth day of hospitalization, and the subsequent course of the illness was uneventful. The patient was discharged after three and a half weeks in the hospital.

This patient's history demonstrates the value of careful monitoring of the cardiac rhythm in those with acute myocardial infarction and the usefulness of drug therapy in preventing the recurrence of ventricular tachycardia and ventricular fibrillation in these patients. The fact that this was a small hospital that did have an oscilloscope and nursing personnel who understood the implications of progressive changes in ECG arrhythmias and notified the physician, and the fact that the cardiographer reinforced the personnel through rapid interpretation and reporting of the original ECG events are to be commended.

In acute myocardial infarction, death may be sudden but it is not unannounced (1). Arrhythmias probably account for about 40 percent of the deaths, and of these about two-thirds are due to ventricular fibrillation (1,2). Ventricular premature beats are the most frequent rhythmic abnormality and may be prodromata of ventricular tachycardia and ventricular fibrillation. In order to prevent these serious arrhythmias, therapy should be promptly initiated when ventricular premature beats occur early in the cardiac cycle at the vulnerable time or period, which has been demonstrated in mammalian hearts to coincide with the apex of the T wave of the ECG (3).

An electrical impulse falling in the vulnerable period may provoke ventricular fibrillation. In the experimental animal with acute myocardial infarction, as opposed to normal animals, the electrical energy of sporadic ventricular premature beats falling in the vulnerable period is sufficient to trigger repetitive bouts of arrhythmia and ventricular fibrillation (1).

In addition to their occurrence near the apex of the T wave, other ominous characteristics of ventricular premature beats are salvos of two or more, multiform configuration (multifocal), and the occurrence of more than five per minute. Some would prefer to eliminate all ventricular premature beats in the patient with acute infarction (2).

## Treatment of Premature Ventricular Contractions

In coronary units, intravenous lidocaine has become the treatment of choice to suppress ventricular premature beats. A bolus of 50 mg or 1 mg per kilogram is given intravenously. Within 90 seconds to three minutes one will either see no effect or an immediate effect. If the first dose of 1 mg per kg does not work, half the initial amount may be repeated within a few minutes and five minutes allowed to elapse before making a further decision. If there is a beneficial effect, a continuous intravenous infusion of from 1 to 4 mg per minute is started and may be continued for several days. Depending on individual dosage requirements for effectiveness and the need to restrict total fluid intake, various intravenous lidocaine solutions may be made up. An example would be a mixture of 2,000 mg of lidocaine added to 1,000 ml of 5 percent dextrose in water, to drip at a rate of 1 ml per minute and therefore deliver 2 mg of lidocaine per minute.

The duration of action of a single intravenous bolus of 1 mg per kg of lidocaine is from 10 to 20 minutes (5,6,7). Lidocaine, like procainamide (Pronestyl), has been shown to cause an elevation in the electric stimulation threshold of the ventricle during diastole, and it would appear that this effect may be related to the antiarrhythmic effect of both drugs. In contrast to procainamide, it has little hypotensive effect in the effective dose range and is decidedly less toxic than any intravenous preparation of quinidine (6). The total permissible dose has not been established, but an anesthetized patient (adult) has been given 500 mg within a one hour period without detectable signs of toxicity (7).

Toxic reactions to sufficiently large doses of lidocaine comprise hypotension, sweating, vomiting, muscle twitching, confusion, convulsions, medullary depression with apnea, peripheral vasodilation, bradycardia, and diminished cardiac output (8A).

If lidocaine proves ineffective, procainamide may be given intravenously, in a dose of 50 mg every two to three minutes, up to 1,000 mg, until the arrhythmia is abolished. Constant monitoring not only of the ECG but also of the blood pressure is essential while the drug is injected. It is best to have established a secure intravenous infusion beforehand and to use a 3-*way stopcock* to which is already attached a bottle containing a pressor agent which can be given at once if significant hypotension occurs. If the initial dose of procainamide is effective, it can be followed by an oral or intramuscular maintenance dose of 1 to 3 g daily, divided into four equal doses. Slow intravenous infusions of procainamide with total doses up to 6 g a day have been used, although hypotension is a constant danger (2).

Quinidine sulfate may be used in an oral dose of 0.2 to 0.4 g every two hours for five doses, or every six hours. Quinidine hydrochloride or gluconate may be given intramuscularly in doses similar to the oral dose and will become effective within five to 15 minutes, with a peak plasma level in 90 minutes as opposed to the oral peak level in two to three hours. Maintenance doses are usually 0.2 to 0.4 g orally or intramuscularly every six hours. Adequate quinidine blood levels must be obtained to achieve a significant antiarrhythmic effect, and patients vary greatly in this regard. Diminished renal function, manifested by a BUN of 25 mg per cent or greater, decreases dose requirements, and high body weights increase dose requirements (2). Since the intramuscular route may be deceptive in shock due to poor absorption from the injection site, intravenous quinidine can be used. This route should only be employed when other measures have failed because of dangerous toxic effects. The intravenous dose is 0.3 to 0.5 g dissolved in 100 ml of saline and given over five to 15 minutes under electrocardiographic and blood pressure control.

Intravenous diphenylhydantoin (Dilantin) has been used successfully to control ventricular premature beats in doses of 100 to 250 mg given within a few minutes. There may be local problems at the site of injection, and toxic effects are similar to those of quinidine. Diphenylhydantoin has largely been replaced by lidocaine. Clinical experimentations involving the use of propranolol are also proving that this drug is effective where others fail in treatment of ventricular premature beats.

A more indirect approach to the control of ventricular premature beats may be necessary in some patients. If significant hypotension is present, pressor therapy may abolish the arrhythmia. Treatment of congestive heart failure with digitalis and/or diuretics may control premature beats secondary to inadequate cardiac output. In the patient who has survived recent acute circulatory arrest, or in the deteriorating patient, correction of metabolic acidosis by intravenous injection of an ampule of 40 mEq sodium bicarbonate, repeated if necessary in five to eight minutes, may be effective. One must watch for sodium overload producing congestive heart failure with this treatment. Premature beats secondary to digitalis intoxication may respond to the intravenous infusion of 40 mEq of potassium chloride dissolved in 1,000 ml of 5 percent dextrose in water, or 50 mg per kg of the chelating agent ethylene diamine tetra-acetic acid (EDTA) in 200 ml of 5 percent dextrose in water infused over 30 minutes.

Finally, premature beats may occur in the patient with acute myocardial infarction from an inappropriately slow heart rate such as sinus bradycardia. Increasing the heart rate with atropine, 0.3 to 1.2 mg intravenously or intramuscularly every two hours, may be effective. If atropine is effective, isoproterenol (Isuprel), 1 mg diluted in 500 ml of 5 percent dextrose in water administered by controlled intravenous drip, may achieve the same results but is also capable of increasing cardiac irritability. If these two drugs fail to produce the desired effect of rate control, there are occasions when transvenous cardiac pacing at a rate depending on the patient's need can produce the desired rhythm control.

## *Treatment of Ventricular Tachycardia*

In patients with acute myocardial infarction, ventricular tachycardia may be of two types (1). The more common type comprises brief, self-limited paroxysms of from four to 20 successive beats at rates from 70 to 250 per minute. Observation of even a single episode of this type requires immediate reporting—for immediate antiarrhythmic therapy, which is essentially the same as that already discussed for ventricular premature beats.

The second type of ventricular tachycardia is rapid and sustained, producing serious compromise of circulatory dynamics often manifested by declining blood pressure, pulse pressure, evidence of congestive heart failure, and occurrence of ventricular fibrillation. This arrhythmia should be terminated immediately. Lown and coworkers (1) recommend that a 50 mg bolus of lidocaine be given intravenously at once, followed in a few minutes by an additional 100 mg if the initial dose is not effective. If lidocaine is not successful, synchronized electrical cardioversion is carried out, usually without general anesthesia; it may be started with 5 watt-seconds and gradually increased to 50 watt-seconds, interspersed with further doses of lidocaine or other measures according to the needs of the particular patient. Some physicians prefer to use 400 watt-seconds routinely (2). In the latter range, precordial shock is quite painful and requires the use of a light general anesthesia with a short-acting barbiturate sufficient to produce amnesia if possible.

## *Treatment of Ventricular Fibrillation*

For ventricular fibrillation, electrical cardioversion at 400 watt-seconds should be done immediately, if possible. If the patient is not in a coronary care unit when this arrhythmia occurs, closed-chest cardiac massage and artificial respiration are carried out in the interim until cardioversion is possible. Repeated injections of 40 mEq of sodium bicarbonate intravenously every five to eight minutes are necessary to help combat acidosis if resuscitation must be continued for any length of time. Once the fibrillation has been corrected, the prophylactic drug therapy to prevent a recurrence is essentially the same as that already described for ventricular premature beats.

## *Summary*

This case demonstrates
1. The importance of monitoring all patients with acute myocardial infarction
2. The significant danger of premature ventricular contractions, especially those occurring in the "vulnerable" phase of the cardiac cycle
3. The successful control of arrhythmias through the use of lidocaine

# D CASE STUDY OF W. J.

Case Study edited and included by permission of American Heart Association from "Diagnosis and Treatment of Arrhythmias."

## Case Data

A 62-year-old male was admitted to the hospital complaining of diffuse anterior chest pain of two days' duration. He had remained in bed at home until the day of admission. He appeared acutely ill with pulse 50, diffuse rales in both lung fields, and blood pressure 190/70. Admission complete blood count and urinalysis were within normal limits. The SGOT reached a maximum of 220 units (normal range 8–40) 24 hours after admission, and the LDH reached a maximum of 3,400 units (normal range 150–500) on the third hospital day.

The admission ECG and chest x-ray are illustrated (Fig. 1).

## Discussion

The chest x-ray shows some abnormality with moderate congestive changes and left ventricle enlargement. The ECG shows abnormal finding indicative of complete AV block, atrial rate of 80, ventricular rate of 52. Typical changes of acute posterior wall infarction by marked ST elevation in leads 1, 2, and aVF; the broad R waves in $V_2$ are probably also secondary to the posterior wall infarction.

While still in the emergency room, after notation of the initial cardiac rhythm, the patient was immediately given atropine, 1.2 mg intravenously,

372

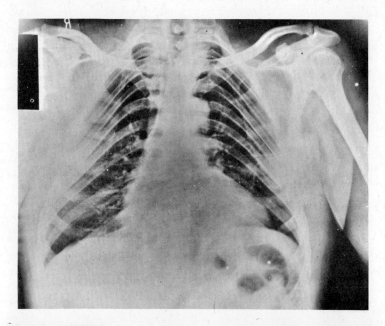

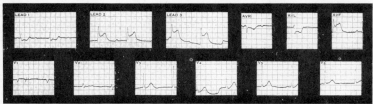

*FIG. 1* Patient W. J.: 62-year-old male with a two-day history of diffuse anterior chest pain. Patient appears severely ill.

(From Diagnostic Aids. Courtesy of American Heart Association.)

hydrocortisone hemisuccinate (Solu-Cortef), 100 mg intravenously, and iso-proterenol (Isuprel), 0.2 mg intravenously, all of which failed to improve his cardiac rhythm. Because he was in congestive heart failure as manifested by early pulmonary edema, he was then given lanatoside C (Cedilanid), 1.2 mg intravenously. He was taken immediately to the x-ray department for passage of transvenous bipolar pacemaker through the right superficial jugular vein under fluoroscopic observation. Over the next hour his rate was gradually increased from 80 to 100 beats per minute by use of the pacemaker, and over the next several hours he was more fully digitalized.

The ECG on the first night, with the pacemaker on, was uneventful. On the second, the ECG, with the pacer off, showed the ventricular rate had increased to 68 beats per minute. On the third day, without the pacemaker, the patient's ventricular rate had increased to 88 beats per minute, with complete heart block continuing. When the pacemaker at 100 beats per minute was turned off, despite a spontaneous rate of 88 beats per minute, his blood pressure declined from 130/80 to 110/80, his respiratory rate increased from 24 to 44 per minute, and his extremities became cool and moist within a few minutes. *Resumption* of pacing promptly reversed all these changes.

The patient's temperature rose to a maximum of 103°F on the third day, and throughout the first two weeks in the hospital he required continuous therapy for congestive heart failure, with additional doses of digoxin (Lanoxin) and diuretics. The pacemaker made it possible to "push" digoxin without fear of increasing the AV block.

On the seventh hospital day, the patient showed second-degree AV block with Wenckebach conduction, which could be converted to 1:1 conducted transiently with atropine. One the ninth day, he showed spontaneous and continuous 1:1 AV conduction. The pacemaker was left in place for an additional ten days.

The incidence of complete or third-degree AV block as a complication of acute myocardial infarction has been reported variable at 2 to 5 percent (1,2,13); in two-thirds of the cases it is noted within the first 24 hours (13). In three-fourths of the cases of AV block the infarction is diaphragmatic (posterior, inferior), since a branch of the right coronary artery supplies the AV node in 90 percent of human hearts. In the remaining one-fourth, complete AV block is associated with anterior wall infarction and carries worse prognosis (13). Reported mortality figures for complete AV block complicating acute myocardial infarction vary from 39 to almost 100 percent (2,14), making studies of comparative treatment methods difficult. There is no doubt, however, that certain patients display transient complete AV block, which reverts to normal conduction either from drug therapy or spontaneously within a few hours or by the end of two weeks.

Catastrophic complications which may occur in the presence of complete AV block include not only ventricular standstill but also ventricular irritability, progressing rapidly to ventricular tachycardia or ventricular fibrillation. In addition, important reduction of cardiac output resulting in congestive heart failure may result from an inappropriately slow heart rate in the presence of associated myocardial disease (15,16).

Some authorities prefer to give drug therapy a trial before inserting a transvenous catheter pacemaker (1). A medical method of treatment comprises the use of atropine in intravenous or subcutaneous doses of 0.3 to 1.2

mg, repeated every four hours if necessary. This drug is effective when vagal influences are contributing to the problem and may be useful in first-degree AV block (prolonged P-R interval) associated with sinus bradycardia, and in some cases of second-degree AV block (intermittent dropped beats). The most important side effects are difficulties with micturition and central nervous system effects including restlessness and delirium.

Isoproterenol may be effective in second- or third-degree block. It may be given sublingually or rectally in doses of 50 to 15 mg every one to six hours (available in 10 and 15 mg tablets). In an acute situation, parenteral administration of 0.2 mg subcutaneously or slowly intravenously may be used. However, results can best be obtained with dose titration of an intravenous infusion in which 2 mg are added to a bottle of 1,000 ml of 5 percent dextrose in water and dripped in at varying rates, often 2 ml per minute (20 to 30 drops per minute depending on the type of infusion set used). It is very important for constant monitoring during titration of an isoproterenol infusion because of the propensity of this drug to increase ventricular irritability. Another disadvantage is the unpredictable and sometimes erratic response of the AV block to this drug (2).

If a sympathomimetic drug with some peripheral pressor effect is desired, the physician might choose epinephrine rather than isoproterenol. Initial dose titration may be accomplished by placing 4 ml of 1:1,000 epinephrine (4 mg) in 1,000 ml of 5 percent dextrose in water in which the effective dose is often in the range of 1 mg per minute. Careful monitoring for increased ventricular irritability is also important with this drug (17).

Adrenal steroids have been reported useful in treatment of AV block complicating acute myocardial infarction (18,19), presumably due to the anti-inflammatory effect on injured conducting tissue. For rapid onset of action in the acute situation, hydrocortisone sodium succinate (Solu-Cortef), 100 mg, or methylprednisolone sodium succinate (Solu-Medrol), 40 mg intravenously, will be effective in one hour. High blood levels can be maintained by repeated intravenous or intramuscular injections every four to six hours or, the physician may elect to continue steroid therapy, orally with prednisone (Deltasone), 10 to 15 mg every six hours, if the treatment is initially effective. Potential hazards and side effects of continuous steroid therapy are well known and will not be repeated here. Just as is true with atropine and sympathomimetic drugs, the effectiveness of steroid therapy is unpredictable in the given patient and has the added disadvantage of requiring a period of hours rather than minutes to be effective during the most critical phase of therapy of acute myocardial infarction.

Indications for the use of transvenous catheter pacemakers for treatment of AV block are not yet universally agreed upon. The obvious disadvantage is the necessity of transporting the patient to the x-ray department for fluoroscopic placement of a bipolar catheter through a jugular venous cutdown; this can only be circumvented by mastering the technique of threading a flexible wire through a needle blindly into the right ventricle, under electrocardiographed control at the bedside. In the skilled hands of an experienced physician, the latter technique is successful in 80 percent of the cases (2,20). Serious ventricular arrhythmias may be induced during placement of the catheter. Infection and ventricular perforation by the catheter tip are rare complications.

Despite these potential problems with catheter pacemakers, there are a significant number of patients, such as the one described here, in whom transvenous catheter pacing during the initial period after infarction is imperative for survival. The decision to put in a pacemaker is made as early as possible to permit adequate mobilization of the necessary equipment and personnel before the patient is in marked distress and requires true emergency management. Once the pacemaker has been inserted, there is considerable security in knowing that the heart can be effectively paced, when and if necessary, and that digitalis can be used when necessary to treat congestive heart failure in the face of complete AV block.

Many cardiologists experienced in coronary care unit work would put a catheter in patients with acute infarction if either complete (third-degree) or second-degree (Wenckebach, 2:1, or occasional dropped beat) AV block is present. Some would add first-degree block with P-R interval greater than 0.30 second to this list of indications (2). The presence of AV block associated with anterior wall infarction would reinforce these criteria because of the poorer prognosis. In instances of first- and second-degree block, the catheter may be kept off and serve as a stand-by to be used should drug therapy fail to prevent the development of complete block or to maintain a sufficiently rapid ventricular rate. The cather tip in the right atrium may be useful in diagnosing complex arrhythmias (20).

Once the catheter is being used to pace the patient, the rate will need adjustment to achieve optimal benefit. The optimal rate varies not only from patient to patient but also in the same patient from time to time, depending on such associated factors as fever, infection, hypotension, and congestive heart failure (15,21). Ventricular arrhythmia may be suppressed by increasing the heart rate in some patients. If the rate is too high, cardiac output and blood pressure will fail (21). Therefore, it is best to start pacing at rates of 75 to 80 beats per minute and titrate the rate by observing closely for signs of improvement in congestive heart failure, hypotension, mental depression, peripheral vasoconstriction, and sweating. The energy level of the pacemaker impulse should be set at the lowest level that will be effective in capturing the ventricle.

The pacemaker is turned off when complete AV block is replaced by either 1:1 conduction or second-degree block that can be controlled by drug therapy. Following return of a stable pattern of 1:1 conduction, the pacemaker catheter is preferably left in place for another 7 to 10 days by many physicians as a standby in the event of recurrence of complete block. So-called *demand pacemakers* are now available which are able to sense a momentary pause in cardiac electrical activity and drive the heart until the normal pacemaker returns. These demand pacemakers avoid the potential danger of competitive normal sinus rhythm and fixed pacing, a form of parasystole in which there is a real danger of precipitation of ventricular tachycardia or fibrillation, should the pacer impulse fall on the apex of the T wave of the preceding beat (the vulnerable period) (22).

If the complete heart block persists beyond 2 weeks, it may be necessary to implant a permanent pacemaker before the patient leaves the hospital.

## *Summary*

This case illustrates a complete AV block complicating posterior wall infarction, which failed to respond to drug therapy initially. Prolonged pacing with a transvenous catheter was successful. Variable control of ventricular rate to meet current circulatory demands was clinically useful.

# E   CASE STUDY OF M. Y.

Case Study edited and included by permission of American Heart Association from "Diagnosis and Treatment of Arrhythmias."

### Case Data

A 39-year-old female came to the emergency room complaining of "heavy palpitation." She had been in the hospital previously, at which time she gave a history of a heart murmur since the age of 23. At that time she was told that her heart was small and that she was "hypothyroid and anemic," and she was threated with thyroid extract and "iron pills." She had noted short bouts of palpitation since her days in high school. Occasionally such attacks had lasted for long periods of time, during which times she noted polyuria, and at the end of these long bouts of palpitation she was quite thirsty. On her previous admission a presystolic apical murmur had been noted. An ECG was read as normal.

Physical examination in the emergency room revealed a heart rate of 170 per minute, blood pressure 110/70, and no additional physical findings of significance.

The chest x-ray and ECG are illustrated (Fig. 1).

### Discussion

The roentgenologist first interpreting the chest film declared it normal. However, one can note the slight prominence of the left atrial appendage in this otherwise small heart with a straightening of the left cardiac border.

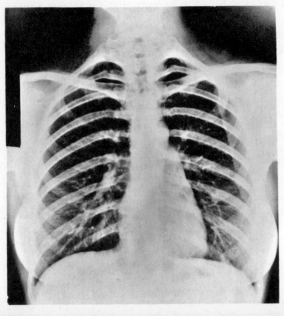

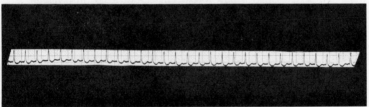

*FIG. 1* Patient M. Y.: 39-year-old female complaining of "heavy palpitation" and "heart murmur" since the age of 23.

(From Diagnostic Aids. Courtesy of American Heart Association.)

This may arouse suspicions that there is early enlargement of this chamber of the heart.

The ECG revealed supraventricular tachycardia.

When this patient presented herself in the emergency room the customary methods of vagal stimulation were utilized: pressure on the carotid sinus, Valsalva's maneuvers, and gagging, none of which reverted the patient's rhythm to normal.

It was then decided to try a pressor drug in order to determine its effects; 0.5 mg of phenylephrine (Neo-Synephrine) was given intravenously. Seen in serial tracings, blood pressure rose from a starting pressure of 105/70 to a level of 190/110. Suddenly the rhythm changed to a sinus mechanism. It was noted that, in the first few seconds after conversion when the heart rates slowed precipitously from a very rapid to a more normal one, there were two ventricular ectopic beats. This is not unusual under these circumstances, since the heart is more vulnerable to ectopic contractions after long R-R intervals. It was also interesting to note that the rhythm sped up as the blood pressure fell in first tracings to 180/100 and finally to 125/90, thus demonstrating the relationship between vagal stimulation and the heart rate.

Many physicians would not use pressor drugs as the drug of choice in these arrhythmias, although in the experience of some this method terminates the attacks most rapidly and thus returns the patient's heart to a normal rhythm with the least side effects from the drug used. It is well recognized that the effects of supraventricular tachycardia are not devastating and that patients can tolerate such rhythms for long periods of time.

Bellet (8B) points out the following as guides for therapy for this arrhythmia:

Most of the paroxysms are of short duration; paroxysmal atrial tachycardia is usually relatively well tolerated; deaths due to this arrhythmia are rare; simpler measures should be tried first, and, if drugs are necessary, those that are relatively innocuous and manifest minimal toxicity should be used. Such measures will terminate the paroxysm in about 90 percent of the cases; intravenous medication and heroic measures should be avoided except in cases of real emergency, and such occasions mean they should be given slowly and the effects followed with the electrocardiogram.

Although this last injunction is important to remember, it is the belief of others that certain uses of intravenous medications can be helpful. In this particular case vasopressor drugs did indeed end the attack quickly, thus alleviating the patient's discomfort. Side effects are few if the dose is carefully regulated. Although there may be danger in raising blood pressure to the levels indicated in this case, most often this has not been a factor fraught with danger. Certainly the vagal response under these circumstances can in certain instances be extremely strong. In an experiment in human pharmacology, a medical student's blood pressure was raised using leverterenol (norepinephrine). The blood pressure rose, the vagal nerve was stimulated, sinus arrest occurred, and cardiac rhythm was resumed with ventricular beats followed, after what seemed an interminable time, by a normal sinus rhythm. The student was *unaware* of this arrhythmia until after the experiment.

Many different methods are employed in the treatment of paroxysmal atrial supraventricular tachycardias. Frequently, the stimulation of the vagus nerve by manipulative means has been helpful either in converting the rhythm or in helping to make the diagnosis; for, even if the rhythm does not convert to normal, there are often periods with vagal stimulation during which the rhythm is slowed and P waves, if present, can be seen to emerge as the rate slows.

Quinidine, procainamide (Pronestyl) and, more recently, propranolol (Inderal) have been used both to terminate the attacks and to control them before they start. It usually takes a fairly large dose of quinidine or procainamide to restore normal rhythms in many of these patients. Propranolol in doses ranging from 15 to 150 mg has proved effective in preventing recurrence of paroxysmal atrial supraventricular attacks as well as proving effective in controlling the attacks when digitalis, quinidine, or procainamide is ineffective. There is a lag period between oral administration of these drugs and their therapeutic effect of about half of three-quarters of an hour. Sometimes vagal stimulation after their administration is effective, whereas it had had no effect prior to their use. Cholinergic drugs have been employed to treat this arrhythmia, in particular, neostigmine (Prostigmin) to block hydrolysis of acetylcholine by cholinesterase, acetyl-beta-methyl-choline (Mecholyl) and acetylcholine. All of these substances have unpleasant side effects. Digitalis has also been effective in some instances, although again, there is a lag period between administration and conversion to normal rhythm. Electrical cardioversion can be utilized, although the necessity for anesthesia makes this procedure somewhat less desirable than those methods which allow the patient to remain conscious.

Long-term treatment of paroxysmal tachycardia is a difficult problem and must be tailored to suit the individual patient. In many, a maintenance dose of quinidine, procainamide, or propranolol will be helpful. Difficulty arises in regulating the dose if the paroxysms are few and far between. Under these circumstances, it is probably best to start with a relatively standard dose of quinidine in the range of 0.2 g three to four times a day. If the paroxysms recur, the dose can be gradually increased either until the paroxysm is controlled or toxic manifestations appear. Several patients observed have needed large doses of quinidine to maintain normal rhythms. Doses of 1.6 to 2.4 g are not unusual for such patients, and it is interesting to note that when the dose is decreased but slightly the paroxysmal arrhythmias recur.

If the paroxysms are usually short-lived, it is probably not necessary to maintain continued antiarrhythmic drug therapy over long periods of time. Often patients taking these drugs do not feel completely normal, although frequently this feeling of malaise is vague and somewhat indefinable. Such patients are content to have quinidine with them and to take one rather large dose to interrupt the attack rather than to take maintenance dosage over long periods of time.

Digitalis may sometimes be of help in these cases, although this is not universally true, and it should be tried perhaps only in those instances in which quinidine or procainamide have been unsuccessful in maintaining normal rhythm or in converting the abnormal rhythm back to normal after such therapy has been attempted. Since paroxysmal supraventricular tachycardia is not dangerous, the physician has time to experiment slowly with his patient, explaining to him that although the abnormal rhythm is known to give discomfort it is not life-threatening.

Paroxysms are often provoked by excessive smoking and excessive ingestion of such stimulants as coffee or tea, or sometimes after periods of prolonged fatigue-producing crises in a person's life they are seen to occur.

One interesting aspect of the case presented here, which is not always appreciated by physicians, is the polyuria and dehydration following one of these attacks. They do not occur in all cases, but are present in a significant number of individuals, so that this finding can often contribute to establishing the final diagnosis. This phenomenon is well documented in a recent article (23) in which a careful study of one patient and a review of the literature are presented. The authors conclude that the increased output of the patient was not related to the change in cardiac output but was most likely due to left atrial distention with subsequent antidiuretic hormone inhibition. It is recognized that this is not the total explanation since there was also a solute diuresis, the mechanism for which was unclear.

## Summary

1. Intravenous vasopressor drugs are useful agents in the therapy of paroxysmal supraventricular tachycardia.

2. These drugs should be used only after traditional maneuvers for vagal stimulation have failed.

3. Other agents such as cholinergic drugs, quinidine, procainamide, propranolol, and digitalis can also be employed to convert the abnormal rhythm to normal. Side effects and/or lag periods often accompany the use of these agents.

4. Electrical cardioversions may also be utilized, but anesthesia is necessary in the higher doses.

5. Preventive therapy is often difficult to maintain.

# F REFERENCES FOR APPENDICES A, B, AND C

1. Lown, B., Fakhro, A. M., Hood, Jr., W. B., and Thorn, G. W. The Coronary Care Unit: New Perspective and Directions. *JAMA*, 199:188. 1967.
2. "The Current Status of Intensive Coronary Care." A Symposium presented by the American College of Cardiology and Presbyterian University of Pennsylvania Medical Center, Philadelphia, Pa., July 15, 1966. New York, Charles Press, 1966.
3. Wiggers, C. J. The Mechanisms and Nature of Ventricular Fibrillation. *Am. Heart. J.*, 20:399, 1940.
4. Lown, B., Bey, S. K., Perlroth, M., and Abe, T. Comparative Studies of Ventricular Vulnerability to Fibrillation. *J. Clin. Invest.*, 42:953, 1963.
5. Weiss, W. A. Intravenous Use of Lidocaine for Ventricular Arrhythmias. *Anesth. and Analg.*, 39:369, 1960.
6. Likoff, W. Cardiac Arrhythmias Complicating Surgery (editorial). *Am. J. Cardiology*, 3:427, 1959.
7. Harrison, D. C., Sprouse, J. H., and Morrow, A. G. The Antiarrhythmic Properties of Lidocaine and Procaine Amide. *Circulation*, 18:486, 1963.
8. Bellet, S. *Clinical Disorders of the Heart Beat.* Ed.2. Philadelphia, Lea and Febiger, 1963. (A) p. 912 (B) p. 295.
9. Rytand, D. A. The Circus Movement (entrapped circuit wave) Hypothesis and Atrial Flutter. *Ann. Int. Med.*, 65:125, 1966.
10. Kleiger, R., and Lown, B. Cardioversion and Digitalis: II Clinical Studies. *Circulation*, 33:878, 1966.
11. Castellanos, Jr., A., Lemberg, L., Gosselin and Fonseca, E. J. Evaluation of Countershock Treatment of Atrial Flutter. *Arch. Int. Med.*, 115:426, 1965.
12. Gilbert, R., and Cuddy, R. P. Digitalis Intoxication Following Conversion to Sinus Rhythm. *Circulation*, 32:58, 1965.

13. Friedberg, C. K. *Diseases of the Heart*. Ed. 3 Philadelphia, W. B. Saunders, 1966.
14. Bruce, R. A., Blackmon, J. R., Cobb, L. A., and Dodge, H. T. Treatment of Asystole of Heart Block During Acute Myocardial Infarction with Electrode Catheter Pacing. *Am. Heart. J.*, 69:460, 1965.
15. Judge, R. D., Wilson, W. S., and Siegel, J. H. Hemodynamic Studies in Patients with Implanted Cardiac Pacemakers. *New Eng. J. Med.*, 270: 1391, 1964.
16. Thomas, M., Malmcrona, R., and Shillingford, J. Hemodynamic Changes in Patients with Acute Myocardial Infarction. *Circulation*, 31:811, 1965.
17. Hurst, J. W., and Logue, R. B. *The Heart*. New York, McGraw-Hill, 1966.
18. Dall, J. L. C. Effect of Steroid Therapy on Normal and Abnormal Atrioventricular Conduction. *Brit. Heart. J.*, 26:537, 1964.
19. Aber, C. P., and Jones, E. W. Corticotropin and Corticosteriods in the Management of Acute and Chronic Heart Block. *Brit. Heart J.*, 27:916, 1965.
20. Kimball, J. T., and Killip, T. A Simple Bedside Method for Transvenous Intracardiac Pacing. *Am. Heart J.*, 70:35, 1965.
21. Sowton, E. Hemodynamic Studies in Patients with Artificial Pacemakers. *Brit. Heart J.*, 26:737, 1964.
22. Sowton, E. Artificial Pacemaking and Sinus Rhythm. *Brit. Heart J.*, 27:311, 1965.
23. Luria, M. K., Adelson, E. J., and Lochaya, S. Paroxysmal Tachycardia with Polyuria. *Ann. Inst. Med.*, 65:461, 1966.

# G BASIC ORIENTATION COURSE IN CORONARY CARE FOR NURSES

*Orientation to CCU*

Recommended Hours: 1

1. History
   —Defibrillation
   —Pacemaking
   —CPR
   —Concept of CCU
     —Initial resuscitation
     —Now prevention
2. Administration
   —Organization
   —Personnel needs
   —Continued training plans
   —Delegation of authority
     —Legal implications
3. Physical design of CCU
4. Selection of patients
5. Length of stay
6. Results we can expect

### Anatomy and Physiology

Recommended Hours: 2

1. Great vessels
2. Coronary system
3. Chambers
4. Valves
5. Conduction system
6. Peripheral vessels
7. Starling's Law of the Heart
   —Concept of heart failure
8. Starling's Equilibrium
   —Serum proteins
9. Central venous pressure
10. Blood pressure
11. Cardiac output
    —Fick principle
    —Central venus $O_2$ saturation
12. Concept of coronary blood flow to the ventricles with relation to intra-ventricular and intramyocardial pressure

### Pathology

Recommended Hours: 2

1. Concept of atherogenesis
   —Causes
   —Principles of arterial obstruction—Reynolds formula
2. Infarction
3. Anatomic pattern with relation to coronary arteries
4. Clinical and pathological correlations
   —Pattern of anterior infarction versus posterior infarction
5. Pathologic changes in the infarcted area with time
   —Acute "softening"
   —Fibroblastic infiltration
   —Scar
   —"Aneurysm"
   —Mural thrombosis
   —Possible rupture
   —Collateral circulation

## *Clinical Course of Myocardial Infarction*

Recommended Hours: 2

1. Clinical syndrome including angina, atypical syndromes, and sudden death
2. Time to death after onset of symptoms
3. Laboratory findings
4. Concept of death from various causes
   —Rhythm disturbances
   —Shock (pump failure)
   —Congestive heart failure
   —Other
5. Complications
   —Pericarditis
   —Thromboembolism
   —Rupture
   —Post-myocardial infarction syndrome
   —Gastric dilatation
   —Renal shutdown
6. Convalescence
   —Time period at various levels of activity
   —Rehabilitation
7. Recurrence
   —Death rate through time

## *Respiratory and Renal Physiology*

Recommended Hours: 1

1. Ventilation
2. Perfusion
3. Diffusion
4. Blood gases
   —$pCO_2$ and $pO_2$
   —Hemoglobin dissociation curve
5. Acid-base balance
   —Buffer systems
   —Respiratory effects
   —Metabolic effects
   —Kidney

6. Electrolytes
   —Osmolality
   —Hyponatremia
   —Hyperkalemia
7. Renal physiology
   —Decreased cardiac output
   —Decreased glomerular filtration rate
   —Meanings of intake and output and specific gravity

## *Electrocardiography*

Recommended Hours: 8–10 hrs didactic
8–10 hrs unknown
& practice interpre-
tation sessions

1. Genesis of the EKG potentials
2. P wave
3. QRS
4. ST segment
5. T wave—discuss vulnerable period
6. Intervals—discuss the time relationships of the EKG
7. Lead systems
8. Vectors
9. Intraventricular conduction delay
   —Right bundle-branch block
   —Left bundle-branch block
10. Infarction patterns
11. Ventricular hypertrophy
    —Discuss voltage
12. Atrial hypertrophy
13. Atrial tachyrhythmia
    —Atrial premature beats
    —Atrial fibrillation
    —Atrial tachycardia
14. Atrial bradyrhythmia
    —Sinus bradycardia
    —Sinus pause
    —SA block
15. Ventricular tachyrhythmia
    —Ventricular premature beats
      —Significance of numbers

    —R on T phenomenon
    —Ventricular bigeminy
    —Ventricular tachycardia
    —Ventricular flutter
    —Ventricular fibrillation
16. Ventricular bradyrhythmia
    —"Benign" slow ventricular tachycardia
17. Block
    —First-degree
    —Second-degree, Wenckebach
    —Third-degree
18. Nodal rhythms
19. Techniques of taking electrocardiogram
    —Misplacement of leads
    —Demonstration


### *Pharmacology and Therapeutics*

Recommended Hours: 4

1. Basic principles of pharmacology
   —Route of therapy. Oral versus IM versus IV
     Discuss accumulation of dose related to absorption rate and excretion
     rate, for example, Digoxin versus Digitoxin.
2. Discuss multiple systems of drug disposal by the body
   —Kidney
   —Liver (example glucuronides)
3. Drug interference and potentiation
   —K + digitalis
   —ASA + anticoagulants
4. Specific drugs used on CCU
   —Digitalis
     —Vagal effects
     —Muscle effects
     —Toxic manifestation
   —Quinidine
   —Pronestyl
   —Lidocaine
   —Dilantin
   —Heparin
   —Warfarin
   —Isuprel

        —Aramine
          —Tachyphylaxis
          —Reserpine
        —Levophed
        —Sodium bicarbonate
        —Calcium chloride
        —Morphine
        —Atropine
        —Aminophylline
        —Coronary dilators
        —Antibiotics
        —Oxygen
        —Propranolol
        —Bretylium
        —Diuretics
          —Mercurials
          —Thiazides
          —Furosemide
        —Barbiturates
5. Other therapy
        —Leg exercise
        —Early armchair treatment
        —Elastic stockings
        —Bed positioning
        —Tourniquets
        —Phlebotomy
        —Diet

### Intravenous Therapy

Recommended Hours: 2

1. IV fluids—Types and uses
2. Obligatory potassium loss
3. Fluid overloading
4. Central venous catheter and principles of central venous pressure
5. Hydration with hypotension and low central venous pressure
6. Transfusion
        —Whole blood
        —Packed cells
7. Hypertonic solutions
        —Salt
        —Mannitol

8. Glucose
   —Protein sparing
9. —Therapy with nasogastric suction
10. Electrolyte replacement therapy
    —Body weight
    —Extracellular phase
    —Intravascular phase
    —Total body water
    —Calculation of total deficit

## *Nursing Care*

Recommended Hours: 2

1. Responsibilities
   —Basic knowledge maintenance
   —Application
     —Diagnosis
     —Therapy
     —Rehabilitation
2. Legal implications
3. Nurse-physician relationships
   —What to do when you know more than the physician
   —How to get a consultation when you think it's necessary
4. Teaching
   —Each other
   —Physician
   —Patient
   —Family
5. The "mask" or how to feel bad and not cause ventricular fibrillation
6. Standing orders
   —In premonitory situations
     —PVC's
     —First-degree block
   —In the emergency
     —Standstill
     —Ventricular fibrillation
     —Heart block
     —Congestive failure
7. Physical findings
   —Heart sounds
   —Râles
   —Edema
   —Neck veins

## CCU Equipment

Recommended Hours: 4

1. —Basic electronics
   —DC vs AC
   —$E = IR$
   —Watts, volts, amps., and ohms
   —Grounds
   —Shock hazard
     —Vulnerable periods
     —Skin resistance
     —Hazards with pacemakers
2. Monitoring equipment
   —EKG
   —Ear piece
   —Artifacts and their genesis
   —False alarms
   —Needle electrodes
   DON'T NEGLECT
   —Blood pressure
   —Neck veins
   —Lung bases
   —Weight
   —Intake and output
   —Edema
3. Pacemaking equipment
   —Generator
     —External and internal
     —Voltage
     —Rate setting
   —Pacemakers—unipolar and bipolar
     —External
     —Internal
       —Epicardial
       —Endocardial
         —Fixed rate
         —Demand
         —P wave triggered
     —Transthoracic
     —Floating

4. Defibrillators
   —Electrode Paste
   —Skin resistance
   —DC vs AC
   —What setting
   —Synchronized shock
   —Elective cardioversion
5. Positive pressure respiration
   —Triggering sensitivity
   —Automatic control
   —Pressure control
   —Inspiratory time control
   —Expiratory control
   —Humidity
6. Automatic tourniquet machine
7. Tape loop
8. Chest compressor
9. Newer techniques
   —Central venous saturation
   —Arterial pressure
   —Cardiac output
   —Premature beat monitor
   —Computer monitoring

*Cardiac Arrest*

Recommended Hours: 2

1. Physiology
   —Time limits
   —Acidosis
   —"Cardiac outputs" with resuscitation
   —Results of resuscitation
2. Techniques of cardiopulmonary resuscitation
   —Methods of ventilation
   —Closed-chest massage
3. Production of ventricular fibrillation in dogs
   —Demonstration of electrocardiogram
   —Demonstration of arterial pressure
4. Defibrillation
5. Demonstration of the safety of synchronized shock
6. Passage of pacemaker catheter into ventricle and artificial pacing
7. Demonstration of "crash cart"

## Final Statement

It is recommended that a panel discussion be offered including both physicians and nurses in the panel and that pre-imposed testing be a definite evaluation section of the curriculum. It is also suggested that pathology specimens be used in demonstration of the pathology of myocardial infarction and anatomic relationships.

# H POSITION DESCRIPTION: CLINICAL SPECIALIST IN CARDIAC NURSING

## Definition

A clinical specialist * in cardiac nursing is a registered nurse who holds a leadership role in cardiac nursing.

## Qualifications

- Currently licensed to practice nursing in the state in which residing.
- Master's Degree in Nursing desirable, or special studies in cardiovascular nursing, human relations, nursing education and hospital organization and management.
- Past experience reflects competence in coronary patient care, leadership, teaching, and ability to consult with groups or individuals.
- Demonstrates effective patterns of communication at an interdisciplinary and interdepartmental level.
- Membership and active participation in the professional nurse organization.
- Membership and active participation in civic and/or allied professional groups.

---

* Position specifications similarly set forth by national, regional, and local coronary care nurse groups.

*Representation of Responsibilities*

- Supervises patient care administered by the staff nurse in coronary care.
- With the team approach, assumes responsibility for follow-up nursing consultation with patient and family.
  a. Contributes to assessment of evolving changes in family relationships.
- Assesses the physiologic and psychologic reactions to the stress of the illness.
  a. Identifies the causative factors of stress.
  b. Determines the cause and effects of the stress upon the patient.
  c. Evaluates the patient's adaptation to stress: identifies the methods of adaption, the present results, and the projected outcomes.
  d. Identifies and evaluates the effectiveness of nursing interventions in patient stress situations.
- In cooperation with medical staff, she sets up and coordinates coronary education programs for staff nurses and other members of the health team.
- Is an active member of the coronary care committee in the hospital of employment.
  a. Participates in establishing policy for coronary patient.
  b. Participates in defining new functions for coronary care staff nurses.

# I POSITION DESCRIPTION: STAFF NURSE IN CORONARY CARE NURSING

## Definition

The coronary care nurse * is a registered nurse who functions as a staff nurse in a well-planned coronary care unit or with patients in medical-surgical units who are on monitored surveillance. She is the key to success in medical therapy of these patients because of her preparation and constant attendance. Through continuous assessment of the patient by direct observation and cardiac monitoring, she can immediately detect the first signs of complications and initiate appropriate therapy when feasible.

Although assigned specific nursing responsibilities, she functions as a team member in patient care. The unique role of the nurse and her status on the team need to be clarified with medical staff to avoid friction which may develop, since many of her new responsibilities of medical therapies were formerly seen as responsibilities delegated to the physician.

## Qualifications

- Currently licensed to practice nursing in the state in which residing.
- Graduate of a baccalaureate or associate arts degree nursing program,

* Position specifications similarly set forth by national, regional, and local coronary care nurse groups.

provided the respective nursing programs have included in their curriculum current concepts of coronary care.

- Registered nurse whose basic nursing education predates current concepts in coronary care but who has attended an approved four- or six-week in-depth intensive coronary care course.
- Registered nurse whose basic nursing education predates current concepts in coronary care but who has attended a two-week coronary care nursing program approved by the state heart association.
- Membership and active participation in the professional nursing organization.

## *Representation of Responsibilities*

- Identifies major cardiac arrhythmias, initiates appropriate nursing actions, and evaluates results.
- Given a rhythm strip, correctly identifies the arrhythmia, describes the possible premonitory signs and the treatment.
- Determines the status of a patient's cardiac and pulmonary circulation condition.
  a. Correctly identifies the cardiac and pulmonary status by observation, palpitation, and auscultation.
  b. Identifies affecting hemodynamics within the arterial and venous system.
  c. Knows factors which can increase or decrease blood pressures.
  d. Initiates effective treatment to correct abnormal pressures.
- Effectively administers cardiopulmonary resuscitation and defibrillation techniques.
- Knows actions, indications, and complications of drugs currently employed in coronary care unit and can select appropriate drug for each situation.
- Demonstrates effective and safe use of important coronary care unit equipment.
- Participates in patient and family planning.
  a. Assists the patient in carrying out activities of daily living.

# J PHYSICIAN'S ORDERS

PHYSICIAN'S ORDERS     CORONARY CARE INTENSIVE    S A M P L E

    12773              MEDICAL UNIT

IMPORTANT:   MULTIGRAPHED ORDERS
MUST HAVE PATIENT'S NAME, DATE AND PHYSICIAN'S SIGNATURE

## ADMITTING ORDERS

Patients admitted to a coronary observation bed having
either a suspected, impending, or proven myocardial
infarction shall automatically have standing orders for
"coronary care" as indicated below unless specifically
changed by order of the admitting physician.

           Cross out those not applicable

           Fill in blanks, and sign

## STANDING "CORONARY CARE" ORDERS

1. Bed rest with head of bed elevated if dyspneic, lowered if in shock and not dyspneic.

2. Bedside commode for bowel movements with assistance.

3. Oxygen by mask or cannula.  4-5 liters/per min.

4. Temperature four times a day orally; axillary temperature if taking oxygen. Rectal temperature if ok'd by physician.

5. Radial and apical pulse, blood pressure, respiration every 30 minutes for four hours, every one hour for eight hours, every two hours for 48 hours and every four hours thereafter.

6. Call physician

   a. When blood pressure is 90 systolic or lower
   b. When frequent premature ventricular beats occur
   c. When pulse is irregular
   d. When any degree of heart block occurs
   e. When pulse is 50 or lower, 120 or higher
   f. When chest pain reoccurs
   g. When sudden dispnea or cyanosis occurs
   h. When ECG arrhythmias appear (as instructed)

7. No bed bath for 24 hours. After that bed baths daily only with specific physician approval.

8. Patient may feed self after proper positioning by nurse and after food has been cut into bite-sized pieces.

## Diet

9. Oral fluids                ad lib_____
   no iced water    Limited to_____forced to_____

10. I.V. fluids may be started by nurse at specific request of physician.
    Type_____
    Rate_____
    Medication added to bottle_____

11. Record intake and output.

12. No telephone, TV, or radio at bedside.

13. Passive flexion of legs every two hours while awake 48 hours.

14. Skin care whenever necessary.

15. Not to brush teeth for 24 hours.

16. Visitors, only immediate family; no more than two at a time.  Hours - 1:00 - 1:30 P.M.; 7:00 - 7:30 P.M.

17. Cardiac monitor on.  Call physician for abnormalities as per instruction.

18. Sedation_____

19. Analgesia_____

20. Laxative_____

21. For sleep_____

22. Cardiac drugs_____

23. Anticoagulant orders_____

24. Laboratory work_____

25. If any arrhythmias or other electrocardiogram abnormality occurs, record rhythm strip STAT and exact time.

26. Twelve (12) lead electrocardiogram.

27. Electrocardiogram rhythm strip every four (4) hours if awake for 48 hours.  Record date and times.

28. If cardiac arrest occurs in absence of physician, RNs will institute standard resuscitative procedures, including assisted ventilation, pacemaking, and defibrillation as outlined by the committee and call "Code 99" and notify physician.

# INDEX

Aberrant conduction, 291
Acceptance of illness by cardiac patients, 91
Ace bandages, 96
Acetylcholine, 49
Acid-base, 123
Acid phosphate, 124
Acidosis, 23, 116-123
  definition, 121, 122
  drugs for, 319-321
  and shock, 319-321
Actions
  of digitalis, 232-236
  of lidocaine, 239, 240
  of propranolol, 241, 242
  of quinidine, 238, 239
Active exercises in care of cardiac patient, 90, 91
Acute myocardial infarction; see Myocardial infarctions, acute
Acute pulmonary edema, 110, 111
Acute pulmonary embolus, 145
Adams-Stokes attacks, 240, 244, 323, 324
Adaptive syndrome, 5
Adenyl-pyrophosphate, 39
  antidiuretic hormone, 115, 116
Adjustment of patient to myocardial infarction, 88
Adrenaline, 329
Adrenergic, 48

Admission sheet for patient with myocardial infarction, 87
Advanced CHF, 184
Air passages, 40
Alarms
  false, in monitoring system, 16
  and monitoring system, 15
Alkaline phosphatase, 104, 112, 126
Alkalosis, 117, 122, 123, 125
Alveoli, 43
American Heart Association, 140, 312
Amine, 329
Aminophylline in acute pulmonary edema, 63
Amphetamine, 324
Amplitude for adequate pacing; see Electrocardiogram
Amylase, 103-111
Anaerobic, 39
Analgesia in myocardial infarction, 94, 29
Anasarca, 329
Anatomy and physiology of heart, 29-33
Anemia, 57
Aneurysm, 100, 329
Anger in patients with myocardial infarction, 91
Angina, 54, 111, 112, 144, 163
  pectoris, 54, 64, 228, 329
  and propranolol, 241, 242
Angiography, 164, 329

Anion, 125-128
Anorexia, 330
Anoxia, 32, 330
Anterior surface of heart in physical examination of cardiovascular system, 28, 29
Antiarrhythmic drugs, 23, 232-246, 244
Antibiotics, 63
Anticoagulation, 63, 96, 144-157, 177, 178, 330
Antidiuretic hormone, 130
Antihistamines and anticoagulation, 148
Antihypertensive agents, 330
Anxiety, relief of, in myocardial infarction, 4, 94, 95, 330
Anxiety states, 4, 8, 9
Aorta, 330
  anatomy and physiology of, 32
  and atherosclerosis, 32, 33, 35, 48
Aortic insufficiency, 330
Aortic stenosis, 330
Aortic valve, anatomy and physiology of, 330
Aortitis, 331
Apex, 331
Apnea, 331
Apoplexy, 331
Aramine; see Metaraminol
Arrest, sinus; see Sinus arrest
Arrhythmias, 182, 323, 244, 275, 331
  cardioversion in, 23, 24
  and diphenylhydantoin, 240
  evaluation of, 211
  and lidocaine, 239, 240
  monitoring system and, 21
  after myocardial infarction, 182, 183
  and permanent pacemakers, 350
  prevention of, in care of cardiac patient, 183
  and quinidine, 238
  and shock, 271
  sinus, 255, 256, 278
Arterial blood, 331
Arterial system in physiologic role of circulation, 35
Arteries, 189
  in anatomy and physiology of heart, 29, 35
  in arteriosclerotic disease, 51, 53
Arteriography, 25, 37, 161, 162, 163, 331

Arteriolar sclerosis, description of, 51
Arterioles, 331
Arteriosclerotic disease, classification and description of, 53, 55, 57
Artery, coronary, 52
  clinical syndromes in diseases of, 53
  pressure, 163
Artificial respiration, 326
Aschoff bodies, 332
Assisted ventilation, 24, 326
Asystole, 22
  and idioventricular rhythm, 293, 307, 347
  ventricular, in temporary pacing, 309
Atherosclerosis, 48, 51, 55, 99, 139, 332
  in etiology of heart disease, 48, 99, 134, 140
  intimal, description of, 51, 99, 134
Atherosclerotic aneurysms, nondissecting, and pulmonary hypertension, 55
Atrial contractions, premature; see Premature atrial contractions
Atrial fibrillation, 22, 63, 240, 264, 267, 269, 270, 279, 294
  in contraindications to Demerol, 94, 95
  and digitalis, 236, 267
  and propranolol, 268
  and quinidine, 268
Atrial flutter, 240, 264, 265, 266
  and digitalis, 234, 235
  and dilantin, 240
  and propranolol, 265
  and quinidine, 265
Atrial gallop, 345
Atrial hypertrophy, 159
Atrial septal defect, 332
Atrial septum, 332
Atrial standstill, 278, 279
Atrial tachycardia, 57, 260, 261
  and digitalis, 260
  in digitalis intoxication, 242
  paroxysmal, 261
  and quinidine, 238, 239
Atrioventricular block; see AV block
Atrioventricular bundle, 332
Atrioventricular dissociations; see AV dissociation
Atrioventricular node, 333
Atrioventricular valves, 333

Atrium, 200, 333
anatomy and physiology of, 29, 30
Atropine, 25, 66, 324
Auenbrugger, Leopold Joseph, 333
Augmented leads, 201, 202
Auscultation of heart in physical examination, 333
Automaticity of fibers, 29
Autonomic system, 47, 333
Autorhythmicity, 249
Auxiliary personnel, 99
AV block, 25, 286, 307, 311, 332
and digitalis, 286
in digitalis intoxication, 286
and diphenylhydantoin, 241
electrocardiogram tracing of, 281, 286
first-degree, and temporary pacemakers, 25, 48, 237, 288
and propranolol, 241, 242
and quinidine, 221
second-degree, and temporary pacemakers, 25, 287, 289, 290
AV bundle, 49
AV dissociation, 48, 295, 296
with block, 295
with interference, 299
and quinidine, 221
AV nodal rhythm and quinidine, 282
AV node, 209, 268, 281
and propranolol, 281, 282
Axes, lead, 189
definition of, 203
and measuring spatial vector, 203, 204
in triaxial figure, 205

Backward theory of CHF, 184
Bacterial endocarditis, 333
Ballistocardiogram, 334
Barbiturate, 334
Batelli, 314
Beck, Claude, 314
Bedrest, 88, 90-92
in myocardial infarction, 171
in right heart failure, 180
Benzothiadiazine, 334
Bicarbonate sodium, 65, 121, 319
and shock, 319
Bicuspid, 334

Bigeminy, 291, 334
and digitalis intoxication, 301
ventricular, and digitalis intoxication, 301
Bleeding time, 112
Block, 282-291
bundle branch; see also Bundle-branch block of heart
and AV dissociation, 294, 295
complete, 293, 345, 373
development of, and PVC count, 286
first-degree, 345
and lidocaine, 275
second-degree, 345
third-degree, 345
transient, and temporary pacemakers, 274
Blood
count in diagnostic tests, 112
flow of, 129, 130, 169
in congestive heart failure, 35
in kidneys, 35, 129
pH, 328
in physiologic role of circulation, 35
volume of, 116, 130, 169
and congestive heart failure, 35
in shock, 35
Blood pressure, 35, 65
arterial, 125, 334
checking of, in myocardial infarction, 88
dyscrasias, 108
venous, 36, 125
monitoring of, in shock, 130
Blood vessels, in arteriosclerotic disease, 51-53
Boehm, 314
Bowel care, 98
Bradycardia, 277, 334
complications with, 254
and digitalis intoxication, 254
drugs for, 239, 240
and lidocaine, 239, 240
and propranolol, 241, 242
Bright, Richard, 334
Bronchi, 159, 173
Buffers, chemical, 124
Bundle-branch block, 296, 297, 334
and electrocardiogram, 297

Bundle-branch block (*cont.*)
  left, 297
    conduction of, 298
  right, 296, 297
    conduction of, 296
Bundle branches, 297
Bundle of His, 335

Calcium, 119, 120
  as emergency drug, 24, 319
Calculation, 197
  of heart rate, 208, 210, 216
Calories, 335
  reduction of, in diet for myocardial
    infarction, 92, 335
Cannon, 49, 50
Capillaries, 335
Capillary pressure, pulmonary, in left
    heart failure, 130, 170
Carbohydrates, 97
Carbon dioxide in physiologic role of
    circulation, 122, 124, 158
Carbonic acid and acidosis, 121-123,
    125-128
Cardiac arrest, 312-324, 326
  atropine and; *see* Sinus arrest
  history, 313
Cardiac arrhythmia; *see* Arrhythmias
Cardiac auscultation, 326
Cardiac care unit, 72
  rhythm strip, 210
  transfer from; *see* Patient, cardiac care
    of
Cardiac cells, polarized, definition of,
    190-198
Cardiac cycle, 130, 335
  electrical pattern, 190-198
  vulnerable period in, with pace-
    makers, 251, 252, 299
Cardiac death, 327
Cardiac dilation in compensatory mech-
    anisms of heart, 339
Cardiac disorders, therapeutic drugs for;
    *see* Heart disease and Patient,
    cardiac care of
Cardiac enlargement; *see* Hypertrophy
Cardiac failure; *see* Heart failure
Cardiac hypertrophy; *see* Hypertrophy
Cardiac impulse in premature ventricu-
    lar contractions, 297, 298,
    368

Cardiac output, 32, 130, 165, 182, 335
  and diphenylhydantoin, 240, 263,
    275
  inadequate, 129, 130
  inefficient, 129, 130
  reduction of, in bradycardia, 277
  in ventricular fibrillation, 321
Cardiac pacemaker, artificial; *see* Pace-
    maker, artificial cardiac
Cardiac patient, care of; *see* Patient,
    cardiac care of
Cardiac rate; *see* Heart rate
Cardiac rhythm, observation of; *see*
    Arrhythmias
Cardiac tamponade, 335
Cardiac tissue, 277
Cardiac vectors, 209
  origin of, and placement of electrodes,
    198
  reference for plotting, 203
Cardiocentesis, 335
Cardiogenic shock, 178, 327
Cardiopulmonary resuscitation, 80, 312,
    326
  complications of, 327
Cardioscope, 336
Cardiotonic, 336
Cardiovascular decompensation, early
    treatment of, 171
Cardiovascular collapse, 327
Cardiovascular drugs, 23, 336
  acute drugs in, uses and approximate
    dilutions of, 319-342
Cardiovascular function, improvement
    of, in acute pulmonary edema,
    130, 179
Cardiovascular system, physical exami-
    nation of; *see also* Heart
  arterial blood pressure in, 182
  venous pressure in, 182
Cardioversion, 240, 268, 271
Carditis, 336
Care of cardiac patient; *see* Patient,
    cardiac care of
Carotid arteries, 336
Carotid body, 337
Carotid pulses in myocardial infarction,
    36
Carotid sinus, 337
Carotid sinus massage in angina pectoris,
    262

Catecholamine actions on heart, blocking of, 24, 25, 237, 241, 246
Catheter, 163, 164, 337
Cations, 114-120
  percutaneous pacing, 163
  transvenous pacing, 130
Cedilanid; see Lanatoside C, 245, 263
Cells, 104
  pacemaker, 253
  red blood, 129, 130, 169
Central venous pressure, 130
Cerebral vascular accident, 337
Cerebral vessels and atherosclerosis, 337
Cessation of heart action, 338
Change, dynamics, 81
Chest auscultation and pulmonary embolus, 105
Chest pain, 54, 66
  in coronary artery disease, 99, 144
Chloride, 123
Chlorothiazide, 338
Cholesterol, 134, 140, 338, 346
Cholinergic, 48
Chordae tendonae, 338
Chronotropic, 137, 246
Circulation, 28, 338
  physiologic role of, 28
  systemic, and shock, 28, 178
Circulatory deficit, 339
Claudication, 339
Clinical syndromes in coronary artery disease, 51-63
Clotting factors, inhibiting synthesis of, 156, 177
Clotting time, 112, 147, 150
$CO_2$, 124, 125
$CO_2$ combining power, 113
Coagulation time, 112, 339
Code "99", 312, 326
Code "Blue", 312
Colace, 97
Collateral circulation, intercoronary, 36, 37, 339
Commissure, 339
Committee, planning, 71
Compensation, state of, 339
Compensatory mechanisms of heart, 339
Compensatory pause, 258
  in premature atrial contractions, 258
  in premature nodal contractions, 286

Compensatory pause (cont.)
  in premature ventricular contractions, 298
Complete bedrest in myocardial infarction, 171
Complete heart block; see Block, heart
Complications
  of cardioversion, 240
  in coronary heart disease, 11
  of myocardial infarction, goals in prevention of, 229-231
  of thrombus or embolus, 56
Concepts of resuscitation, 80, 312, 326
Conduction, 195-200, 216
  disturbances in, in electrocardiogram intervals, 187, 207
  of left bundle-branch block, 298
  of normal ventricular conduction, 196, 207
  of right bundle-branch block, 296, 297
Conduction system, 188-200, 277
  damage to, 15
  and digitalis intoxication, 234, 242, 243, 245
  and lidocaine, 239, 240
Conduction velocity and quinidine, 238, 239
Congestive heart failure; see also Heart failure
  aims, 183
  and diet, 174
  and digitalis, 175
  edema formation in, 130, 172
  heart sounds in, 169
  left heart failure in, 130, 170
  rest, 174
  right heart failure in, 170, 171
  symptoms, 184
  treatment of acute pulmonary edema in, 169
Constrictive pericarditis, 340
  and congestive heart failure, 170, 171
Continuing education, 81, 82, 83
Contractility of left ventricle in cardiogenic shock, 178
Contractions of heart, 250
  and lidocaine, 239, 240
  normal, 340

Contractions of heart (*cont.*)
premature atrial, 258, 260
and ventricular tachycardia or fibrillation, 270, 303, 304, 323, 370
premature nodal, 271
premature ventricular; see Premature ventricular contractions
Contraindications
to lidocaine, 239, 240
to quinidine, 238, 239
Controlled fat diet, 138, 139
Cooking, 137, 138
Coping responses of patients with myocardial infarction, 4, 8, 9, 91
Cor pulmonale, 216, 340
Coronary arterial system, 60, 340
Coronary arteries, 60, 218
and atherosclerosis, 58, 60
Coronary atherosclerosis, obstruction and, 51, 53, 132
Coronary care
committee, 81
director, 80, 83
objectives, 84, 315
Coronary care unit
care of patient in, 7, 10, 12-14, 315
design of, 12-24
Coronary heart disease; see also Heart disease
cardiogenic shock in, 327
clinical syndromes in, 59
and complications, 60
congestive heart failure in; see Congestive heart failure
incidence and predisposition in, 145, 229
myocardial infarction in; see Myocardial infarctions
pathology in, 60
Coronary insufficiency, chest pain in, 58, 105
Coronary sinus, anatomy and physiology of, 29, 285
Coumadin, 63
Coumarin, 149-151, 340
Counter shock, 22, 237, 307
CPK in myocardial infarctions, 109
Creatine phosphokinase in myocardial infarction, 39, 104-106, 109
Crile, 314

Cyanosis and pulmonary embolus, 341
Cytologic, 341

Danger to patient with pacemaker, 27
Day, Hughes, 70
DC shock in cardioversion, 22, 237
Death, 182
of myocardium, electrocardiogram changes in, 218
sudden
in coronary artery disease, 321
in digitalis intoxication, 242, 243
Decompensation, cardiovascular, 341
description of, 341
early treatment of, 132
Defibrillation, 8, 23
Defibrillator, use of, 17, 18, 341
Definitions in basic electrocardiography; see Appendix A
Deflections, electrocardiographic, 196
in measuring spatial vector, 199
vector leads and, 209
Deformities of myocardial infarction, characteristic, 221-225
Delegation of nursing functions, 89
Denial as response to myocardial infarction, 89
Depolarization, 189, 191, 207, 249, 309
definition of, 189
of heart, pacemaker cell and, 207
of myocardium, cardioversion in, 309
phases, 309
of ventricles, 207
deflections on leads and, 207
Depressant, 341
Depression in patients with myocardial infarction, 6, 8
Dermatomyositis, 107
Diagnosis
criteria for, in acute myocardial infarction, 220-225
differential, in chest pain, 229
of heart disease, electrocardiogram in, 65, 206
and resuscitation, 312
Diaphragmatic myocardial infarction; see Myocardial infarctions, diaphragmatic
Diastole and heart sounds, 32, 33, 65, 127, 168, 169, 341

Diastolic threshold and pacemakers, 32, 127
Dicumarol, 157
Diet in myocardial infarction, 62, 91, 97, 128-143
Differential diagnosis in chest pain, 229
Digitalis, 63, 112, 181, 232, 341
  in acute pulmonary edema, 130, 179
  and cardiogenic shock, 312
  in right heart failure, 63
Digitalis intoxication, 234, 242, 243, 245, 267
  changes in rhythm in, 242
  and electrocardiogram, 242, 243
  and potassium depletion, 63
Digitalis lanata, 234
Digitalis leaf, 234, 235
Digitalis purpurea, 234
Digitalis toxicity, 63, 233, 236, 245
  and diphenylhydantoin, 241
  and lidocaine, 239, 240
Digitoxin, 235, 245
Digotoxin, 235, 245, 262
Dilantin; see Diphenylhydantoin
Dilatation, cardiac, in compensatory mechanisms of heart, 341
Diphenylhydantoin, 240, 263, 275
Direction of electrical force of heart in electrocardiography, 200
Director, medical, 72
Displacement of heart, physical examination in, 44
Distention, 98
Disturbance in conduction in electrocardiogram intervals, 197
Diuretics, 174, 237, 342
Diuril; see Chlorothiazide
Dosages
  for digitalis preparations, 232-236
  of lidocaine, 239, 240
  of propranolol, 241, 242
Dramamine, 66
Drugs, 232-236
  acute, uses and approximate dilutions of, 232-246
  cardiovascular, 232-246
Duration of pain, 95, 96
  in angina pectoris, 54
  in myocardial infarction, 54, 95, 96
Dyspnea, 230, 342

Ectopic beat, ventricular, 292
Ectopic focus in heart, 276, 341
  circus rhythm, 276
Ectopic rhythms, supraventricular, 239-261
Ectopic tachycardias and quinidine, 238, 239
Edema, 169, 342
  acute pulmonary, 130, 342
  formation of, 130, 342
  and congestive heart failure, 130
Edrophonium, 242, 262
Education, public, in care of cardiac patient, 1, 82
Ehrlich, S. Paul, 70
Einthoven, 186-190
Ejection power, 169, 170
Elastic bandages, 172
Elastic stockings, 172
Electric countershock, 328
Electrical activity of heart in electrocardiographic lead, 102, 187
Electrical blocking circuit, automatic, in pacemakers, 342
Electrical events in heart, sequence of, 102
Electrical field in depolarization, 194, 195
Electrical hazards, 27, 80
Electrical impulses in physiology of heart, 195, 196
Electrical pattern of cardiac cycle, 196
Electrical potential, 187
Electrical requirements in equipment, 17
Electrocardiogram; see also Rhythm strip
  and arrhythmias, 65
  and artificial pacemakers, 18, 271
  with asynchronous cardiac pacing, 18
  cardioversion of ventricular fibrillation in, 2, 240
  in coronary artery disease, 65
  and determining pacemaker function, 268, 307
  in diagnosis of heart disease, definitions in, 65, 206
  diagnostic purpose of, 65, 215, 226
  and dissecting aortic aneurysm, 102
  and gastric or duodenal peptic ulcers, 97, 98

Electrocardiogram (*cont.*)
intervals of, 258
meaning and significance of, 258,
286, 298
lead of, in electrical activity of heart,
102, 186
location of cardiac vectors and, 203,
204
monitoring system and, 17, 102
in myocardial infarction, characteristic deformities in, 65
placement of electrodes in, 198, 199
for augmented leads, 201
precordial leads and, 201, 202
in series, 207
standard limb leads in, 201-206
time lines of, 215
and transvenous pacing catheter, 102
twelve-lead, 206
Electrocardiographic deflections, 201-
206
Electrocardiography; *see also* Electrocardiogram
basic, 206, 207
in myocardial infarction, 21
Electrodes, 14, 198-227
on external chest wall as pacemakers,
15
ground, 17
placement of, 227
in augmented leads, 201, 202
in electrocardiogram, 227
and monitoring system, 14
position of, for V leads, 202
types of, in monitoring equipment,
14
Electrolytes, 114-128, 236, 342
Elevation of temperature in myocardial
infarction, 87
Elimination, facilitation of, in cardiac
patient care, 97
Embolism, 343
Embolus, 102, 155, 343
prevention of, 63, 96
pulmonary, 155, 156
Emergency cart on coronary care unit,
21
Emergency drugs, 319
uses and approximate dilutions of,
319
Emotions, 3, 21, 76

Empathy, 343
Endarterium, 343
Endocarditis, 343
Environment
for patient with myocardial infarction, 84-99
during resuscitation, 312-325
safe, in care of patient with pacemaker, 27, 80
Enzymes, in myocardial infarction, 11,
103, 104, 111
others, 109, 274, 343
Epicardial electrodes as pacemakers, 130
Epicardium, 343
Epimysium, 37
Epinephrine, 6, 23, 323, 324, 343
and cardiogenic shock, 319
Equipment, monitoring, 14-18
Escape beats, ventricular, 294
Essential hypertension, 344
Evaluation of patient status in myocardial infarction, 84-89
Examination, 86
nurse's role on admission, 87, 88
Excitability of myocardium, 194
quinidine and, 239, 240
Exercises, 54, 80, 91
in care of cardiac patient, 88
Explanations, 86-88
of care and equipment for cardiac
patient, 87, 88
for patients with myocardial infarction, 87, 88
Extracellular fluid, 116, 126
Extracorporeal circulation, 344

False alarms and monitoring system, 14,
15
Family of patient with myocardial infarction, 88
Fascia, 37
Fatigue, 40
Fatty substances in intimal atherosclerosis, 158
Fears of patients with myocardial infarctions, 95
Feeling state of patient with myocardial
infarction, 95, 96
Fibers, automaticity of, 249

Fibrillation
  atrial; see Atrial fibrillation
  ventricular; see Ventricular fibrillation
Fibrin, formation of, 156, 177
Fibrinogen, 344
Fibrosis, 36
  atherosclerotic process, 36
Fick principle, 165
Fluid administration in myocardial in-
    farction, 88, 92
Fluoroscopy, 161, 336, 344
Flutter, atrial; see Atrial flutter
Footboard in care of cardiac patient, 91,
    172
Forward failure in congestive heart
    failure, 184
Fowler's position in congestive heart
    disease, 182
Friction rub, pericardial, 183
Frontal plane projection of mean QRS
    vector, 203, 204
Frustration, 4
Fusion beat and premature ventricular
    contractions, 299-301

Gallop rhythm, physical examination
    in, 345
Ganglion, 345
Gastrointestinal disorders, 97
Gitalin, 235
Glycerin suppositories, 97
Glycogen (glucose), 39, 117
Glyconeogenesis, 5
  glutamic-oxalacetic transaminase, 103,
    106
Goals, 84, 100
  in patient care with myocardial in-
    farction, 84, 85, 86
  of rehabilitation in myocardial in-
    farction, 85
    in acute phase, 85, 86, 88, 89
    in later phases, 85
Ground electrode, 14, 15
G-Strophanthin; see Ouabain

Heart
  anatomy and physiology of, 29, 129
  block, 345
  compensatory mechanisms of, 129

Heart (cont.)
  decompensated, 141
  depolarization of, 188-200
    deflections on leads and, 196
    pacemaker cell and, 194
  digitalis and, 232-236
  effects of stimulation of sympathetic
    and parasympathetic nerves
    on, 253
  electrical activity of, 206
    in electrocardiography, 204
    sequence of, 204
  lidocaine and, 239, 240
  in physical examination of cardio-
    vascular system, 29, 129
  propranolol and, 241-242
  quinidine and, 238, 239
  rupture of, 183
  size of, 29
  work load of, 29-31
Heart block; see Block
Heart disease
  coronary, and complications; see
    Coronary heart disease
  diagnosis of, with electrocardiogram,
    206
  disease control program, 80
  etiology, 53
Heart failure; see Congestive heart fail-
    ure
Heart rate, 197
  and electrocardiogram intervals, 215,
    216
  increase in, in compensatory mecha-
    nisms of heart, 339
  isoproterenol and, 319, 323, 324
  risk factors, 136
Hemoglobin, 346
Hemoptysis and pulmonary embolus,
    65, 185, 186
Hemorrhages, 145, 148
Heparin, 107, 146-156, 177, 346
Hepatic necrosis, 107
Hepatitis, 107
Hexaxial figure, 205
"High output failure" in congestive
    heart failure, 169
His bundle, 216
Homeostasis, 49, 50
Hooker, 314
Hypaque, 163

Hypercapnia, 346
Hyperkalemia, 118
Hyperlipidemia, 135, 346
Hypertension, 141, 167, 239, 346
Hypertrophy, 130, 166-168, 346
    cardiac, 130
        in compensatory mechanisms of
            heart, 130
        in coronary artery disease, 52
Hyperventilation, 123
Hypervolemia, 346
Hypoglycemia and tromethamine, 132
Hypokalemia, 66, 118, 119
    and digitalis intoxication, 118
    and symptoms of, 118
Hypotension, 66, 346
Hypotonic state, 117, 127, 128
Hypovolemia, 347
Hypoxia, 347

Iatrogenic, 347
Idioventricular rhythm, 293, 307, 347
Igelsrud, 314
Impulse, 188-206
    in conduction system of heart, 196
Indandione, 149
Inderal; see Propranolol
Infarction, 218-231, 347
    myocardial; see Myocardial infarctions
    and pulmonary embolus, 347
Infection, prevention of, in care of patient with pacemaker, 166
Inferior vena cava, anatomy and physiology of, 45-47
Injury of myocardium, electrocardiogram changes in, 218-220
Innominate artery, 347
Inotropic, 137, 246
Insufficiency, 347
Intake and output
    in care of cardiac patient, 100, 131
    in right heart failure, 132
Integration of experience of myocardial infarction, 84-100
Interatrial septum, 347
Intercoronary collateral circulation, 36, 37
Interfered beat and AV dissociation, 299
Intermittent claudication, 140

Intermittent positive pressure, 100
Interpersonal relationships in care of cardiac patient, 84-99
Interpolated premature ventricular contraction, 293, 300, 301
Interstitial fluid, 115, 116, 123
Intervals, 209, 211
    of electrocardiogram; see Electrocardiogram
    in regular ventricular rhythm, 212, 213
    P-R; see P-R interval
    R-R; see R-R interval
Interventricular septum, 348
Intimal atherosclerosis, description of, 348
Intracellular fluid, 126
Intravenous fluids, 128
Ions, 114-127, 189, 190
IPPB in treatment of acute pulmonary edema, 18, 94, 172
Irritation of pacemaker site, 276, 341
Ischemia of myocardium, electrocardiogram changes in, 218
Ischemic attacks, transient, 348
Ismelin, 62
Isoelectric, 211, 216, 281
Isoenzyme, 104
Isoproterenol, 319, 323, 324
Isuprel; see Isoproterenol

Kidneys, function of, 124, 125
    and cardiogenic shock, 62
    and congestive heart failure, 62, 184
Kouwenhoven, 314

Lactate dehydrogenase (LSD), 105, 107
Lactic acid, excessive, and shock, 39, 107-109
Lanatoside C, 235
Langworthy, 314
Laxative, 63
LDH in myocardial infarction, 107, 108, 110
Lead I, 198
    placement of, 196-198
    tracing of, 196
Lead II, placement of, 196-198, 281

Lead III, placement of, 196-198, 281
Lead axes, and measuring spatial vector, 196-198
Lead of electrocardiogram, 196-206
  augmented, 203
  bipolar, 227
  deflection on, source of, 196
  in electrical activity of heart, 180-196
  precordial, 202
  standard limb, 198
    and augmented, 203
    measuring spatial vector from, 204, 205
  unipolar, 227
  wave changes in, in myocardial infarction, 220
Left bundle-branch block, 107, 297
  conduction of, 298
  electrocardiogram tracing in, 298
Left heart failure, 170
Left ventricular failure, 170
Left ventricular hypertrophy, physical examination in; see Hypertrophy, ventricular
Levarterenol, 62
Levophed; see Levarterenol, 62, 182-230, 245
Lewis, Sir Thomas, 200
Lidocaine, 25, 237, 239, 275
Limb leads, standard, 196-206
  and augmented leads, 203
  measuring spatial vector from, 204, 205
Linoleic acid, 348
Lipid, 348
Lipoprotein, 348
Liver, disease, 105, 108, 109
Location
  of heart, 44
  of myocardial infarction, 112, 218-226
  of pain
    in angina pectoris, 54
    in myocardial infarction, 95, 96
"Low output failure" in congestive heart failure, 170
Low salt diet in right heart failure, 174
Lumen, 348
Lung, 105
Lymph circulation, 38, 44

Maas, 314
Magnesium, 121
Magnitude of electrical force of heart in electrocardiography, 198
Malignant hypertension, 166
Management of acute pulmonary edema, 172-174
Manometer for venous pressure readings, 101
Mean QRS and T vectors, plotting of, 204-206
Measurement, of venous pressure, 101, 130
Medulla, 31
Memory tapes of monitoring systems, 21
Mephentermine, 62
Mercuhydrin in right heart failure, 174, 237, 242
Mercurial diuretic, 348
Metabolic acidosis, 122, 124, 328
Metabolism, 348
Metabolites, essential, in circulation, 124
Metaraminol, 62, 182, 245, 262, 319
Milk of magnesia, 97
Mineral oil, 97
Mitral insufficiency, 348
Mitral valve in anatomy and physiology of heart, 349
Monitoring system, 14, 80, 84, 200
Morphine sulfate, 95
  in treatment of acute pulmonary edema, 96
Mouth-to-mouth breathing, 20, 326, 327
Multifocal ventricular contractions, 302
Multimedia instruction, 76
Mural thrombus, 349
Murmurs in physical examination of cardiovascular system, 349
Muscles, 37-40
Musculoskeletal disorders, 106
Myocardial failure and shock; see Heart failure
Myocardial infarctions, 54, 59, 112, 349
  acute, 54, 99, 144
    anterior wall, 222, 227
    antero-basal, 223
    antero-lateral wall, 221, 367
    apical, 223
    and arterial blood pressure, 163

Myocardial infarctions (*cont.*)
acute (*cont.*)
  inferior, 224, 227
  and lidocaine, 239, 240
  posterior, 224, 373
  postero-basil, 225
  postero-lateral, 225
  care of patients with, 66, 84-99, 229-231
  changes in pulse and blood pressure in, 66
  characteristic deformities of, 65, 66, 102, 108
  chest pain in, 54, 66
  diaphragmatic, 224, 227
  electrocardiogram in, 99
  in differential diagnosis, 111, 112, 229
  electrocardiogram tracing in, 65, 99
  monitoring system and, 14
  predisposing factors, 99, 229
  rehabilitation of patient with, 66
  revascularization, 164
  threats, 231
  topographic regions of occurrence of, 135
Myocardial necrosis, 60, 64, 218, 349
Myocarditis, 349
Myocardium, 50, 168, 182, 220
  anatomy and physiology of, 50, 99
  depolarization of, phases of, 220
  dilated, in compensatory mechanisms of heart, 339
  healing process, 100
  irritability of, and diphenylhydantoin, 240, 263, 275
  ischemia, injury, and death of, electrocardiogram changes in, 64, 99, 108, 228
  lidocaine and, 239, 240
  mirror effect, 229
  propranolol and, 241, 242
  quinidine and, 63

National Diabetic Society, 116
National Diet-Heart Study, 135
National Heart Institute, 80
Necrosis, 349
Needle electrodes, placement of, on anterior chest wall, 198

"Negative" deflection, 191
Negative electrode in monitoring device, 191
Negative pole, V leads and, 199
Neo-Synephrine, 262
Nervous system in physiology of heart, 38, 44-46
Neurocirculatory asthenia, 349
Neurologic changes, 118
  and digitalis intoxication, 234, 242, 243, 245, 267
  and lidocaine, 239, 240
  and quinidine, 63, 238, 239
Neuromuscular irritability, 124
Niehaus, 314
Nitrites, 246
Nitroglycerin, 91, 96
Nocturnal dyspnea, paroxysmal, 242
Nodal contractions, premature, 285, 286
Nodal escape beats, 282-286
Nodal rhythm, 282-284
Nodal tachycardia; see Tachycardia
Nodes, sinoatrial and atrioventricular, 282
Normal pacemaker, 350
Normal sinus rhythm, 253, 254
Normal V lead electrocardiogram, 202
Nursing, 22, 26, 94
Nursing personnel, 68-70, 80, 244, 306
Nutrition, 91, 92

Obesity, 130
Observation of cardiac rhythm, 81
Obstruction, 350
Occlusion, 350
Organic mercurial diuretics in right heart failure, 174, 237, 342
Orthopnea and left ventricular failure, 350
Oscilloscope, 15, 27
Osmolality, 115
Osmotic pressure, 115, 123, 128
Osteoblastic bone lesions, 105
Ouabain, 263
Oxalate, 107
Oxygen, 61, 65, 99, 172
  in acute pulmonary edema, 172
  in physiologic role of circulation, 29, 39, 42

Oxygen (*cont.*)
  and treatment
    of myocardial infarction, 61, 93
    of shock, 62


P wave, 188, 208, 210-211, 215, 252
  in arrhythmias, 258
  definition, 208
  diphasic, 211
  location of, in normal electrocardio-
    gram, 209
  notching, 211
  and precordial leads, 202
  peaking, 211
  and quinidine toxicity, 268
PAC; *see* Premature atrial contractions
Pacemaker, 18, 271, 350
  runaway, 293
  sinoatrial node as, in cardioversion,
    240
  site of, 294
  wandering, 257, 258
Pacemaker cells, 188
  and depolarization of heart, 188-206
Pacing, modes of, 18
Pacing catheter, 130
Paddles, placement of, in cardioversion,
  322
Pain
  of angina pectoris, 54, 64
  in myocardial infarction, 95
    relief of, 95
    syndrome of, 4, 95
  in pericarditis, 159
Palpation, 350
Pancarditis, 350
Papillary muscles, anatomy and physiol-
  ogy of, 350
Paramedical, 73
Parasympathetic nervous system in phys-
  iology of heart, 47, 351
Parasystole, 299-301
Paroxysmal atrial tachycardia; *see* Atrial
  tachycardia, paroxysmal
Paroxysmal nodal tachycardia; *see*
  Tachycardia, nodal
Paroxysmal tachycardia; *see* Tachycardia
Paroxysmal ventricular asystole and
  temporary pacemakers, 307

Passive motion exercises in care of
  cardiac patient, 54, 90, 91
PAT; *see* Atrial tachycardia, paroxysmal
PAT with block, 263
Patency, 351
Pathology in coronary heart disease, 51-
  64
Patient, cardiac, care of, 87, 88, 172
  cardioversion in, 240, 268, 271
  objectives in, 172
  public education in, 1, 2
  rehabilitation in, 133
  resuscitation in, 80, 312, 326
Peptic ulcer, 105
Percutaneous pacing catheter, 130
Pericardial cavity, edema formation in,
  158, 159
Pericardial effusion, 159
  and congestive heart failure, 159
Pericardial friction rub, 159
Pericarditis, 63, 102, 351
Pericardium, 351
Perimysium, 37
Peripheral circulation, anatomy and
  physiology of, 140, 351
Peritrate, 63
Permanent pacemakers, 377
Personality, 68, 69
Phenergan, 66
Phenobarbital, 63
Phenomenon, Wenckebach, 289, 290
Phlebitis, 351
Phonocardiogram, heart sounds and, 3
Phosphates, 123
Phosphocreatine, 39
Physical examination of cardiovascular
  system, 44-49
Physical findings in myocardial infarc-
  tion, 229, 230
Physical therapy, in care of cardiac pa-
  tient, 98
Physiology of heart, 44
Placement, 200-206
  of electrodes; *see* Electrodes
"Plaque" formation in intimal athero-
  sclerosis, 55, 56
Platelets, 112, 150, 177
Pleural effusion in edema formation,
  158, 159
Plication, 351
PNC, 271

Point of maximum impulse, 251, 252
Polarized cardiac cells, definition of, 48, 190
Polybrene, 148
Position of patient
  in cardiogenic shock, 321
  with myocardial infarction, 87
"Positive" deflection, 190
Positive electrode in monitoring device, 190
Positive pole, V leads and, 200
Post myocardial syndrome, 183
Postoperative care with permanent pacemaker, 272, 273
Postoperative complications of permanent pacemaker insertion, 272
Postresuscitation care, 24, 328
Potassium, 117, 122, 189, 237
  depletion of, 117, 125
    and digitalis intoxication, 118
    and diuretics, 118, 119
  elevation of, and electrocardiograms, 119
Power source of pacemaker, 207
P-R intervals, 208, 209, 215, 216, 252
  in arrhythmias, 211
  calculation of, 211
  meaning and significance of, 211, 281
  prolonged, and digitalis intoxication, 211
  shortened, 211
Precordial reference figure, 202
  plotting of, 202, 203
Predisposition to coronary heart disease, 99, 102
Premature atrial contractions, 258-260
Premature beats, 310, 352
Premature nodal contractions, 271
Premature ventricular contractions, 297, 298, 368
  and bigeminy, 2
Pressor, 352
Pressure
  arterial blood, 32
  venous, 32
    in physical examination of cardiovascular system, 32
    in right heart failure, 32
    in shock, 32
Prevost, 314

Procainamide, 63, 237, 239, 263, 275, 351
Pronestyl; see Procainamide
Propranolol, 24, 25, 237, 241, 246
Prostatic carcinoma, 105
Prostigmin, 98
Protamine, 148
Proteinase, 123
Prothrombin, 96, 147
Prothrombin time, 96, 113, 147, 154
Psychologic reactions with myocardial infarctions, 89, 90
Public education in care of cardiac patient, 4, 5, 89-96
Public health, 80
Pulmonary capillary pressure in left heart failure, 170
Pulmonary circulation, anatomy and physiology of, 29, 32, 34, 351
Pulmonary disorders, 108
  acute edema in, 130, 179
  embolus in, 105
Pulmonary vessels in left heart failure, 184
Pulse, 353
  deficit, 279
  pressure, 6, 353
Pulse generator, 16
Pulsus alternans, 353
Purkinje system, 353
PVC; see Premature ventricular contractions
Pyruvic acid, 107, 123

Q wave, 189
Quadrigeminy, 293
Quinaglute; see Quinidine
Quinidine, 63, 238, 245, 263, 353
Quinine, 63
QRS complex, 189, 208, 209, 212-216, 252, 298
  abnormalities of, in myocardial infarction, 221-226
  bizarre, and quinidine toxicity, 238
  definition of, 212
  duration, 216
  location of, in normal electrocardiogram, 196
  precordial leads and, 200
QRS intervals, 208
  meaning and significance of, 201, 212

Q-T duration, 214
Q-T intervals, 208


R on T phenomenon, 291
R wave, 186-206
  deflection of, 212
  in myocardial infarction, 221-226
Radiography, 159-165
Rate, of heart, 44-46, 197, 208-210,
    216
  in arrhythmias, 253
  calculation of, 197, 210
  change in, in pacemaker failure, 208,
    251
Rauwolfia, 353
Reactions of patient, psychologic, with
    myocardial infarction, 89, 90
Readings, venous pressure, 130
Reassurance for patients, 87, 88
Receptors, 49
Recording
  leads of electrocardiogram and moni-
    toring system, 188-206
  venous pressure, 130
Reentry theory, 310
Reference
  for plotting cardiac vectors, 199-203
  for zero potential, 188, 189
Refractory, 251, 252, 299
Regurgitation, 353
Renal blood flow, normal, 353
Renal hypertension, 353
Renal ischemia and cardiogenic shock,
    167, 168
Renal tubular necrosis and shock, 167,
    168
Repolarization, definition of, 190, 191
Reserpine, 62, 354
Respiration of patient, 40, 101
  aids, 18
Respiratory acidosis, 122
Responses, coping of patients with myo-
    cardial infarctions, 95, 96
Rest for patient, 171
  with myocardial infarction, 95, 96
  with right heart failure, 174
Resting membrane potential, definition
    of, 188, 190
Resuscitation, 23, 24, 80, 100
Rheumatic fever, 354

Rhythm; see also Rhythm strip
  changes in, 39
  disturbances of, 354
  interpretation of, in monitoring sys-
    tems, 212-216, 248, 249
  nodal, 282
  normal sinus, 196
  regular ventricular, intervals in, 196
  regularity of, in arrhythmias, 196
Rhythm flow sheet, of cardiac care unit,
    210
Rhythm strip, 248, 275
  in atrial fibrillation, 267
  in atrial flutter, 266
  in bigeminy, 291
  in complete heart block, 287
  diagnostic purpose of, 248
  in first-degree heart block, 287, 295
  with fusion beat, 299-301
  with idioventricular, 209
  with interpolated premature ventricu-
    lar contraction, 299-301
  with multifocal premature ventricular
    contractions, 302
  in nodal rhythm, 252
  in normal sinus rhythm, 253
  in paroxysmal atrial tachycardia, 261
  in paroxysmal nodal tachycardia, 285
  in premature atrial contraction, 260
  in premature nodal contraction, 285
  in second-degree heart block, 287
  in sinus arrest, 257
  in sinus arrhythmia, 256
  in sinus bradycardia, 254
  in sinus tachycardia, 254
  with unifocal premature ventricular
    contractions, 297, 298
  in ventricular fibrillation, 305
  in ventricular tachycardia, 302, 303
  in wandering pacemaker, 257, 258
  in Wenckebach phenomenon, 289,
    290
Right bundle-branch block, 296, 297
  electrocardiogram tracing in, 296,
    297
Right heart failure; see Congestive heart
    failure
Rigor mortis, 40
Roentgen studies in viewing coronary
    arteries, 159-165

S wave, 201
SA block, and temporary pacemakers, 268
SA node, 208, 251, 354
Safety in environment for patient with pacemaker, 27, 80
"Sagging" of S-T segment in digitalization, 242, 243
Salt, 131, 139, 167
Scarring
  in atherosclerotic process, 56
  after myocardial infarctions, 220
Scherlis, Leonard, 73
Sclerosis, medial and arteriolar, description of, 354
Second-degree heart block, 345
Secondary hypertension, 354
Sedation in myocardial infarction, 63
Sedimentation rate, 112
Semilunar valves, 354
Septum, 355
Sequence of electrical events in heart, 200, 201
Serum enzymes, 103-111, 274
  in myocardial infarction, 104
Serum glutamic oxaloacetic transaminase in myocardial infarction, 103
Serum lactic dehydrogenase in myocardial infarction, 107, 108, 110
SGOT in myocardial infarction, 103-111
SHBD in myocardial infarction, 109
Shielding process, 298, 299
Shock, 355
  cardiogenic, 178, 378
  causes and classification of, 378
  after myocardial infarction, 178
Shunt, 355
Side effects
  of lidocaine, 239, 240
  of propranolol, 241-243
  of quinidine, 238, 239
Significance of arrhythmias, 187-189
Signs of death of heart muscle, 218
Sinoatrial bradycardia and temporary pacemakers, 255
Sinoatrial node, 253, 355
Sinus arrest, 256, 257, 278
  atropine for, 256
  and temporary pacemakers, 256

Sinus arrhythmias, 255, 256, 278
Sinus bradycardia, 254
Sinus block, 256
  and analgesia, 254
  and diphenylhydantoin, 240
  with premature atrial beats, 256
Sinus node arrhythmia and diphenylhydantoin, 254
Sinus rhythm, normal, 253
Sinus tachycardia, 255
Sinus of Valsalva, 355
Skeletal muscle, 105
Social scientist, 81
Sodium bicarbonate, 116, 119, 122
Sodium ions, movement of, in depolarization, 115, 116, 122, 189
Sodium-restricted diet in right heart failure, 116, 132, 141-143
Spatial vector, measurement of, from standard limb leads, 198, 200, 202, 204
Spontaneous discharge cycle, 249, 299, 309
Staff, medical, nursing, 71
Standard limb leads, 201
  and augmented leads, 203
  measuring spatial vector from, 204, 205
Starling and Lane, 314
Starling's curve, 130
Stasis, 355
Status, 70
Stenosis, 355
Stimulation of sympathetic and parasympathetic nerves in effects on heart, 253, 309
Stokes-Adams syndrome, 345, 355
Stress, 3
Strip, rhythm; see Rhythm strip
Stroke, 356
Stroke volume, 356
S-T segment, 208, 212, 252, 309
  abnormalities in, in myocardial infarction, 218, 219
  depression of, 228
Subintimal hemorrhages, 356
Supraventricular tachycardia, 239-261
Sympathetic nervous system, 6, 47, 356
  blocking agent for, 47
  in physiology of heart, 31, 47
  and shock, 309, 310

Symptoms, 356
  of acute pulmonary edema, 130, 179
  of angina pectoris, 64
  of cardiogenic shock, 178
  of hypokalemia, 118
  of myocardial infarction, 229
Syncope, 356
Syndrome, 356
Systemic circulation, 30, 356
  anatomy and physiology, 33
  and shock, 33
Systole
  in anatomy and physiology of heart,
    32, 33
  and heart sounds, 32
Systolic hypertension, in physical ex-
    amination of cardiovascular
    system, 32

T wave, 189, 208, 209, 214, 252
  abnormalities in, in myocardial in-
    farction, 219
  definition of, 189
  location of, in normal electrocardio-
    gram, 196
  notching, 214
  pointed, 214
  precordial leads and, 199
  tall, 214, 226
Tachycardia, 56, 277, 278, 356
  atrial; see Atrial tachycardia
  paroxysmal, 351, 381
    atrial, 260
    nodal, 285
    and Wolff-Parkinson-White syn-
      drome, 267
  sinus, 255
  supraventricular lanatoside C and,
    379
  ventricular; see Ventricular tachy-
    cardia
Tapes, memory, of monitoring system,
    21
Team, health, 69
Tensilon; see Edrophonium
Terminal connections in monitoring de-
    vices, 17
Tetralogy of Fallot, 356
Therapeutic drugs for cardiac dis-
    orders, 232-242

Thiazide therapy in right heart failure,
    324
Third-degree heart block, 345
Threshold potential, 249-251
Thrombophlebitis, 357
Thrombosis, 56, 64, 102, 155, 172, 175-
    178, 357
Thrombus, prevention of, 51, 96, 156,
    176, 357
Thyroid, 57
Time lines of electrocardiogram, 197
Tonus, 39
Tournade, 314
Tourniquets in retarding venous return,
    118, 181
Toxic effects
  of lidocaine, 239, 240
  of quinidine, 238, 239
Tracings; see Rhythm strip
Training program, 74, 78, 79, 81
Tranquilizers and anticoagulation, 145
Transfer from cardiac care unit, 81
Transient heart block and temporary
    pacemakers, 289
Transvenous pacing catheter, 130
Treatment; see *particular disorder*
Triaxial figure, 204
Tricuspid valve, 357
Trigeminy, 292, 301, 357
Twelve-lead electrocardiogram, 206
T-P segment, 212

U wave, 208, 214
Ulcers, gastric or duodenal peptic, 97
Unifocal premature ventricular con-
    tractions, 302
Unipolar leads in augmented leads, 202
Uremia, 357
Urine, output of, and cardiogenic shock,
    101

V leads, electrode positions of, 202
Vagal, vagus effect, 253, 309
Vagus nerve in physiology of heart, 31,
    357
Valsalva maneuver and venous pressure
    readings in shock, 175
Valves
  in anatomy and physiology of heart,
    31

Valves (*cont.*)
  of heart and congestive heart failure, 33
Valvular stenosis and thrills, 33, 357
Vascular disorders, 169-172
Vascular insufficiency, intermittent symptoms of, 169
Vasoconstriction, 182, 245, 357
  center, 36
  compensatory, and shock, 101
Vasodilatation, 96, 357
  and nitroglycerin, 96
  in shock, 96
Vasodilators in cardiogenic shock, 178
Vasoinhibitor, 358
Vasopressors, 23, 241, 245, 262, 276, 358
Vector
  cardiac, 204
    frontal plane projection of, 204
    on lead axes, 205
    plotting mean, and augmented leads, 204
    reference for plotting, 204
  definition of, 205
  spatial, measurement of, 203-205
Vena cava, anatomy and physiology of, 358
Venous circulation, 125, 358
  in physiologic role of circulation, 101
  pressure in, in right heart failure, 101
Venous pressure, 101, 102, 358
  central, monitoring of, in shock, 101
  in physical examination of cardiovascular system, 101, 353
Ventricles, 358
  anatomy and physiology of, 188
  depolarization of, 196
    deflections on leads and, 196
    sequence of, 196
  function of, in cardiogenic shock, 178, 327
  left, 183
  as pumps in heart function, 29
Ventricular arrhythmias; *see also* Arrhythmias
  and lidocaine, 239, 240
Ventricular asystole, 22, 23, 307, 320
Ventricular bigeminy and digitalis intoxication; *see* Bigeminy

Ventricular conduction, conduction of normal, 196
Ventricular contractions, premature; *see* Premature ventricular contractions
Ventricular depolarization, definition of, 207
Ventricular ectopic beat, 294, 297, 298
Ventricular failure, left, and rales, 321
Ventricular fibrillation, 321, 371
  calcium and, 119
  and circulatory arrest, 327
  in digitalis intoxication, 233
  procainamide and, 239
  and quinidine, 238
  and vulnerable period of cardiac cycle with pacemakers, 237
Ventricular hypertrophy; *see* Hypertrophy, ventricular
Ventricular premature beats and propranolol, 239
Ventricular premature contractions, 303, 309
Ventricular rate
  artificial cardiac pacemakers, 272, 323
  in AV block, 274
  and permanent pacemakers, 309
Ventricular repolarization, definition of, 194
Ventricular septal defect, 358
Ventricular standstill, 307, 327
Ventricular tachycardia, 270, 302-304, 323, 370
  in AV dissociation, 295
  in AV block, 306
  and bradycardia, 277
  and cardioversion, 309
  and defibrillation, 304, 308
  in digitalis intoxication, 234
  lidocaine and, 239
  procainamide and, 239
  and quinidine, 238
Vesalius, 313
Vinberg, 37
Visceral nervous system, 47
Vital signs, checking of, in myocardial infarction, 87, 88
Vitamin K in anticoagulation, 150, 151
Vitamin supplement, 132
Voltage, in polarized cardiac cells, 190-196

Vomiting, hazard of, in myocardial infarction, 91, 92

Wandering pacemaker, 257, 258, 358
Warfarin sodium, 150
Water, 114, 116
Water balance, 127
Weight, checking of, in care of cardiac patient, 130
Wenckebach phenomenon, 289, 290
Wheeler, Dorothy, 73
Wolff-Parkinson-White syndrome, 107, 267, 279

Work load of heart, reduction of, 92
WPW, 107, 267, 279
Wyamine; see Mephentermine

X-ray studies in pericarditis and myocardial infarction, 158
Xylocaine; see Lidocaine

Zero point, 191
Zoll, Paul, 314